TALES FROM
THE TRENCHES,
A LIFE IN PRIMARY CARE

TALES FROM THE TRENCHES,
A LIFE IN PRIMARY CARE

GEORGE F. SMITH, M.D.

Table of Contents

Dedications

This book is dedicated to my son, who hopefully will have a better understanding of what his dad did during his worklife; my parents, who fully supported my educational pursuits and gave me enough genes to get through the schooling; my colleagues, who gave my patients expertise that I didn't have and provided me with learning opportunities and a welcoming, friendly, inclusive medical community; and most importantly, my patients, who were the reason for my career, my work and my passion while providing me with an understanding of the workings and misworkings of the body and the human condition and for whom I remain eternally grateful for their trust in my doctoring.

Prologue

Walking back to our offices after lunch in the doctor's dining room chatting with Felix, one of the interventional cardiologists at the hospital where we work, I commented on what great satisfaction and fun he must get from his procedural work—busting clots in patients with heart attacks and inserting stents into clogged coronary arteries. This was amidst talking about the Bay Area sports teams, the Giants and the Warriors. He then turned to me and said: "It must be tough in your job doing all that triaging." Hmmm, I thought for a moment after being taken aback by this off-the-cuff assessment of my professional life. "Well, that's not really how I spend my day" I started to explain and reminded him that I manage all the medical cardiology problems and the other medical specialty problems that my colleagues do in a similar way as them. I just don't do the fancy procedures and tests that they have in their tool box and playground. That might be the best and simplest description of my work as a General Internist in the modern world. Yes, of course, when patients need specialty care and consultation I guide them to those more knowledgeable and experienced for a specific complex problem. But, mostly my job is to evaluate and care for any and all health problems encountered by humankind adults.

I stick to my age range of patients: 15 to 115, starting with the fully actualized adult physiology in the teen years and then to the endpoint where it seriously declines and "death do us part". No, I have not yet had a patient make it to 115 but I do have a couple of "rules" for those that make it to a century, of which I've had many. Rule number one is to invite me to their 100th birthday party and rule number two is to ascribe their making it this far in life to "all my good doctoring". In reality, those centenarians don't need to follow any rules and can just do whatever they want with each extra day of living. While the job I do can be labeled as a "family doctor", my training and experience has been specific to encompass all the medical problems of physically mature humans. My training differed significantly from those who did a specific Family Medicine residency even though the duration of post medical school residencies were the same, three years. Internal Medicine residents do *not* spend any time in Obstetrics, Pediatrics or Surgery as my Family Medicine colleagues have done. Although as medical students we have all done many months rotations on those services. In the modern world of medicine, it is rare that a Family Medicine trained physician does any delivery of babies and certainly no true surgery but they often will do some pediatrics. In more rural medical settings this can be a huge benefit to the community. I spent nearly all my training working in a hospital setting taking care of a variety of the very ill but also spent time in outpatient clinics and a significant portion in the emergency room. The last year of my residency was also for taking medical specialty electives such as pulmonary, cardiology, rheumatology, gastroenterology and even dermatology in order to fine tune a greater understanding and experience of those difficult and specific problems. I spent nearly a third of my residency working in the Intensive Care Unit, the most fascinating, difficult and demanding area of medical care. Honestly, I loved that experience more than anything. Going out into the real world after training felt somewhat easy and was a surprising mild letdown after all that intensity.

There was this moment right after the end of residency when the feeling of being unmoored to a specific future of not knowing what I would be doing in the next year(s) was all a bit anxiety provoking, unsettling and somewhat exhilarating. Finished were college, medical school and three years of torturous but glorious internship and residency. Now what do I do with my life? I had offers to join internists in the Boston area in their private practices but that seemed so definitively grown up and a very deterministic life path. In the back of my mind was to move to the West Coast after an awakening vacation to Northern California a few years prior. It seemed best to focus on the short term—make a few dollars and study for my board certification exam upcoming in three months. This would at least complete the pathway until now. Also the consideration of doing more training in either a cardiology or pulmonary fellowship tugged at me. But the concept of two or three more years of a grinding fellowship kept me from jumping into it. So, for the first time in my life I stepped off the treadmill of pushing forward for some future goal and decided to work and to experience life as others do, freeform style, at least for a year before deciding what was next. This was 1985 and I was 30 years old. It was relatively easy to find shift work at either an emergency room or an urgent care clinic back then as my credentials were acceptable. This allowed me the flexibility of working as much as I needed but also the ability to take a significant amount of time off without constraint and loss of job. I signed up with a couple of clinics and sought work in a couple of local hospital ERs in the greater Boston area to give variety and security to a schedule that fit my life.

My first real job after residency was in the ER at Falmouth Hospital on Cape Cod starting two days after my residency was over on June 30th. They needed summer help as it was one of only 2 hospitals on the entire Cape and it was such a pleasant area with beaches, bike paths and local restaurants and the nearby Woods Hole Observatory for scientific study. I subleased my Boston apartment and found a studio for rent from one of the other ER docs. Working twelve-hour shifts three times per week felt so luxurious after all the hundred-hour weeks during residency. As I spent a good deal of my time studying on the beach, life felt somewhat relaxed and unpressured. I was used to everything that the ER could throw my way but my first day there shocked me in a unique way. In the late morning an ambulance brought in a 40-year-old woman who had fallen off her horse. She was paralyzed from the neck down and yes, a severely tragic event. Quickly word spread around the ER that the woman was the head nurse there! Soon all the physicians of the hospital were crowding into the department and trying to help with her care. The neurosurgeon was on the way and a new treatment for spinal cord injury, high dose intravenous corticosteroids, had been given but the prognosis was terrible for any recovery. I worked hard that day to get her transferred to Massachusetts General Hospital in Boston, but I had to keep working to see all the other patients that were needing care. Life and medical care goes on. That is the way it is. Many times in the ER when a serious life-threatening problem comes in, personnel and resources are directed to stabilizing the patient but then all the others that have been waiting will get their evaluation and treatment in time. It's one of the big reasons patients wait 6 hours to have their non-emergent sore throats checked.

While the life of a shift worker physician certainly was enjoyable for a couple of years after my residency, I began to collect a dossier on my older ER colleagues as my job experience grew from working at two ERs in the Boston area to then three different ones when I moved to Southern California with some friends the following year. There became a somewhat consistent life story of those colleagues doing years of ER work. Many had either completed an internship or residency and like me were unclear on the next professional step to take—private practice or more training. What happened was the pleasant lifestyle of working two or three twelve hour shifts a week carried on for these guys until middle age at which point life, family and habit prevented any other path to a different work life. With no responsibilities other than working a schedule, getting paid a decent amount and having no other business duties seemed easy and pleasant, I began to give thought to if I really wanted to work a 12-hour Saturday night shift in an urban ER when I was fifty. The answer to that question became increasingly no. So what was I going to do with my life?

Well, forty years later that question has been answered and like most it would not necessarily have been predicted to happen in the manner that unfolded. But isn't that everyone's life path? A bit in one direction than in another and another seems to be normal for most and mine was no different. As my "regular" professional life has turned into mostly retired, it's not the end of my experiences as a physician. For the past few years, I have been doing part time work at a clinic and also volunteering at a free clinic in San Francisco but I am only doing about 1 day a week of doctoring these days.

My professional life has taken me to experience nearly every work situation possible for an American physician. Initially, I was a contracted shift worker for emergency rooms, outpatient clinics and hospitals. This was the life I lived in the first few years after my training. This work confirmed that I was reasonably prepared for the various problems of acute care medicine, but also expanded my exposure to new medical problems and the intricate structures that are part of the medical working world. These structures are vast and complex. Because medical care in the U.S. is rendered as a business—either as a for-profit entity, a non-profit organization, or a government agency the structures have some similarities and significant differences. The variety of different healthcare settings are particular to each entity. I will explore these backstory components of medical care as it's crucial to how medicine is practiced in the US.

After my first 3 years as a journeyman acute care doc, the need to "settle down" and find a real job became an imposing life force and I searched for good jobs where everyone at the time looked—the classified ads in the *New England Journal of Medicine*, the most prestigious and widely read medical journal in the world. During my training, I briefly dated the assistant to one of the main editors of the journal and felt almost close to this bastion of cutting-edge medical knowledge although I remained several degrees separated. Such was the importance of this journal and it was produced in the hub of modern medical care, Boston. Even having a letter published in response to an article or editorial was considered a major feat. It was joked among doctors that this was the "brown journal" because it arrived each week in a brown paper covering and if you didn't open it, the stack of brown paper journals awaiting you would build up to an almost untenable, guilt-ridden height on one's desk. At the back of the journal were the job offers divided into specialties and listed in order with the proximity to Boston first and then expanding out to the rest of the country. I write about the "Brown Journal" in more detail in one of the following essays. At the time, I had moved to the L.A. beach town, Manhattan Beach, with some friends and was working at two different ERs and an urgent care clinic and had determined this was not the life for me either workwise or location-wise. I was drawn to the beauty of Northern California and to San Francisco in particular. Having lived my entire adult life in an urban setting, I couldn't imagine any other scenario. There were not many positions offered for an internist outside the Kaiser system but I applied and interviewed and accepted one that was a little tangential to my field. It was working with two other internists who were involved in a spine center and included inpatient and outpatient evaluation and treatment of patients undergoing surgery and issues of management of chronic pain. Not really the intense ER or ICU care I had been more accustomed to but it seemed like an interesting setting working with many other physicians as well—orthopedists, rehabilitation specialists, anesthesiologists and psychiatrists in a team format. The patients were complex and many had prior spinal surgeries, disability issues, psychological problems and pain medication issues. Many came from all over California to seek a comprehensive consultation and treatment plan. There was an inpatient month long chronic pain rehab program as well as a very active surgical program where patients would undergo these extensive and complex procedures involving fusions and hardware placement of the spine. This was a new world for me and an adjustment of thinking about medical care. Soon after I joined these two guys they merged into one large multispecialty group and moved to a nearby hospital lured by a capital outlay. I found myself employed in a fairly large new organization of about 20 physicians with an extensive bureaucratic administration attempting to be modeled after the famous Cleveland clinic. Interestingly, this was new to all involved and the power politics and personality wrinkles of a new organization was in play especially after the initial financial backing from the hospital was used up. This was a complete learning experience of not only a new paradigm of medical care but of how a new business evolves and the difficulties of each process. I would go on to work with this group for many years and was involved not only with the complexities of evaluation and treatment and caring for thousands of patients that underwent spine surgery but also with various research projects and even authored a couple of chapters in a textbook of spinal care that the group published. After a few years I began to see myself evolving to become an expert in spinal problems and chronic pain management even though I spent a fair amount of time taking care of the medical problems of patients who had surgery. Eventually, however, there was a significant shift to push more patients to surgery even though it was apparent there was little benefit. It became clear that this work life was not compatible with my ethics of the financial pressure being put upon me and that I needed to return to good old fashion general medical care. I go through this part of my professional life in "My Stint as a Back Doctor".

My path into the world of private practice took on a somewhat patchwork quilt of work. I needed to sustain enough income to pay a mortgage and to live in the Bay Area. For over a year, I worked part time at Kaiser in their clinics as well as signed up to be a consultant to our hospital's wound care clinic while subleasing office space from another internist. At the same time getting up to speed about the business aspect of medical practice that included insurance contracting, billing procedures, payroll and various components of a small business. It helped to build my practice by taking ER calls at our hospital for patients that needed admission but did not have a designated physician on staff. Many of these patients were elderly and had complex problems. Being used to taking care of hospital patients, this felt quite natural. After that first year I had the opportunity to take over a practice of a local internist that died suddenly. This propelled my private professional life to fill up significantly in a short period of time and secured my ability to focus on my role as primary care internist.

I recall quite vividly the pleasant and real feeling of seeing patients in my office that had a variety of medical issues that largely did not involve disabling spinal pain. What a great relief to be away from that extremely difficult world of chronic pain and recurrent unsuccessful surgery! My practice felt like a breath of fresh air and I enjoyed meeting and interacting with all the new patients that needed a primary care physician.

Learning as you go is the nature of all life and starting a de novo medical practice and running a business for the first time was challenging and exciting. When an older established doctor died of a massive heart attack at the racetrack there was no one to take over his busy practice. Encouraged by colleagues who helped me contact his widow, we created a definitive transition that helped his patients continue their needed care. Most of the patients were pleased not to be left without someone they could quickly and easily see as I had plenty of time to open up my schedule. One important cultural aspect was in play, however. The doctor who died, Joe Muscat, was Maltese and had the largest group of Maltese patients in the Bay Area. I was about to become immersed in a genetic and cultural pool of folks I had no previous contact or knew much about except that Malta was an island somewhere south of Sicily in the Mediterranean and that there was a famous movie starring Humphrey Bogart with the name Maltese in it. Turns out that this group of hard working, close knit, family-oriented folks were like any other immigrant group that struggled to make a life in the new land of America. They worked in various trade jobs, bought homes, sent their kids to college and had a few genetic traits that would distinguish them physically and medically. There was a definite physical resemblance to southern Italians. Dark olive skin and dark haired with the men being of small, roundish stature with a propensity for male pattern baldness. The women also resembled many of the traits of southern Italian women. This was quite familiar to me having had my maternal side of my family all of Italian descent. Somehow, many of these patients seemed to be like my aunts and uncles from South Philly with a similar temperament and strong spirit. It was a good fit for both of us. My essay "Private Practice" reviews the details of setting all this up and its evolution.

While this would be exposure to a new group of patients with a specific ethnic origin, it was only the beginning to all the ethnic diversity that inhabits northern California. The world came to my office and sat in my waiting room for an appointment with a guy that grew up in New Jersey. At times I looked out to my waiting room and saw the U.N. there—Filipinos, a large and growing group in Daly City, South Pacific islanders from Fiji, Tonga, and Samoa, Asians from China, Burma, Korea, Vietnam, Japan war brides and their husbands and all the other smaller south Asian countries. Also sitting in my waiting room were folks from Russia, Ukraine and the Middle East—Palestinians, Arab Muslims and Christians, Persians (as Iranians referred to themselves), and, of course, Indians, Pakistanis and Afghans. These various immigrants mixed with those that came to the Bay Area before and after WW2—Italians and Irish farmers and, of course, Mexicans that crossed the border to work extremely hard jobs as gardeners, housekeepers, restaurant help and laborers in construction. Whew, what a mix. The common factor is that medical illnesses are the same across all ethnic, cultural and religious lines. The body is the body but the response to illness and difficulty is reflected by individual and cultural factors. This appreciation of the cultural aspect evolved over the course of my career and was as important as keeping up with all the vast, complex medical advances over the past 30 years.

Solo private practice was my professional life for nearly twenty-five years. I've witnessed and endured all the various changes in healthcare and hospital care and did my best to keep current with treatment and policy and regulations and the vagaries of the adversarial reimbursement industry known as health insurance. In California, the evolution of health insurance over the past 30 years had all the permutations and difficulties in dealing with a fragmented, competitive, for-profit world of deliberate obfuscation and opacity. My colleagues and I have been forced to join various physician groups to maintain the ability to see our patients being switched from one HMO to another almost yearly and now to a system that is focused on significant out-of-pocket expenses and limited networks a.k.a. Obamacare. No movement has improved the difficulty for either patients and physicians in navigating this morass of near impossible disconnectedness. I'll explore this and how it relates to actually caring for patients.

While solo private practice has been my primary focus, I also began working in the San Mateo County medical clinics, a government system, and gained a broader experience with different and more challenged clientele. I signed up for a part time position after many of my patients lost their insurance in the aftermath of the 2008 financial crisis. I worked half day a week at one of the half dozen outpatient clinics around the county for six years. Many of these patients didn't speak English and some were severely challenged psychologically, financially and had serious substance abuse issues. The wide range of unusual medical problems expanded my experience beyond a stable private practice environment, all adding to my forty years in primary care medicine enriching my opportunity to see all sides of the medical profession. I don't regret a single second as it has seemed an appropriate fit for my personality and temperament. My life in medicine has been fulfilling in so many ways that I could not have anticipated or predicted and now compels me to tell its story.

The purpose of this book is to explore my career in a reflective and honest way. It includes perspectives on medicine from various viewpoints as well as many complex patient stories of their lives and diseases. My experience reflects a specific period in the history of medical care and hopefully accurately represents the time from the later 20th century into the early 21st century. Contained in these essays are a significant amount of medical information and I have painstakingly done detailed research to be certain it is factually correct but I have decided to not include references or footnotes as this is a first-hand account and not a medical reference work. However, I do invite anyone who has uncovered incorrect medical information (specific for this time period) to send me corrections so that I may modify the information for future editions (email me at drneogeo@icloud.com). Also, I should make mention in this current era of artificial intelligence, that none of the writing here was done with any AI programs so I am completely at fault here. The book is not constructed as a continuous narrative and therefore the essays can be read one at a time and in any order. The longest chapter is the "The Brief History of Medicine" which is included as a background to where medicine has come from before its current advanced scientific status. Although in 50-years time, this time period will likely appear as primitive as those in the past. Many doctors and people do not have the perspective of how severely limited care has been until the modern era and it seems crucially important to understand the contrast so it might be best to read that chapter first if so inclined. Thanks for reading and cheers!

PART 1

The Journey

CHAPTER 1

Why Become a Doctor in the First Place?

All I can do here is relate my own experience. There are no health care workers in my immediate or extended family. I had no early childhood experience or natural inclination that I recall to go into medicine. I don't think that I am particularly drawn more than others to selfless altruism and didn't necessarily have a strong innate drive to "help others". So how did I get here and spend my entire adult life studying, training and then practicing general medicine?

My best guess is that there were several factors that formed in my mind's desire by the time I reached college that put me on this path. One influence was that I did have an old fashion, old school, family practitioner that saw me when I was banged up or sick as a kid. Dr. Schwartzchild had a calm pleasant demeanor that was truly comforting the times I needed doctoring as a child and teen. His office was located on the ground floor of a split level New Jersey suburban home that had a small waiting room and a couple of exam rooms that were accessed by his large driveway. He was able to efficiently convert part of his home to his office. His wife was the receptionist and assistant, an exotic and beautiful Egyptian woman, who answered the phone, greeted you and took payments which were all cash back in the 1960s and '70s. The various health issues that brought me to Doc Schwartzchild included stitches for scalp and hand lacerations, strep throats, ear aches, knee bangs, rashes and other common ailments. Those visits usually occurred after hours or on the weekend and he would always fit me in somehow. His steady, relaxed manner would take care of the problem completely and efficiently. Primary care physicians in the 1960s and '70s were all encompassing treatment centers. Somewhat like a modern urgent care center. He could perform a variety of minor surgical procedures including suturing a laceration, lancing boils, or cutting off benign growths and he dispensed medicines for infections and pain in his office. There were large brown glass bottles filled with the common medications one needed for infections (penicillin, tetracycline), rashes (antihistamines, prednisone) and pain (codeine and aspirin). He would fill up a small paper envelope with each of the ones you needed and write on them how to take them. Medical care was simpler, straightforward, effective, efficient and much less expensive back then. Of course, there were limitations of treatments and diagnostic tests that have since evolved over the past 50 years. His wife would tally the bill for my mom to pay on the way out. Rarely did one go to the ER unless it was a real life threatening emergency. So medical care was a stable presence in my youth that I only needed on a rare occasion. He was middle aged then and represented the natural template of a family doc. However, I didn't think more about his life or was particularly curious about it at the time or even later but now it seems like such an ideal way to practice the profession. When I was accepted to medical school, he reached out and congratulated me and it felt like a warm embrace to adulthood and the start to my then chosen vocation. He, at that time, had retired from the hectic life of private practice to do insurance physicals which he said was more relaxed and he liked the work.

The other more direct influence I had was from Coach Cathers, my sophomore high school biology teacher. This guy was smart, nerdy and highly motivated to learn and teach. The only teacher I ever had who was able to plainly and openly discuss aspects of human sexuality from a biological and hormonal perspective. Fascinating stuff to male teenagers. He didn't actually coach any sports but got the name because he was always playing sandlot sports with his students: basketball, touch football, softball, etc. He was a poorly paid young man recently graduated from college and newly married without kids and was re-applying to dental school during his time teaching. I found myself in his advanced placement science class relaxed and having fun while learning all this cool stuff. It was a relatively small group of about 10-12 kids rolling along at a fast pace. During that year, we learned about him and he about us and we could all sense a pleasant, natural kinship in this pursuit of knowledge and understanding of biological processes. At some point mid-year, we heard of his aspirations to go to professional school and how it was a dream and life goal. He was obviously dead set on this being the most important thing in his life. He then began to talk to us about what we should consider in life. Something no teacher ever spoke of during high school. Pointing out our natural abilities to be able to grasp complex topics easily, he encouraged us to use that talent in life. He pushed us to consider either medical or dental school or an academic professorship. I remember distinctly the first time a little light bulb went off in my young, confused, teenage head that this is something important to consider. So, the seed was planted and began to take shape as I progressed through high school. Of course, I had no real idea what it meant to be a doctor, dentist or professor. Coach Cathers' dream was fulfilled when he entered dental school after my senior year of high school. We all gave him a big hug and high five when he proudly told us the news. His wife was pregnant and he was moving away and I would never see or hear from him again. But his encouragement and inspiration struck me and when I entered college it was with the conclusion that I would be "pre-med" as would a good portion of my classmates in my major. To me at the time, the concept of being a doctor was not with any real knowledge of the path to get there or the reality of the work itself. It largely was an academic goal. One that had a beginning and path forward to focus on with the end being a true unknown. This I found was a typical mindset of my friends in college working toward med school admission and my subsequent medical school friends who went along with the same vague concept. Also, I had no specific inkling what "type" of doctor I wanted to be.

Work in the medical professions can include huge differences in experience and work life. One can go from psychiatry, which includes the bizarre human details of the mind's inner workings to the bizarre inner workings of the abdomen as a surgeon or even to sitting in a dark room reading X-rays and scans of the body and having little patient contact. One friend of mine remarked as she entered her radiology residency with the disdain of physical contact "How can you stand touching patients?" She obviously picked the right field for herself. So the world of medicine includes many "different strokes for different folks".

When I made my life decision to go to medical school, I didn't have a specific specialty in mind either. Maybe, that is how I ended up as a general internist in primary care. However, being a student-athlete for my entire scholastic career, I was naturally interested in understanding the physiological processes of physical training especially as an endurance athlete in track and field and later as a marathon runner. The field of exercise physiology was just coming into being in the mid-1970s. The first great, comprehensive textbook came from the Karolinska Institute in Sweden and was edited by the world's most prominent exercise physiologist of the time, Per-Olaf Astrand. The book *Textbook of Work Physiology* covered all aspects of exercise physiology from muscle, hormonal adaptation and the latest science on training techniques that produced the greatest effects. Professor Astrand served on the Nobel prize committee and was generally regarded as one of the founding fathers of exercise physiology. When I received my copy of his book in 1977, I was working in physiology research at the medical school I would eventually enroll in the following year. I recall pouring over every detail in each section many times, fascinated that there was such knowledge of what was going inside the body under physical strain. At the time, I was training for the New York City marathon and subsequently the Boston Marathon six months later. I applied the knowledge of the smartest training techniques to my own training and attributed some of my success with running a 2-hour 28-minute Boston Marathon to that book. During that year, there seemed to be a true alignment of my life activities. I was working in the rehabilitation department research lab doing experiments on immobilization and nerve damage and its effects on muscle physiology while training for marathons, intently studying the most advanced knowledge in human exercise physiology and applying to medical school. No wonder then when asked during one of my medical school admission interviews about my motivation, desire and special skill that should be considered for my application I gave a lengthy answer about understanding the body under extreme physical stress can be viewed as a parallel to understanding the body afflicted with disease processes. My interviewer looked at me oddly and moved onto another question. I felt at the time that I totally blew the answer and was looking at another year of research. However, now at the end of my career, I see clearly that observation, even though it was all conjecture at that time, was a decent way of looking at medicine as physiology under various stressors. Whether those stressors are battling cancer, metabolism out of control with diabetes or severe asthma creating attempts to compensate. In a way, I was physically and intellectually involved with how the body responds to difficulty and how that adaptation can make the body work in a better way. It seemed clear to me at that time there was a congruence, connection and straightforward path from my scholastic attraction to the sciences, my athletic interests as an endurance athlete and my future to the practice of medicine even though I had little to no real knowledge of what was involved. My life was in seemingly blocks of four years from high school to college and another four years of medical school felt like a natural extension. After all, what else was I to do?

Another aspect of life also influenced the direction I took. I didn't see much inspiration in other walks of life. My father was an accountant and what I could discern from his work didn't appeal to me. Likewise, other aspects of business life did not have any pull. I worked various part time jobs in high school and summers of college and all seemed such drudgery: restaurant work, construction work, store clerk and delivery person. I had uncles who were car mechanics, electricians and other trade and business types and none seemed to be a job I wanted to do. Essentially, by process of elimination it was natural to keep to a life of science with all this cool stuff to learn. As science and math were fun, challenging and interesting, I seemed to naturally do well in the course work. I also found I wasn't drawn to an academic career of teaching or research. I got the most scholastic enjoyment in mastering a topic and doing well on tests and moving onto the next phase. I also didn't have a particularly long view of life then, in that

I really couldn't imagine or fantasize about my life at the age of 40 or older, for example. That concept was too distant and never entered my mind. As mentioned, my life was defined in blocks of time and during those times I was in a sort of cocoon working on completing that segment while keeping a balance of athletic and social involvement and going through the aspects of living all young folks seem to need to go through. Many of my classmates were more focused on life after completing school and had more definite plans but many others were like me and just went from one task to the next and growing up along the way in the seams of academic calendars without a true inkling of what was the end game in all this.

While there were many in my college major, biology, that declared themselves "pre-med" or "pre-dental" school, there was no specific designation from the college for this. There was a set of course requirements to complete in order to apply to medical school and, of course, the dreaded long, arduous, difficult and significantly decisive MCAT (medical college admission test) in senior year that we all prepared diligently for months in advance. This standardized test carried a significant weight to the admissions offices and ranked higher than one's GPA (grade point average). So there was lotsa fretting over this important standard.

What was lacking during college was any true career counseling or real-life experience placement to have students get a true understanding of what they were committing their body and soul to during their college years. Interestingly, none of us in "pre-med" actually ever talked about what we could expect from a life in medicine. The vast majority like myself had no direct interaction with the medical field and nearly no-one had a direct relative that was a physician. All we were focused on was obtaining the best grades from the required science courses. Enormous time and fretting were spent trying to master organic chemistry and comparative biology without any regard of where this was taking us. Possibly we were like Coach Cathers in that working on the goal was the point and the endgame could be figured out later. Certainly, that was my case. It was so difficult and competitive to gain admission that nothing after that could be imagined. This is in contrast to many other countries in Europe. There, many students enter a 6-year medical degree program when starting at the university level and the weeding out occurs along the way so that only a minority graduate. In the US, with very little exception all students who are admitted complete the four years of medical school and nearly everyone goes on to a specific internship and residency training in the field of their choice. Some go on to also obtain a PhD and move into the academic world of research and teaching.

So yes, it is odd looking back that the majority of us had no idea what we were really getting into and very few had a definitive plan of what type of physician we wanted to be when we "grew-up". That was the nature of the beast back then in the late 1970s but has changed now as most pre-med students do volunteer or paid positions at clinics, hospitals, ERs or offices to gain a line of experience on their applications. The big prize was getting an acceptance letter to any medical school. During my application time in the late 1970s was the peak for applicants. Only about one in three applicants were admitted. Tough times indeed. Fortunately, the year of research at the medical school I would attend did help me attain admission.

A career as a doctor can take many different forms and even a career change is possible if one doesn't like what one chooses. Many medical students don't make up their mind on a specialty until after the 3rd and 4th year clinical rotations when one gets a real life view of what's involved in each world. Also, I've known several classmates and residency mates that went on to entirely different fields and residencies after completing one and finding it was not for them. Certainly, a career path change from being an engineer to a carpenter or financial expert is much more difficult. In medicine, one can complete another several year training program of whatever specialty or subspecialty and be able to have a new life of one's choosing.

Like most then, I went blind into the healing arts, intent on completing the final segment of classroom learning in the first two years to proceed onto the real-life experience of hospital life and bedside learning and doctoring. I'm glad and grateful it has worked out, as I still have no idea what else I would or could have done!

CHAPTER 2

Internship

8 a.m., July 1st, 1982—the start of my internship in Internal Medicine at the Faulkner Hospital in Jamaica Plain, Boston. Three weeks earlier on the day after my 27th birthday, I received my diploma from Thomas Jefferson Medical College, the largest private medical school in the US with our class graduating 230 freshly minted doctors. We listened attentively to the commencement speech by the first woman to sit on the US Supreme Court, Sandra Day O'Connor. Her appointment that previous year by Ronald Reagan was a significant step pushing forward gender equality in the professions. Our medical class reflected the slowly but progressive changing demographic makeup of medical school students with about 15% of our class being female, up from a couple decades previously of about 1%. Currently and for some time, there have been more women than men in nearly all medical schools in America.

A few months earlier on the infamous "match day" (when all the medical students in the US find out where they will be doing their professional residency training), I found myself scrambling for a position after not matching to any of the programs I had picked. I was accurately counseled to only pick a spot that was acceptable as one could get forced into an undesirable program and location. As I had only chosen two, it was not a big surprise to find myself "unmatched" on match day. Many good programs did not completely fill up because high level students chose them down their list. As there was a ranking by both the students and the programs according to preference, a program could find itself not filling its quota. My decision turned from fretting about the lack of a residency training program to negotiating with several pleasant program directors of smaller programs in Boston. I chose one that seemed to suit me after chatting with several of the interns and residents. It turned out to be an excellent choice! The Faulkner Hospital was a smaller modern teaching community hospital on the western side of Boston and was affiliated with two medical schools, Tufts and Harvard. Being a less prestigious, smaller community-based teaching hospital unlike the many behemoth medical institutions of Boston (e.g. Massachusetts General, Beth Israel, the Deaconess, etc.), the Faulkner gave the interns and residents a hands-on direct care experience of caring for common medical problems of sick patients. This was in contrast to following a parade of senior faculty, fellowship doctors and senior residents seeing more obscure, rare diseases at the tertiary referral centers Boston is known for. This appealed to me greatly and my new colleagues conveyed that I would be able to handle all the aspects of modern Internal Medicine and at the same time have some fun. The Faulkner had been rebuilt less than 10 years earlier and was a modern, concrete structure that had recently gained a minor amount of fame by being in the 1981 film *Who's Life Is It Anyway?* starring Richard Dreyfuss in a story of the complexities of assisted suicide. Several of the medical staff had cameo roles in the film.

There is a somewhat true saying of "don't get sick and go to the hospital on July 1st!" This is due to the fact that at teaching hospitals the residents and interns are at their lowest level of experience and practical knowledge. For interns in particular, it is the first time one is really responsible for the care of patients, this includes trusting one's judgment in the diagnosis, interpreting and ordering appropriate tests, and deciding on specific treatments. Of course, this is not done in a vacuum as the second-year residents oversee the interns and senior/third year residents are at the top of the pyramid to help guide care. However, the weight of decision-making falls heavily and definitively on July 1st for the newbie "real" doctors. After a couple of mornings of orientation in the hospital and meeting upper level residents and staff it was time to dive into the profession.

I recall that getting used to being in a hospital all day was quite an adjustment when I started my clinical rotations in my third year of medical school. After literally a lifetime of classroom and lab work and studying, it was a shock to arrive at 6 or 7 a.m. everyday for rounds on sick patients with a group of students, residents and faculty staff physicians or while in surgical rotations getting scrubbed in for assisting for a surgery. My first six months of hospital clinical experience were a difficult and disorientating apprenticeship of learning how hospitals "worked". From the physical layout, to the rhythm of the day, and even for simple tasks such locating a patient chart or the radiology department and even finding the cafeteria it seemed impossible to know what to do and where to go. As a medical student, being the lowest on the totem pole of care as well as being the most annoying and least helpful of everyone in the hospital meant no respect and obviously no confidence. Even the nurses had little time or patience for the fumbling medical students although at times they could be quite instructive in most aspects of hospital life. I learned to try to stay out of the way and do whatever "scut" work was asked while at the same time trying to learn any useful tidbit. Most late afternoons were an experience of aching feet from standing most of the day and extreme mental fatigue from trying to be an alert sponge.

The process of starting an internship is really in the "handoff". What this means is that the patients from the previous day need to be transferred to the new team taking care of them. The various floors of the hospitals are divided into sections, e.g. north or south. The other areas such as the ICU (intensive care unit), SICU (surgical intensive care unit), telemetry (where patients are on heart monitors or other monitors are watched closely but not as closely as the ICU) and the ER (emergency room) are also cared for by those specific teams of residents, interns and students on that rotation. Each rotation can be 4-8 weeks at a time and then one switches to a different team so that throughout the year each one has obtained experience in all the different parts of the hospital.

The handoff between teams as occurred on that fateful first day of July is one of extreme relief for the outgoing team and extreme anxiety for the incoming team. My initial assignment was with a team of 4 interns, one second year resident and 2 medical students on the south side of the 4th floor. There also was a senior resident (3rd year of training) that oversaw our entire floor. We had about 30 inpatients to care for and listened attentively as we first heard the morning report from those who were on-call the previous night. This included the basics of each patient's diagnosis and progress at that point as well any new patients that had been admitted from the previous night. While our first jitters were kept hidden as well as could be, the newly advanced second year resident who just the day before was an intern felt the pressure of being in a position of overseer not only of large caché of patients but of making sure the newbies didn't screw up and at the same time trying to teach the ropes of medical care to both interns and students. That position I remember being nearly as difficult as the start of internship. After hearing about the patients and having them split up equally among us, we proceeded to "rounding", the process of going to each patient room and assessing their status and deciding on their care. With the rolling cart and the nurses accompanying us with all the charts, we went first to the patients who were admitted the previous night to check their status, confirm their treatment was correct and make any further decisions on treatment or tests that were needed. Because we would be rotating on-call every 4th night, it was crucial to have knowledge of all the patients on the team as complications could and did occur at night. Morning rounds took a good deal of the morning but could easily be interrupted by a call from the ER for a new patient that needed admission to our team or from the ICU transferring an improving patient to the general medical floor. Those patients were then assigned in rotation to each of us to go do the "work up" or the admission history and physical and orders for treatment. Late mornings we gathered in the radiology department to review all the X-rays, CT scans, ultrasounds of other radiologic tests done on the patients. Here we would get to see the films with the radiologists and begin to get a sense of those black, gray and white images from various body parts. Afternoons were spent going over test results that were performed in the morning as well as a re-evaluation of the patients' status and response to care and ordering additional treatment or evaluation tests. Of course, there were often new patients being admitted as well. Some of them came from the private physicians' offices who then entrusted us to deliver proper treatment after a brief discussion on their problems. Some patients needed a specialist to evaluate and help guide their care and we would also go over their written consults or talk with them about a case to be clear of the plan. Our second year resident was around to help out with the more difficult patients and to provide guidance on the rationale of certain treatments and evaluative steps. We were all familiar with the workflow of the day from being medical students but now actually needing to make the decisions and not look too dumb in front of fellow interns and senior residents explaining one's thinking process was a big step up in the hierarchy and part of the personal journey to becoming a "real" doctor.

While I don't recall all the specifics of that first day of internship, I can say that the terror of anticipation quickly gave way to the reality that work needed to be done and that one did not want to miss any significant factors or make any grave mistakes which upped the ante to be super compulsive. The next level of anxiety was, of course, the first night on-call. The anticipation of spending all night in the hospital with little prospect of sleep and having to evaluate and order all the treatments needed for a new acutely ill patient easily led to less sleep the night *before* call. So, it was common to already be sleep deprived when one's call night started. At that time we had a primitive beeper that we wore which was similar to a one-way walkie-talkie radio. We received direct voice messages from the hospital operators to call a certain number when we were needed. These could come from nurses, the X-ray department, other interns or residents or departments such as the ER passed through to the hospital switchboard operators. The messages came in a combination of vibration and a quite loud, scratchy voice such as "call 5203, call 5203". Occasionally, a call would be announced overhead but this was frowned upon as it could be heard throughout the entire hospital.

"Code Blue" calls (patients discovered suddenly without a pulse or were not breathing) were announced by room number and floor level by an overhead announcement indicating a possible cardiac arrest that needed an urgent response. The word "blue" is used because it designates finding a patient with bluish colored skin which indicates a general low level of oxygenated blood instead of having a normal pink hew. When a code was called on the floor, the team of interns and residents working closeby were the first to respond, but also the senior resident would join the mayhem trying to make sure that procedural items like intubation and possible need for a special IV line to be placed appropriately in order to deliver resuscitation medications and monitoring devices. A "Code Blue" could be quite variable in that it was called usually by the nurses who found a patient simply unresponsive, other times in patients with no blood pressure, respirations or pulse or even having continuous seizures. Quickly hooking up an EKG machine after CPR was started was the first order of business in a true cardiac arrest situation. Sometimes "Codes" were quite short when in reviving an overmedicated patient with supplemental oxygen or in a patient that needed to be put in "trendelenburg" (where one lowers the head and elevates the legs in order to facilitate blood flow to the brain when blood pressure is low). In-hospital cardiac arrests have a much higher rate of successful resuscitation (25%) as compared to out in the real world (<10%) due to quickness of response and advanced technical and medical availability.

There is a common set of medical problems one encounters on a general medicine floor including: congestive heart failure (backup of fluid into the lungs due the pumping of the heart not being sufficient); pneumonias either bacterial or viral or rarely fungal; acute asthma not requiring a ventilator assist; gastrointestinal bleeding, which can be from the esophagus, stomach or lower intestine; strokes from blood clots or bleeding; diabetic ketoacidosis from prolonged very high blood sugar levels resulting in metabolic derangements; blood clots in the lungs or legs; severe infections of the skin; complications of cancer or cancer treatments; respiratory decompensation related to COPD in smokers (chronic obstructive pulmonary disease); and septicemia which is due to blood stream infection. Certainly there are many more acute diagnoses that get patients a bed in the hospital which can be uncommon such as kidney failure or deteriorating neurologic status of multiple sclerosis. Some acute admissions require the patients to be in the ICU or heart monitoring units such as heart attacks or cardiac dysrhythmias, those with very low blood pressure or if in need of a ventilator for respiratory failure. After initial improvement these patients are often sent to the medical floor for less intensive treatment. Also, teaching hospitals have a specific area for surgical patients that may to be treated before or after an operation. Surgical problems include: intestinal blockage, gallbladder disease, bowel resection due to cancer or disease, or vascular surgery for a blocked artery in the neck, abdomen or legs. Many of these patients also have multiple medical problems that require the medical team to evaluate and stabilize before and after their surgeries. There is a lot of cross-over of care in a hospital between the surgical and medical teams.

After the first couple of days on internship, I found myself in the dread of the first night on-call. This meant answering calls from nurses, the lab and radiology department after 5 p.m. This also meant doing the "H+P" (literally, the history and physical report for the medical chart) on the new admissions from the ER. One of the newer excellent innovations that our residency program started was a "night float". This was a rotation where one of the interns for a month would work 6 nights a week from 10 a.m. to 8 a.m. and help do some of the admissions that occurred deep in the night to relieve the workload of those on regular call. Being on-call meant staying in the hospital for nearly 36 hours straight before going home the following evening. There was an on-call room with a bed where one could try to get some rest between calls from the nurses and admissions from the ER. There was never much sleep to be had and often if one did get to sleep the sudden, loud interruption of a call jolted one back to a fully awake but disoriented state.

My first night on-call included admitting an elderly man who had become increasingly short of breath for a few days and was brought to the ER by his family. He was wheezing, had hypoxia (low oxygen) and his chest X-ray had a few hazy patches scattered around. The ER intern thought all his problems were related to pneumonia which sounded like a reasonable diagnosis. Since he was not sick enough for the ICU as his oxygen level came up with supplemental oxygen via nasal cannulas, the second-year resident assigned him to the floor. He was a scruffy looking 74-year-old man, unshaved for a few days, a tattered undershirt and stained overshirt but was reasonably comfortable from a breathing standpoint when I saw him on the ward. I had reviewed his old chart which was not large but did include a prior history of smoking which he stopped several years ago. There was mention of a diagnosis of COPD (chronic obstructive pulmonary disease from smoking) and a tendency toward mild heart failure determined by an echocardiogram showing a lower than normal ejection fraction (heart muscle pump measurement). When I examined him, I found that he was wheezing throughout his lungs and had a minor amount of edema (swelling) of his ankles. At this point, I became concerned that this patient could have other significant medical diagnoses besides pneumonia. It was quite possible that he was also having an exacerbation of his COPD with the wheezing and had fallen into heart failure as well with his low oxygen straining his heart. The problem was that all three conditions are treated quite differently and if I just treated the pneumonia with antibiotics and oxygen and if these other two conditions were more of the reason for his shortness of breath, his condition could worsen overnight and he could, well, die. Also, I didn't want to look like an idiot if he worsened and had to go to the ICU and didn't want to look bad at the morning report with the Chief of Medicine, Dr. Huevos. Mulling over this expanding list of issues, I decided to talk to the second-year resident about this case, pleading that I "didn't want to get burned on my first on-call night". We agreed to address all the potential threats and treat him with bronchodilators to relieve his wheezing, start an appropriate antibiotic and to give him a diuretic to reduce any fluid overload. He was a typical pneumonia patient, unable to cough out his phlegm instead swallowing it.

The next morning after a near sleepless night, I sat nervously, constantly checking my notes in Dr. Huevos' office with the other interns and residents as a brief summary of each admission from the previous night was presented. The relaxed, well rested chief listened attentively to each and incisively offered a pertinent question regarding a missing data point or examination finding. In my case, he asked in his low pitch, Hungarian accented voice at the end of the presentation, "well, …

and what was the BUN?" I scrambled a bit to find the result and then knew why he was asking and said, "35". The BUN is an acronym for the blood level of urea, a waste product. When elevated it can indicate lower blood flow to the kidneys such as occurs with congestive heart failure. He made this point in a simple and non-judgmental manner but in such a definitive way that it would never be forgotten.

That patient ended up improving with this combination of treatments that included "covering all bases". In about 48 hours he was able to breathe without the need for supplemental oxygen and his chest X-ray looked a bit better. It was still a bit unclear what the leading underlying diagnosis was, but improvement is always welcome. This case turned out to be emblematic of much of acute care hospitalization treatment. While doctors are usually well schooled in defining a specific disease entity, patients come to the ER or office with a symptom that can indicate many possible diagnoses. We call this the "differential diagnosis" meaning in the chart at the end of the history and physical it was common to include a large list of possibilities under the label "DDx". This is stressed in medical training in order to keep a broad view of the possibility of various diseases. One then whittles down the list to only a few or hopefully one main contender. However, patients often have more than one medical issue going on at the same time that doctors and especially interns need to keep an open mind while treating and gathering more data.

The above description of the nuts and bolts of internship does not nearly tell the complete story of the personal experience of learning the healing trade. Internships which started only in the 19th century are based on the concept of apprenticeship. Being immersed in learning skills while trying to do them is the basic way humans learn anything. Medicine is no different. One starts with a bit of knowledge and a lot of determination, motivation and time to dedicate to the process. In this way, one's entire day and life becomes one of learning. Being completely immersed allows familiarity and then the experience to predict what can occur in a variety of situations. The combined experience of observing and participating in the care of 30 patients a day, discussing the details and plans in our small group of various diseases and their treatment and then seeing directly the good and bad results of how events play out and how their treatments can be effective or not (including side effects and bad outcomes) builds an experiential gestalt that creates the physician. No matter how difficult or physically taxing or emotionally draining, an internship molds one into a doctor who is soon comfortable and informed with being around very sick individuals. The enhanced power of this type of learning is in the repetition in seeing the common and some of the uncommon serious medical problems many times over. We could easily have a handful of patients with congestive heart failure, pneumonia, stroke, or gastrointestinal bleeding on our team at the same time as well as various cancers in different stages and responding to different treatments. By getting a direct insight into the nuances of how diseases can have variations of symptoms, testing results and responses to treatment builds a true understanding of severe illness processes. It still amazes me that after several months of this immersion, I too had a real feel for the common hospital problems and developed a growing comfort level of seeing sick patients under my care.

All acquired skills require that mistakes are made on an ongoing and progressive level and then understanding the corrections needed. Proficiency takes a certain period of analyzing the process, obtaining the knowledge necessary and understanding the fine points of potential events. However, in medicine there is little room for mistakes. A small mistake of misreading a lab report, X-ray, or physical sign or symptom can cost a person's life. This concern sits constantly on the shoulders of all interns at all times. This is not like learning to be a blacksmith, where one might make some very poorly constructed horseshoes until the senior tradesman goes over the details of properly hammering the metal into the correct shape becomes ingrained in which the misshapen shoes can be discarded, reshaped or used for a short time. The horse never dies from a bad fit. Fortunately, the process of oversight in internship with its various levels of checks that go up the ladder of experience and expertise is present. Interns learn mostly from second and third year residents and from the medical staff assigned to oversee and teach. The collectiveness of all this exposure quickly broadens one's knowledge base, understanding and toolbox of skills. In parallel, the medical staff that sends their sick patients to the hospital, often give a broader insight into the life background of the patient's current illness. This aspect of the patient is often downgraded in the intern's mind as somewhat trivial in comparison to treating the severe problems present in the moment but becomes more important later in training and working in the field of medicine. In the hierarchy of experience and knowledge in a teaching hospital, interns learn to impart knowledge to fledgling medical students that hover around with book knowledge but no context. Fascinately, one of the best ways to solidify one's understanding of a complex issue that is not completely understood is to explain it to someone else. In this way, interns learn a significant amount by simply teaching students the hows and whys of hospital life, reasoning behind ordering certain tests and treatments and how to begin thinking like a doctor focusing on the important stuff instead of in a tangent typical of medical students. The old saying "when you hear hoofbeats, think horses not zebras" applies significantly to medical student thinking as one has just studied all the various diseases and they are all blended together without any ranking when they enter the hospital. So on rounds, when they reflexly pipe in with an obscure disease such as "idiopathic pulmonary fibrosis" or "sarcoidosis" for someone who is short of breath in middle age instead of the common causes such as pneumonia or asthma or COPD it is fun to listen to the thinking that the interns had just 1 or 2 years prior.

It is often asked of interns "how do you keep all that information about the drugs, dosages, tests, interpretations, etc. in your head especially when you're chronically sleep deprived?" Well, one doesn't have that much working memory and interns are no different. Many commonly used medications are easily recalled (e.g. intravenous furosemide 40 mg every 6 to 12 hours for diuresis in heart failure) while many combinations and sequences of various medications are not. Therefore, in my era of training (mid-1980s) one always had the invaluable *Washington Manual* tucked safely in one of the coat pockets of a clinic jacket along with one's stethoscope and various tools for examination like an otoscope, ophthalmoscope, reflex hammer, pin for testing sensation, etc. The *Manual* as it was called was the only pocket size source of all the important information available in a portable and easily accessible format. It was spiral bound so one could look up a topic and keep it flat in a 5" × 7" format. The pages had a mild plastic coating so it was not easily torn or ruined with water or clumsy fingers. It included all the up-to-date treatments as it was revised every 3 years (corresponding to the length of an internal medicine residency). It was first written by a senior resident of Washington University medical center in St. Louis in 1943 and quickly became the crucial "on the ground" reference for acute hospital medical care. Everyone had one and most of them were marked with notes from their owner. Interns and their manuals were inseparable and a quick look up of a dose of medicine or disease was as often as checking the time on one's watch. The manual was brilliantly written in that it gave a short, concise description of each disease and the evaluation and specific treatments. While it could be described as somewhat like a cookbook, it gave quick insight and directions to the full panoply of medical diseases. While medicine was and is considered an "art" and a science, the use of the underpinnings of its science are the basis of modern medicine. The art of the field comes in more when the diagnosis is less clear from a scientific standpoint or when the problems the patient has are at the margins of known medical treatments. The crucial aspect of the Washington Manual was that it gave instant reference to *current* scientific treatments and understandings, so it was at times even more trustable than advice given by other residents or senior physicians. Medicine was entering the era of more rigorous scientific treatment in the '70s and '80s so to be at the leading edge of this wave with this little book gave one the proper distilled knowledge known at that time. While this book continues to be revised, other online references have taken its place. Namely, the reference known as *UptoDate* has a vast database of disease information and treatments written for clinicians. It has become the goto reference over the past 15 for most as it is updated regularly (sometimes every few months) as new research and data become published and is authored often by many of the world's experts on a particular topic and is available as an app on smartphones.

No-one can become a good doctor just by knowing what is known. Clinical observation and experience in complex situations gives physicians insight into what are known as "pearls". A clinical pearl is a particular small bit of advice that can be crucial to a particular situation which has been observed by many doctors or over a long course of experience. A clinical pearl when imparted to an intern is a little gift of gold from a senior physician that lifts the level of understanding to a higher level immediately. Interns and actually all doctors are on the lookout for "pearls" of clinical wisdom. I heard one of these pearls early in my internship from the chief of pulmonary medicine, Dr. Brockman. "All that wheezes is not asthma" has stuck with me since and has been passed to other interns, students and colleagues over the years. Simply put, even though a patient has audible wheezes, which are typical in asthma patients, it does not mean exclusively it is due to asthma. Asthma is a common problem and is due to the constriction of large, medium and small bronchioles which transmit air deep to the lung tissue. Asthmatics can have "attacks" triggered by allergies, cold air, or infections and are treated with inhaled medicine that dilate the constrictions. Other medicines are also used in severe cases to stabilize the reaction such as cortisone. However, there are various other problems that can also cause the lungs to wheeze such as congestive heart failure or lung damage from smoking or even viral or bacterial pneumonias which are all treated differently.

I'll give a sample of some of the pearls we learned along the way. One of the best and simplest pearls of identifying someone with severe anemia is when their creases in their palms are no longer pink (also their whole hand is whitish due to low volume of red cells). Another is when low white cells are seen in patients with a viral infection. In patients with joint pains, morning stiffness that lasts for at least an hour can indicate rheumatoid arthritis, a serious inflammatory disorder. An important pearl in considering if someone is having a heart attack (myocardial infarction) is that "chest pain from a heart attack is never fleeting, symptoms lasting less than a minute are usually not related to ischemia (lack of blood flow to the heart from a blockage)". Another bit of modern and important wisdom is "you can't make an asymptomatic patient feel better".

There was also another important underground source for interns on how to survive and get perspective. This was contained in the bitingly accurate and comically satirical book *House of God* written in pseudonym by Samuel Shem (later to be discovered to be psychiatrist Stephen Bergman) in 1978. The novel follows the course of the year of medical interns in a fictionalized version of a famous Harvard teaching hospital. The book immediately developed a cult following and became "required" reading for all interns of any specialty soon after its release. By the early 1980s it had attained mythical status for physicians in training. It was released to scandalous reviews for its frank portrayal of hospital life for young doctors, patients, administrators of a dehumanizing medical system and its psychological harms. It formed an important anchor for medical interns to have the abuse and difficulties so humorously articulated and stirred important societal discussions of humanistic care and the ethics of medicine training. The story follows a naive and poorly prepared intern for the travails that await him. He is introduced and instructed into the "Laws" by his massively overweight senior resident which will allow for his psychological survival. The premise of the Laws is that medical care only causes more suffering and death and by doing nothing one finds that patients get better faster. The author brings to light the derogatory term for patients "gomers" (an acronym for "get out of my emergency room"). The various episodes in the book show the conflicts and paradoxes of hospital care from an insider's perspective. While the book was derided by the older medical establishment, especially in Boston where I was doing my residency, it provided an important psychological and humorous buffer to what we were going through. At lunch, we interns often referred to one of the "Laws" or brought up a parallel experience we were having that was documented in the book. I'm not sure if it is still read today, but it provided sympathy and humor as a survival guide during a time of extreme physical and psychological exhaustion using dazzling humor and horror. Concepts of the book have crept into modern culture and sitcoms as depicted in the popular series *Scrubs*.

While working 100 hours per week was a grind, it did not mean that we didn't squeeze out social time when there was an opportunity. Young men and women in their late 20s have an irresistible need to socially connect with each other. The lack of time and the urgency made our free time even more precious than ever. A teaching hospital has an ample supply of both sexes working closely together. Boston was somewhat famous for having scores of young Irish women in the nursing and ancillary services. Our intern group of fifteen included five women of which nearly all were married in contrast to the ten men of which only one was. The daily interactions of all the teams and the rotations to the various departments gave everyone exposure to each other. Naturally, there was bound to be pairings. My first introduction to the potential social life was after the first week when there was a pool party at the nurses residence next to the hospital. Yes, it seemed a bit odd that there would be a pool and affordable housing for nursing but it was one of the attractions that brought staff away from the bigger more famous hospitals in Boston. The chief resident and the senior residents were all there, ready to give us the inside tips to getting along with the attending physicians and specialists as well as the inside scoop on the social side of the hospital. Stories were told of various hilarious exploits of previous interns and residents that were passed down to each new group.

The socialization of our group evolved slowly. We were all too wrapped up in just getting by without killing our patients that it took nearly 4 months or so to get comfortable with being an intern, to get to know each other somewhat and to get to know the hospital staff to be able to pick a night out for a drink together. Our first get-together which included those not on-call and some of the nurses on the floor was at a local bar-restaurant near Boston Circle on Commonwealth Ave near where I lived, The Tam. There was music and dancing on Thursday nights. This was the first unleashing of built-up energy to just have fun with a few drinks to chat and laugh and dance. As happens when young men and women commingle, there was the end of the evening pairings and make-out sessions at cars before going home. All so innocent and needed after months of stress-racked work. While the group mix changed depending on the call schedule, there was a regular get-together every couple of weeks to keep and expand the social structure of the hospital. This gave an outlet to the bonding during work that was able to be expressed and enjoyed out of the restraints of hospital life. Later in the spring, we were able to get together for sunny, warm New England evenings for an informal softball game and beers afterward. Of course, eventually a few of the single interns ended up falling in love and pairing off with a nurse or radiology technician. This seemed the natural result of such intense experiences shared. A couple of these turned into long-term relationships and marriages. However, for me it was inconceivable to consider a serious relationship in the midst of this process. Honestly, I couldn't handle any other responsibilities other than getting to the hospital every day and finishing my work. These occasional escapes were great but there was a price to pay for every missed hour of sleep that was consumed by drinking beer.

Along the way, we got to know the teaching senior staff of experienced physicians that gave us some insight and entertainment as well as pearls of wisdom. A small group of specialists spent a good amount of their time in the hospital such as the chief of cardiology and pulmonary medicine as well as infectious disease, gastroenterologists and neurology. They were consulted on very ill patients in the ICU frequently and offered their expertise on care as well as performing procedures such as special monitoring vascular lines for patients with low blood pressure, bronchoscopy for unclear lung problems and endoscopies for intestinal bleeding and possible cancer diagnoses. These procedures were beyond the scope of what we were going to learn as interns and residents as one would need to complete a specialty fellowship of an additional 2-3 years to become proficient in these. However, we were to learn and become proficient in many important emergency procedures during our training and internship. The beginning of the infamous method of "see one, do one, teach one" is heard throughout teaching hospitals as skill and confidence is passed down.

The important procedures we learned to save lives or to monitor very ill patients were many. Intubation is done by placing a breathing tube accurately into the upper trachea to assist with breathing and to give oxygen. The need for intubating a patient is obvious when she is not breathing, for example after a cardiopulmonary arrest, or when measuring blood oxygen and carbon dioxide the levels become dangerously out of range to continue to support life. Commonly, during a "code blue" it is needed to assure that oxygen can be delivered to best assist the resuscitation. However, in the "heat of the moment" it can be extremely difficult. In this example the patient is undergoing chest compressions for cardiac resuscitation, she could have loose dentures in her mouth, she could have vomited and have food in her upper esophagus and airway, she could be very thin or very obese or have a very short neck that makes tilting the head back to see the airway difficult. Also, time is of the essence in an arrest situation.

I remember clearly the first time I saw a senior resident grabbing a laryngoscope in one hand, which is foldable curved blade with a light at the end, then quickly and precisely guiding it down the throat to visualize the larynx which was quickly followed by a smooth, controlled sliding of the endotracheal breathing tube in the other hand into the correct position followed by inflating the balloon at the lower end to secure it in position. This act amazed me in a way few others had in my life. The resident was calm and almost matter-of-fact during the task, indicating he had done this scores of times. Literally, this person's life was rescued in a few seconds of technical skill. The patient was an enormously overweight man who had overdosed on heroin and was in the ER after having a respiratory arrest. He was blue with a faint pulse and had a very low oxygen level in his blood. This was an extremely difficult intubation situation. It took practicing on a dummy at least a hundred times before I felt I had an idea of how it could be done. My best learning experience was after a code blue death when my second-year resident said to give it a go after the nurses had left and the curtains were drawn. It was difficult for the senior residents to have the interns try a procedure at such an urgent time but there were sometimes when a patient was going into respiratory failure and was sedated that made the attempts more controlled. These are where we developed skill and confidence. Of course, there were emergencies in the ER or the ICU where prompt intubation was needed and a more senior resident had not yet arrived and these were the most intense and focused times I remember. To be honest, I and most of us did not really feel comfortable about intubation until sometime in our second year of residency after many tense situations had been encountered and conquered.

The other "big" hospital procedure to get under our belts was placement of a central line. This is a large bore intravenous catheter put into a major vein in the neck or upper chest in order to secure access for administering IV fluids, blood, medications and for also measuring what is known as central venous pressure or the CVP. With a central line one can administer large amounts of fluid or blood quickly, give certain cardiac medications and by reading the CVP determine if the patient is dehydrated or has too much fluid in her body. It has become the most useful tool in severely ill patients for decades. The other reason needing a central line placed is because the patient no longer has any usable veins in her extremities. Mostly IVs are put in the hands or arms of patients and quite rarely in the legs. Many patients have tiny veins or veins that have been used up with previous IVs that are not able to be cannulated. Having a working IV is indispensable in the vast majority of patients in the hospital. We were exposed to this technique and indications early in our internship. One example was an elderly, frail woman who had lost a significant amount of blood from a stomach ulcer overnight after being admitted for vomiting blood was then experiencing a lower blood pressure on rounds the next morning. Her one small, barely functioning IV in her hand was blown. Our second-year resident called for the "central line kit". There are generally two technical approaches to place a large bore catheter. One is from the side of the neck behind the muscles that attach from the lower skull to the clavicle (the sterno-cleido-mastiod muscle) so that one can place a large needle into the internal jugular vein. This is generally thought of as the easiest and safest approach. The other approach that was favored by the surgical residents was to enter at the upper chest just under the outer collarbone to place the needle and then catheter into the subclavian vein. This had more potential downside if one misdirected the needle and entered the lung causing a pneumothorax. However, it likely is more stable in that it allows the patient to move her neck without a big catheter taped. We learned the first approach first.

Simply, one disinfects the area with betadine, opens the kit, puts on sterile gloves, then one hand identifies the landmarks on the neck while the other hand holds the large, long needle with a syringe. Some local anesthetic could be used but if the patient was unconscious it was unnecessary. Passing the long needle slowly into the neck with light backward pressure on the syringe until there was a gush of veinous (dark) blood coming into the syringe indicating one was in the correct spot. Then the syringe was removed and the plastic catheter was fed into the syringe for several inches to secure a proper deep placement in the large vein. The end of the catheter was attached to an IV bag and easy passage of fluid through the catheter confirmed it was in the correct place. One needed to secure the line by a suture tied around the catheter and to the underlying skin to keep it from coming out. Of course, bad things could happen such as not finding the vein after several pokes, or putting the needle into the nearby carotid artery (which is deeper in the neck) causing a pulsing of bright red arterial blood or even piercing the lung from above. Of course, we would be aware and frightened to not have such a mishap.

Seeing a senior resident place a central line under duress in a quick and adroitful way was inspiring, giving us hope we could get to that skill level. It would take most of the year to get enough opportunities and practice. While there were occasional mistakes, none of the complications were severe, permanent or fatal, as I recall. It was a procedure that we all got excited about doing due to the immediacy and challenge to "strike gold" by placing the guiding needle into the correct vein.

Of course, there were many other procedures we got to do along the way, although less frequently. These included placing an arterial line in a wrist artery (tricky but not so difficult); passing a temporary cardiac pacer wire into the heart of patients whose intrinsic heart rhythm was too slow or damaged and needed immediate assistance (quite tricky technically as one was pacemaking from inside the heart; and even the rare procedure of relieving blood filling up around the heart causing tamponade by putting a large needle and syringe and extracting the blood.

One of the strangest and least frequent was to place a soft rubber tube into the stomach and inflate a balloon at its end to compress against the bleeding lower esophageal varices (swollen veins from backpressure) found in alcoholic cirrhotic patients. This was to stop the patient from bleeding to death. This was in the period before gastroenterologists performed emergency endoscopy where they now cauterize the bleeding veins to get them to stop. This usually occurred in the middle of the night on a semi-comatose, drunk patient but the oddly comical component was that after it was properly placed, the patient was fitted with a football helmet which held the tube in place. An additional benefit was that this tube prevented the patient from vomiting and then aspirating the contents into his lungs. Typically, it remained in place for 48 hours or so to assure bleeding would be stopped. Of course, patients who awoke the next day were typically confused and agitated about all of this and were always trying to pull it out. Sedation and restraints were needed.

During that period of ICU medicine there was a special catheter named a Swan-Ganz catheter (after the two doctors that developed it) that was fed into the right side of the heart and could measure internal pressures and oxygen content in extremely ill and complicated patients from the access of a central line. It could also be "wedged" into a pulmonary artery to measure the pressures of the left side of the heart. While this seemed to be an important way of monitoring some ICU patients, it was eventually found that the information added no great benefit to care and it was quite expensive and technically demanding and it has subsequently completely fallen from use. However, at the time, we all loved playing with the numbers and the emerging high technology of "Swann lines".

Death and dying were a definitive part of that first year of real doctoring. While it was not a daily event, it lurked in the background of every admission we did and every bad turn a patient took. The reality that old, very sick patients died was clear. Mostly, we observed it from a point of view of unchangeable events in the course of the limitations of medical treatment. We could not bring back a non-beating fibrillating heart from a cardiac arrest most times. Even if we were right there when it happened. Even after 30 minutes of electrical shocks, chest compressions, intubation with 100% oxygen, multiple rounds of various cardiac stimulating and regulating drugs delivered via a new central line patients often died. We stood there afterward, our heart rates slowly returning to normal in the quiet after all the hectic activity and machines ceased, gazing at the motionless, peaceful corpse lying on the bed and witnessing directly and definitively that life ends at some point. We confronted the limits of what we could do and accepted them as part of what we were learning. Soon after, explaining the events to the loved ones and attending staff physicians there seemed to be a sense of completion and perspective that allowed us to quickly move back into the world of the ill that could be helped.

Of course, death comes in various ways, sometimes quick, sometimes unexpected and other times slow and drawn out. We were to experience significant doses of all the varieties. Some patients arrive at the hospital already close to death. Cancer patients that have not responded to chemotherapy and came in for an infection or extremely low blood counts for the last time. Heart failure patients that cannot clear the excess fluid that has built up in their lungs and body while the attempts at diuresis with powerful medications are barely improving their condition. Long term stroke patients with paralysis of half their bodies, unable to speak and swallow with bed sores, infections and lungs filled with vomit and a psyche ready to give up. We could not ignore death and had the opportunity to see it happen up close and observe it directly and see the hows and trace the whys. It's a natural event. Of course, we cannot keep all patients alive with treatment. Of course, there is an end to a long life. Most deaths we saw were not unexpected at all. Rather they reinforced the lessons of the limits of medicine and of mortality itself. Of course, for us in our twenties this was something way far in the distant future. While we were directly involved with the care of the dying, these patients were not our family or friends, so it was somewhat easy to keep a professional distance emotionally from the inevitability of life. Medical students are not given much instruction on death and dying. It's all about what to do to keep life going. Interns learn on the job the process of dying. I recall getting some important insight into allowing dying patients to die from several of the attending physicians who knew their patients well and understood that there was a limitation to what could be or *should* be done for them. One example was when a patient with terminal cancer was admitted for increasing pain of metastatic disease and was started on a morphine drip. The attending, Dr. Walls, softly instructed me to

keep increasing the rate until the patient was comfortable, then unconscious and then allowed to stop breathing quietly. He knew this was the
patient's wish and while euthanasia was not technically permitted, a
death such as this was looked on as a natural, kind, human way to limit
suffering. This was way before the current "advance directives" that
patients can sign but there obviously was no conflict with our work
and we recognized that this type of comforting death had to come from
the physicians who knew best. While this was not common, never did
I feel uncomfortable with this gentle acceleration of a patient's death.
There was never a doubt that withdrawing active treatment and giving
comfort care was a bad decision and it was obviously more humane
than continuing futile medical care for a period of time that only prolonged a patient's suffering. Understanding when to stop treatment to
prepare a patient and family for death was one of the crucial lessons I
learned during internship and residency and which I carried throughout my entire career. While it may seem to many to be too complex
and difficult to determine when death is coming, in reality, it has been
nearly always easy to identify the situations where the end of life was
near and that further treatment offered no hope of real recovery or a
return to meaningful healthy life. And so for me (and I would say most
physicians), the situations are obvious to know and discuss end of life
processes with patients and family with assurance and kindness.

An important issue in discussing death, as I've been asked at many
cocktail parties, is "how can you deal with it, psychologically?" and "do
you become numb to it?" Well, the answer is complex as are most. As
mentioned, most of the death that is encountered is expected and it's
not so difficult to separate out an inevitable event from a preventable
one and therefore, as anyone would do, accept the reality and move on.
I will admit and I'm sure many/most other physicians would as well,
that to do the best one can, it is crucial to maintain a certain sense of
emotional distance to keep one's thinking and analysis on track to best
help patients medically. That doesn't mean there isn't compassion and
empathy for what the patient and the family is going through but it is
not best to be stuck in the tragedy instead of looking at the realistic
possibilities for treatment and keeping a balance of level-headed judg-

ment as the primary focus. Certainly, some situations are much more tragic than others. I remember a middle-aged man with a progressive, fatal blood bacterial infection that caused multi-organ damage, coma and brain death over the course of a few weeks. It was quite difficult emotionally to be involved with this situation especially in the context of his wife and children holding vigil in the hospital but it was crucial for the medical team to stay focused on the complexity of this man's medical issues in order to give him the best chance of recovery.

There has been a long tradition in medicine that a postmortem autopsy could help determine the exact cause of death. This practice was fading in the 1980s and has continued to decline today where there are few autopsies done. However, on those occasions where we were privileged to go to the morgue after the pathologist had completed the autopsy was the effect of having an entire review of medical school in an hour! The detail of the pathologist was always quite impressive by discussing the various organs and tissues and the effect the illness had on each as well as putting together a cogent and scientific rationale for the cause of death. Usually the pathologist also found other disease processes some of which were not known and which gave us a deeper understanding of the cause of death beyond what we already knew from lab tests, scans, biopsies and examinations. Autopsies always broadened our view of what to be thinking in the future. Death informed us in a more complete manner.

My internship was transformational. I couldn't have anticipated the growth as a physician and a person due to this immersion. Encountering and understanding common serious medical illnesses found in a community hospital and becoming competent to initiate treatments and to anticipate nuances of illness seemed impossible at the start. I could for the first time call myself a doctor. Certainly, I hadn't learned everything, but there were two more years to refine and expand my fluency in medicine. Of course, there was no fanfare or graduation or anything marking the end of it. On June 30th, 1983 I was ready to become a second-year resident the next morning and continue on. The preciousness of that extremely difficult, stressful year of incredible growth lingers in my mind 40 years later.

CHAPTER 3

My Stint as a Back Doctor

February 1988 and it was time to grow up, find a real job and move away from the cultural and personal wasteland known as Southern California where I had been living and working for the past year in various ERs and urgent care clinics. An important observation surfaced from my work with ER colleagues. Like me, they had roamed around deciding what work to focus on and then after 10 to 15 years of ER life they were trapped to spend the rest of their careers there. Many expressed that it "just happened that way" with a resigned shrug. It was not terrible working a few shifts per week, not having any business expenses, collecting a paycheck and having the flexibility to take a prolonged vacation or break if desired. I thoroughly enjoyed it for over 2 years, but it began to seem like a dead end that could easily become my future. The idea of working Saturday nights in the ER after twenty years looked less and less appealing. Also, I began to sense an indifference and disconnectedness of life in the ER. While it was generally interesting and actually fun, the parade of various patients I saw were nearly never seen again by me and I never found out what happened to the ones I treated. Was this what I wanted in my career in medicine? It began to seem hollow the longer I worked in that world. The harsh reality is that in the "exciting life" in the ER one sees the same dozen or so serious problems and the same few dozen minor problems over and over along with the large number of unnecessary visits due to psychological-social-economic reasons that are not helped at all in the ER.

In many ways, ER work has an easy repetition of stabilizing serious patients and handing them off to the hospital staff for admission or treating minor problems and sending patients home all without a connection to the outcome afterward.

At the same time, a debate within myself was settled to not go back to do several more years of training in a specialty fellowship. It was relieving that these possible career tracts which had played in my head since I finished my residency were fortunately put to rest. My life pattern of having a forward direction of blocks of time of school and training that had defined my life until age 30 was at last broken. This letting go allowed other possibilities to be considered. The experience of a free form life for these couple of years where I could work hard for periods of time but also be able to take a month or so off to travel to Europe or wherever in order get other life experiences while having no long-term work commitments felt to be a very important part of my "school of life" and maturing self. However, the nagging question of "what am I going to do when I grow up?" played in the back of mind continuously. So while in the midst of work that seemed increasingly disconnected, living in a social environment bent on superficialness and at a relationship crossroad, the question needed to be answered.

My wish to live in the San Francisco Bay area was instilled after a vacation there while as an intern. After I finished my residency in Boston, I worked locally in clinics, hospitals and ERs and actually had several job offers to join practices or to take hospital-based jobs on a permanent basis but I declined them all as the west coast was pulling me. I migrated first to the southern California beach town of Manhattan Beach as several medical school friends were relocating there and it seemed like it would be fun and I could easily do the same kind of work. After a short time in the L.A. area, I knew it was not for me from a personal or career aspect. However, I had no job leads or idea to actually get a real job in Northern California except for maybe applying to Kaiser, the large HMO organization based in Oakland. At that time Kaiser was not considered a good place to work and had a reputation of employing substandard docs (not true today). Instead, I turned to the most prestigious medical journal in the world, the *New England Jour-*

nal of Medicine, which ran classified jobs for physicians every week in the last section of the weekly publication. Most jobs were for Internists as it's a journal mostly about my field. There were a small number of jobs listed for the Bay area but I did see one that seemed OK although a bit different than a typical internal medicine practice. There were two brothers in private practice doing internal medicine who were also part of a spine and chronic back pain program. The position seemed interesting enough so I applied via a letter and was asked to come for an interview. I met both brothers in their small office in the sunset district of San Francisco where I noticed immediately how entirely different their personalities were. The older brother, Jerome, was very high energy, fast talking, somewhat loud but friendly and funny while his younger brother, Les, was a pensive, calm, zen-like calculating but engaging man in his early forties. They were both over ten years older than I and had built their practice over many years. Their work life evolved into a large percentage of their time working with a group of orthopedists, physical therapists, rehabilitation specialists and psychiatrists at the recently developed spinal care center at St. Mary's Hospital in San Francisco along with general internal medicine. They explained their work to me in detail that included a seemingly fun and academic aspect of this growing multi-disciplinary world in trying to help these unfortunate back and neck pain patients, many of which had undergone several surgeries without benefit. It seemed like an interesting job although quite different from what I was doing but included general medical care as well as hospital work in the city where I wanted to live. I told them I was very interested. I felt ready to "grow up" and join the real world. They called me a few days later and offered me the job. We agreed to a start date in two months as I had to finish my work schedule, find a place to live and move.

Jerome called me about a month later and explained that they were in negotiations to join this newly formed organization called Spine Care that was being funded by a rival hospital and that I would be folded into this new entity as they would be. He assured me that the job offer was still good. We hadn't discussed salary and benefits and all the other work details but was told this would all become clear soon. So the situation changed from joining their small practice to being an employee of a new large organization. Being a neophyte to negotiating an employment contract, I wasn't clear of the implications or any of the dangers or downsides of employment. I was mostly happy with moving to San Francisco and felt that I would get a fair deal. We spoke a couple of weeks later and set up a schedule to get oriented to the hospital and the work and meet everyone we would be working with and go over the employment agreement when I arrived.

The situation was quite complex when I arrived. This new organization had been set up and all the doctors involved were going to be employed and it included a diverse group of orthopedic spine surgeons (the main one was quite famous for operating successfully on a celebrity football player), internists, pain specialist anesthesiologists, physiatrists (physical rehabilitation specialists) and psychiatrists. Les and Jerome were also the directors of the 30 day inpatient pain treatment program as well as caring for all the patients in the hospital who had spine surgery. I was initially impressed with meeting everyone and was getting a general understanding of this advanced multidisciplinary care. The new CEO I met with shared with me the vision of this center being "state-of-the-art" and projected it being the premier care center on the west coast. These were lofty ideals for sure. I was offered a starting salary and benefits that was at an entry level internist pay for that time which was a not so whopping $78,000 per year. This was similar to what I was earning in the ER but I was only working nine months out of the year!

So I found myself taken in by a newly constructed multidisciplinary corporation and not part of a small group of internists who did consulting work after I had moved five hundred miles and signed a year lease. I wasn't quite sure what to make of this switcheroo that Jerome and Les had been able to do by offloading their offer to me onto the corporation but it seemed somewhat reasonable. Certainly, it was a much better deal for them to not have to bring on a younger colleague and pay a salary before he could "come up to speed" economically. I rationed that at least I was where I wanted to live and I had time to "learn the ropes" of this new endeavor while getting paid a sufficient amount that I could live on.

While I had extensive experience treating spinal pain patients, I was not very familiar with the specific details of diagnostic imaging such MRI scans which were advancing rapidly then. I knew a bit about the various advanced diagnostic and treatment procedures such as precise spinal injections into various structures of the spine from my friend and med school mate, Garrett, who had done a fellowship on this in Boston. I lacked any in-depth understanding of the paradigms of decision making regarding recommending spinal surgery nor even what exactly the surgeons did from a carpentry standpoint. There was a steep learning curve to get through all this new stuff. I quickly became immersed in this world on a daily basis by rounding in the hospital with "the team"— the surgeons and internists and then spending time with the anesthesiologist who did spinal injections and then with the radiologists reviewing spinal images and then in the clinic evaluating outpatients in consultation and culminating in weekly team conferences where everyone met going over the most complex cases to come up with a comprehensive treatment plan.

These team conferences were fascinating in the pulling together of all the different aspects of evaluation and included lively and revealing discussions from the different disciplines. Many of these patients had very complex histories of back injuries, prolonged disability, previous surgeries, other unsuccessful treatments and long-term life difficulties that included the financial, psychological and family stresses that interplay into one's individual experience. It was revealing to hear from the psychiatrists who warned about patients' risky situations for more surgery in the context of their traumatic upbringing, difficult relationships and tendencies to substance abuse.

While the team members worked together and listened to each other, there existed a natural tension between the surgeons and the non-surgeons at these conferences. The general mind of a surgeon is to believe it is possible and want to fix any structural problem especially when others have not been able to. It was easy to see how the hero role was adopted by both surgeon and patient in that "this guy can ride in on the white horse to save the day". In their desperate state, patients are easily taken in by this hopeful fantasy. Particularly when their life has been in shambles and they see a famous surgeon who recently operated on a star football player who returned to play and then win a super bowl title. Because of advances in spinal surgical techniques, nearly any spinal problem could have a surgical approach. Various new ways to fuse the spine with implanted metal hardware were coming on the market rapidly at that time giving the surgeons more tools to work with (some might say "play" with).

Diagnostically, it was new to me that specialists used not only MRI scans to look for abnormalities in the discs and spinal structures (which were becoming more detailed every year) but also pain locating techniques with specific injections of numbing medicine and cortisone of individual spinal nerves or joints. In addition, they were using pain provoking injections directly into individual intervertebral discs (the shock absorbers of the spine between vertebrae) to try to locate which ones correlated with the patient's pain. The internists contribution to the conference included any of the medical issues such as overuse of narcotics or tranquilizers and any other medical conditions affecting their overall health. This along with the feedback from the physical therapists and rehabilitation specialists on the ability of these patients to overcome their pain and disability by improving their strength, stamina, posture and body mechanics gave a complete picture of what was going on and where the treatment should be directed. It certainly seemed to be a true multidisciplinary approach where each component and all opinions were considered and a consensus was agreed upon. The various options included surgery and what type and the risks of a bad outcome, as well as detox from medications, further outpatient rehab, psychological counseling and treatment with intensive rehabilitation. The last was a 30-day inpatient program of all day individual and group physical therapy and psychological counseling. At that time in the late 1980s, these programs were still covered by insurance even though they were quite expensive (although much cheaper than another spine surgery). Chronic pain treatment centers had drastically grown in number and were in vogue then. There were many centers around the country offering similar programs. One quite famous pain program was at the University of Washington in Seattle which was generally the model for chronic pain treatment.

This was quite different from what I was previously doing and certainly a lateral move from standard internal medicine work. However, I felt that I was learning a lot of new stuff while applying my previous medical knowledge. The internists also took care of the post-surgical hospital care which meant treating patients recovering from surgery which was part of the standard hospital work that I was quite used to.

At the same time the new corporate organization was developing its structure. As I began to understand further, the sponsoring entity was a competing hospital just slightly south of San Francisco and they were in the process of completing a new clinic, physical therapy center, radiology suite and injection center at Seton Hospital in Daly City. Interestingly, St. Mary's Hospital, where I started my new job, was run by the Sisters of Charity, a Catholic order of nuns. This was in seemingly slight contrast in name but in complete contrast to the business structure of the Daughters of Charity who ran Seton. Why these Catholic organizations opposed each other and competed with each other for specialty medical services at their various hospitals was beyond my grasp of religious politics. Seton Hospital had previously established a high level cardiac care center which was a bit unusual for a community hospital and they were apparently looking to enhance their status by luring away this spinal care group that had been slowly built up over the previous half dozen years or so offering several million dollars in start-up incentives. However, for the next 6 months until completion of the new facility we were at the old place. The structure of the organization quickly took the form of a large corporation with layers of managers, different departments and supervisors in order to mimic the well-known medical institution, the Mayo Clinic, used as a model. It became known to me that all the different specialties were still in the process of finalizing their relationship with the corporation which had as its goal to bring all the doctors into one group as employees. Previously, all were operating separate medical practices but came together to treat these complex patients at the spine center. The benefits of this arrangement at St. Mary's was in using their facilities without having to pay for the overhead of office space and personnel. The hospital benefited from all the surgeries, procedures and referrals to their other services along the way.

For my part, I felt a need to come up to speed with the scientific information available on this topic which included a great deal of published material in various journals and textbooks. I attempted to speed read all that I could find including 15 years of the journal *Spine* and various texts on spine surgery, rehabilitation and pain management of which, fortunately, there was not a significant volume. At that time medicine was entering into the new age of "evidence based" medical care. This meant that instead of mere "expert" opinion regarding proper decision making on care, there was a focus on rigorous scientific studies giving direction to care. Of course, medical care is quite diverse and nuanced and many areas have been and continue to be poorly researched from a highly regarded scientific standpoint. Most notorious in the lack of well designed modern studies and free of investigator bias was the surgical literature. Most published papers included only a series of patients that one or two surgeons treated in a certain manner and reported their "success" rates. Some of the worst offenders in this category were orthopedic surgeons. It was somewhat comical and common knowledge that orthopedic studies showed at least an 80% success rate while ignoring complications, having no control group and often committing the research crime of looking at their data *afterward* and then deciding on how they would determine the criteria for success. This was no different in the spine surgery literature and in reviewing many years of surgical studies one would conclude almost all patients did great with any surgery! Not the results found in the real world, however. My current work saw a constant parade of patients from all over the west coast that had not only unsuccessful back surgery but many times were worse off than where they started. Looking further into the scientific studies of other components of treatment of back pain there was extreme paucity of well-done studies on the effectiveness of physical therapy, spinal injections or specific medications or the increasingly popular pain programs. This was turning out to be a wide-open field of justifying whatever treatment one was in favor of and no one really knew what worked and why scientifically. No wonder patients sought out any-and-all alternative care treatments such as chiropractic, acupuncture, herbal concoctions, crystals, magnets, faith healers, and various posture maneuvers such Feldenkreis and Alexander techniques as none had been studied in any scientific way to know what did what or helped what type of back condition. It turned out this field of back care was the wild west of medical treatment, anything goes! All the folks I worked with knew of this lack of science behind the treatments and diagnostic procedures and accepted their limitations but were interested in getting at the true answers. It was admirable that they were at least trying to use an approach that took all factors into account and try to come up with a workable paradigm. They were based on assumptions and logic while including checks and balances of having many different physicians look at these complicated patients before launching into another complex spine surgery.

I was along for the ride in this niche world of medicine that many perceived as a lost cause. Most doctors abhor back pain patients and are naturally biased against those in chronic pain. They are often perceived as losers, drug seekers and manipulators and seemingly unhelpable. Therefore, many general practitioners refer them to specialists such as neurologists, neurosurgeons, orthopedics and rehab specialists for care. My own reaction when seeing a difficult back pain patient in the ER or urgent care clinic was one of guarded sympathy and also often accompanied by a sense of something not being right in their life. Frequently, there was a lingering or implied background issue coinciding with the story of their back pain. Of course, I treated them as if their condition was real and needed care.

There seems to be a natural selection in folks that get a backache and in those who then seek care for it. An episode of back pain for humans is a common occurrence, more than 85% of the population experience it at least once in a lifetime. Therefore, for the vast majority of us it is a normal course of living in a world with a mechanical body governed by the forces of gravity. We typically experience it as something that just happens on occasion and resolves with time. Statistically greater than 90% of back aches resolve within a couple of weeks even if nothing is done and greater than 95% in 6 weeks are better. The medical literature is quite clear that it doesn't matter what is done during that time to help improve those odds. What is clear is that trying to remain physically active does help someone return to their normal state of health instead of resting which makes everyone weaker and stiffer quickly. For every 2 days of bedrest, it takes 4 days of activity to return that person to their previous state of physical condition. So unlike in the old days, resting and doing nothing is worse than doing what one can within the limits of one's pain.

The patients we saw at the spine clinic were generally not that 95%, although refreshingly we did see some. Mostly they were folks for which their back pain continued to bother them for long periods and for some permanently. Why they didn't heal up remains the multi-billion-dollar healthcare question. Many patients had a worker's compensation claim because of lifting something, falling or some other physical event that caused their back pain and their inability to work. Others claimed that the accumulation of specific physical activity at work overtime caused their back to start hurting. Many developed a backache that didn't go away or got worse and saw a specialist and ended up with disc surgery or a fusion surgery which didn't alleviate their pain. Some of these went on to have another disc surgery or a fusion operation which also did not help and some even had a series of many surgeries. There also was another group that just developed a backache for no particular cause that ended up ruling their lives causing them disability, financial ruin, divorce, and depression. A good portion of all these patients ended up taking daily narcotic pain medicines, muscle relaxers, tranquilizers for anxiety, sleeping pills and antidepressants all of which didn't help much but only "just took the edge off" as it was classically described. These were the typical chronic spinal pain patients that I saw at my new job. Their stories were usually long and very complicated and often included a difficult life, a terrible boss, stressful working conditions and strange injuries, such as a forklift knocking them over. Some had compounding events such as abandonment by their previous doctors who couldn't figure out why their surgery didn't work. Many experienced the dissolution of their marriages or relationships along with moving to an isolated remote community due to financial reasons, all worsening their misery. It was not surprising then to hear of many of these unfortunate folks left with nothing but taking pain killers and other medications to dull their ruined lives. This was difficult work but by working with a group of physicians and engaged staff, we were somewhat buffered mentally seeing such a constant parade of human misery and suffering. Having a team approach with common goals was important to continue in this work.

While the question "Is it all in my head doctor?" was occasionally asked by a reflective patient, it was more common to hear "There is something seriously wrong with my back and I need to get it fixed to get on with my life." I quickly understood that it was my job to figure out which was more correct but it became apparent that often both were pertinent. The mind is in the body and the body generates the mind. That is the simple truth of humanity as conscious feeling animals. There is no duality or separateness of our mental state and our physical state. They are connected from the beginning to the end of our lives. So, trying to figure out and sort out this interaction in these patients' reporting of how severe their pain was, where it was located, how it affected their lives and how it impacted their emotional state and relationships in the world led me to start exploring, studying and trying to figure out the experience of pain itself. I was increasingly becoming more of a chronic pain doctor than a spine doctor.

Doctors reflexly think of a patient's complaint of pain as indicating something abnormal in the body. Pain in the chest can mean a heart attack; pain in the right lower abdomen can mean acute appendicitis; a sudden, severe "worst headache of my life" can mean a ruptured cerebral aneurysm. We naturally associate symptoms with pathology and there can be many different diseases that cause the same symptoms. This is the core issue of being a physician. Sorting out symptoms in a hierarchical way from life threatening to trivial is the first process and one that is paramount when working in an emergency room. But what about pain that persists long after one would expect it to? In some cases this is explained by nerve damage in which the nerve transmits the signals of pain because it is damaged and can no longer modulate its action and sends continuous messages of pain to the brain. This is seen commonly in neuropathy from diabetes where patients can experience a constant burning and tingling sensation in their lower legs and feet and is seemingly paradoxically associated with the loss of sensation of light touch. Here the damaged nerve not only has lost its normal function of perceiving touch or pressure (which can lead to skin ulcers and infections) but now produces its own firing of pain signals due to the internal damage in the nerve. There are many other forms of nerve injury pain that can cause chronic pain. An extreme version of the body producing pain on its own is found in the syndrome of *reflex sympathetic dystrophy* or as is currently classified as *complex regional pain syndrome*. This strange condition arises from a previous injury, broken bone or surgery and is characterized by persistent pain in the same general area but is *not* attributable to a nerve injury. It is accompanied by other physical changes such as alternations of sweating and swollen red skin in the area of pain. Also, the area is hypersensitive to light touch or pressure setting off a severe bout of pain. Fortunately, this condition is rare but is quite dramatic and disabling. The cause remains unknown but is thought to be due to a combination of factors of released inflammatory chemicals that cause the local and central nervous system to be "revved up" and produce pain signals continuously. Unfortunately, the treatment of this disorder is very difficult and not very helpful for the majority of cases. Since the pain pattern and prolongation of severe pain experienced does not correspond to any specific anatomic abnormality, doctors have traditionally had difficulty accepting the diagnosis leading many patients to be classified as "crazy", manipulating or lying. This view has changed as modern medicine has attempted to research and treat this unusual disorder. But the main question remains: Why should pain persist when the injury or surgery has healed?

In the work at the spine clinic, the focus was to determine if there was a significant identifiable source of the patient's pain a.k.a. the *peripheral stimulus*. Specifically, we looked for potentially correctable problems including: a new or recurrent herniated disc causing nerve pressure and pain; compression of a nerve or nerves from *stenosis* meaning the bones of the spine were compressing the nerves; or *spinal instability* which is a somewhat vague term meaning that segments of the spine move around more than usual and cause either mechanical pain from excessive movement or nerve compression.

How is the spine constructed anyway? This remarkable structure forms a tripod at each level with a large anterior block of bone joined together by the intervertebral discs above and below the vertebrae and two small posterior joints known as facet joints. The spine can move forward, backward, sideways and has partial rotational ability due to its anatomy. Each vertebra has a bridge of bone over the back forming the spinal canal where the spinal cord passes from the head to the level of the upper lumbar spine. From that point the spinal nerves that go to the lower body and pelvis traverse the canal and exit out the side holes between each vertebrae. The spine is divided into three sections: the cervical spine consisting of the 7 vertebrae of the neck, the thoracic spine made up of 12 vertebrae and their connecting ribs protecting the chest and the 5 lumbar vertebrae of the lower back. There is also a naturally fused bone below the lumbar spine known as the sacrum which connects with the pelvis bones. The intervertebral discs are composed of thick rings of cartilage filled with a proteinaceous viscous liquid known as the nucleus pulposus connecting the vertebrae blocks together in front. The discs are the structures that allow the spine to move in all directions while the facet joints give some support and limit rotation.

As far as back pain is concerned, the most common area of complaint is the low back (lumbar region) about 5 times more than the neck (cervical area). The thoracic spine is a rare area of pain and may indicate a more unusual medical condition such as a tumor.

The most common abnormality seen on an MRI scan of the spine is a *degenerative disc* which is due to the natural aging of the spine. As the intervertebral discs age due to normal movement, bending, twisting or compression of the body and spine, small cracks and tears begin to occur in the cartilage rings that make up the disc and these tears just like other cartilage in the body do not repair back to normal. Over time this can cause the discs to become compressed in height (one of the main reasons we all become shorter with age), stiffer and subject to herniation of the internal gelatinous pulp that is at the center of the disc. A herniated disc means that the outer thick wall of cartilage has torn all the way through and the toothpaste like inner material has worked its way out. Usually, a herniated disc occurs in the direction of the back of the disc where the spinal nerves and boney covering are located. This is where problems can occur if a nerve or nerves are compressed significantly which can cause sciatica or nerve injury. Disc herniations are almost always due to a strong force of bending forward or compression pushing the disc and its nucleus to a backwards position. In the modern era of MRI imaging of the spine and other body structures the details of bones, discs, nerves and canals and tissues are seen in extremely fine detail. MRI scanning has found that shrunken, abnormal, damaged spinal discs especially in the low back and neck are very common. In fact, in looking at the general population, nearly everyone has one or several of these findings by the age of 30. And even more revealing, nearly a third of the population has a herniated disc in the lumbar spine without having any back or sciatica pain! So, is this finding of *degenerative discs* or even a herniation actually something pathologic or a natural consequence of being an upright human that moves around the world and lifts and bends and does physical things? This is important in that an MRI cannot tell the difference if someone has a backache or not as the same or worse findings can be seen in those with *no* back pain. Since *degenerative discs* include the usual finding of "bulging discs" as part of the natural deterioration, many surgeons have assumed that these findings are the source of pain in symptomatic patients and therefore many patients have had surgeries based on this belief of association. Unfortunately, this has led to a plethora of "the failed spine surgery syndrome" and to even more surgery. The most common spine surgical procedure is a "discectomy" which literally means removal of an intervertebral disc. However, this is a misnomer. The surgeon doesn't cut out the entire disc but rather "trims" the bulging or herniated part of the disc as a rationalization that the pain and pressure on the nerves will be relieved, and the patient will be better after recovery.

The history of lumbar disc surgery goes back to 1935 when two surgeons William Mixter, M.D., a neurosurgeon, and Joseph Barr, M.D., an orthopedic surgeon, working together at the Massachusetts General Hospital in Boston, reported the first successful removal of a herniated lumbar disc in a patient with sciatica. Since then, the procedure has grown in popularity with both surgical specialties performing it more frequently each decade since. Currently, it ranks as the third most common surgical procedure in the US with over 400,000 being done each year. Both neurosurgeons and spinal orthopedic surgeons perform this surgery and there is not much difference in the way it is done. These days, most surgery for a herniated disc is done with a small back incision and a microscope to minimize surgical injury and reduce healing time. The classical and still accepted indication for lumbar disc surgery is continued sciatica pain for at least 6 weeks from a clinically corresponding disc herniation seen on a modern imaging study, either CT scan or MRI. A more urgent surgical indication is in a patient with progressive nerve injury causing worsening leg weakness, sensation loss or dysfunction of the bowel or bladder due to a corresponding disc herniation.

Fusing the spine is often considered by spine surgeons after a discectomy has not been successful. The thought behind this is that the disc is the direct source of pain itself so by fusing the two vertebrae together with bone and often with metal rods and screws to hold the area in place then the patient's pain will resolve. This rationale is taken from other areas in the body where orthopedic surgeons fuse joints to reduce pain from an arthritic joint. In general, neurosurgeons are not skilled or recommend fusion of the spine as they generally focus only on problems where a nerve compression or injury is involved in the case. Fusing the spine is a big step up in the complexity of surgery, risk of complications and the reduction of successful outcomes and generally remains in the purview of orthopedic spine surgeons.

The general estimates for success of subsequent spine surgeries is that after each one, successful percentages are cut in half or more. The general statistical success after initial lumbar disc surgery is deemed to be about 80%. A second surgery with or without fusion leaves only half of those (the 20%) failures better and the success reduces further with each subsequent surgery. So, after several surgeries, a patient has a low chance of being significantly helped with an additional surgery even if there is something identifiable.

With seeing so many patients who had previous unsuccessful surgery, the intensive and expensive evaluation that they underwent seemed important in order to sort out those that had a reasonable chance of improvement with surgery even though it usually meant a fairly complicated procedure. Many of these patients were not only from the local Bay Area but traveled hundreds of miles from the far reaches of California and even Nevada to get an evaluation and hope of what could be done for them. Many were referred by their primary care doctors or from local surgeons who did not know if any more surgery would help them. Many of them stayed for a few days for a full team evaluation as outpatients before our weekly conference. Afterward the team went over the results and recommendations with each patient and their family. These were often intense discussions going over the details of the scans, medical issues, psychological issues, physical rehabilitation status and ability and the possible surgical options. Most times there was not a recommendation for surgery. Many patients had such physical deconditioning and weakness of their back and the rest of their body from being inactive for long periods that it was determined they needed a "boot camp" style rehabilitation before any other consideration. Still others were so psychologically distressed and depressed and drug dependent that they needed intensive counseling and detox. Many were recommended for the 4-week inpatient pain program described above which depended on insurance coverage. While surgical options were discussed in the team conference, we didn't directly discuss surgery as an option unless there was consensus that it was the only or best option left and that the patient had a clear identifiable spinal abnormality and was deemed healthy enough from a physical and psychological standpoint. This left patients going in different directions after the conference and because of the volume of patients there were still several per week that were put on the surgical schedule. Many others returned later after completing courses of non-surgical treatment and were re-evaluated to consider surgery. Patients were usually relieved with a surgical recommendation as it validated their sense of "something wrong with my back".

Sometime in the fall of 1988, the new facility was finished and there was a bit of a strange transformation to the new offices about a dozen miles south of San Francisco. We still maintained a diminishing presence at St. Mary's but they were a separate entity as two of the original four spine surgeons decided not to join the new corporation and move their professional life down the road. The new spine center occupied 3 floors of a brand-new building with a brand-new MRI and CT scanner along with a suite of fluoroscopy rooms that the injection specialists could do their thing. The second floor was where all medical offices were located and the third floor housed an enormous open floor plan physical therapy center, a large conference room and the business offices. This certainly had the appearance of a well-organized, corporate-appearing, high level center. Unlike at St. Mary's, all the employees were part of the corporation and there were now levels of management such nursing supervisors, pod managers, front office managers, billing managers, medical records managers as well all the staff. It was a very busy place with all these non-physician workers, something I nor any of the other doctors had experienced in their professional life. Some of the logistics were difficult to work out as there was still all this activity at the other center going on. It took another 6 months or so to completely separate all the work from St. Mary's. As a contrast, the hospital we were now working out of was much older than the more modern and sleek one in San Francisco. Seton Hospital was built in the early 1960s and was a 10-story monolithic rectangular block situated on a hill overlooking the freeway. Some had nicknamed it "Our lady of 280".

Life and work went on and we were seeing a lot of patients from all corners of the west coast. Many were there to see this now mythical surgeon, Arthur White, who bestowed a large sense of hope in all the patients he saw. Most patients were there to have him personally evaluate their back, so he would roam around the clinic jointly with the other doctors to go over their case in brief, casting his spell of belief that we could rectify their back problems. It was a remarkable thing to witness in some sense. I would go over all the details of the consultation with the patient, review all their data, examine them and discuss the important points with him and he would spend an energetic, dance-like, intense 10 minutes expounding on his philosophy of spinal treatment, giving advice and recommending treatments and tests while rarely recommending surgery at the first visit. Patients were satisfied with this upbeat and hopeful approach and were given a definite plan. Some were referred for a few days of intensive team evaluation. All came back to review their situation and get further recommendations and to monitor their progress and reassess their plan. As is the normal variable of response, some patients were improved with a conservative approach of specific physical rehabilitation, some improved with an addition of spinal injections of cortisone, and some were unimproved. Many were hampered by a chronic use of narcotics pain medications which paradoxically causes one's pain tolerance to diminish as the body adapts to its use. Some had completed all the non-surgical treatments and rehabilitation and were still subjectively unimproved. This prompted a re-evaluation of whether a surgical intervention was to be recommended. It turned out that many patients ended up in this last situation as there was not much else to offer at that point except for the disappointing advice to "live with it".

As time went on, many of these patients were considered surgical candidates after a prolonged period of many visits with the team members and the surgeons while still unable to live their lives after rehab, injections, medication adjustment and psychiatric counseling. There seemed to be an element of time fatigue and having had these patients "jump through all the hoops" and then it was decided they must be in need of an operation. Also, patients were often convinced it was the only way to fix their back and were generally eager to sign up for an operation as a concrete and validating way out of their pain and disability.

The surgical schedule kept growing and at one point the surgeons were doing about 20 spine surgeries per week. Among my duties was to help care for these patients before and after surgery, so I spent a good deal of the morning at the hospital taking care of all the details of post-surgical hospital care and discharging the patients home when they were ready. Because so many of the surgeries involved a second, third or fourth surgery, many patients underwent an instrumented fusion procedure that also included removing some disc material and opening up the bony holes on the side of the spine for the nerves to have more room. The fusion surgeries also became more complicated as the surgical thinking was to fuse the front of the spine by placing bone where the disc was and to also fuse the rear of the spine by using bone from the patient's pelvis. This surgery was dubbed the "360" which meant an operation from the front and back of the spine. All these patients also had metal rods and screws inserted to keep the whole thing secure until all the bones fused by healing new bridging bone. The time for these operations was several hours and as is the case with any surgery, the longer and more complex the procedure the higher the rate of complications.

Working with the spine center's surgical nurse, I decided to keep track of all our complications over a two-year period. I had discovered that there was a paucity of comprehensive reported data on surgical complications in the literature except for a few small studies reporting rates of infection. It seemed like an important study to do to clarify the issue. This study which we started as a prospective study ended up including over 1000 patients, by far the largest study of its sort. Since not all complications are equal we divided them into major and minor. The major ones included: deep tissue infections that required drainage and prolonged care, pneumonias, blood clots, heart attacks or strokes, nerve injuries or other incidents that were life threatening or required prolonged hospitalization to treat properly. Minor complications were things like a urinary tract infection, skin rash, mild adverse drug reaction or superficial skin infection. In the literature of surgical complications, no-one had categorized serious versus minor either. All the team was in favor of the study in our quest to be at the forefront and do service to the field. At the end we compiled the data and presented it to the annual North American Spine conference. We found that 10% of patients had at least one complication and that nearly 5% had a major one. The most common serious complications were deep tissue infections (2% of all patients) that required opening and draining the incision, prolonged antibiotics, occasional removal of hardware as the source of infection and even occasional skin flap transfer to close the wound. However, other serious complications included pneumonias and deep vein clots each occurring 1% of the time. Two patients died, one from a heart attack and the other from a large blood clot from the legs to the lungs giving an overall mortality rate of 0.2%. The study was well received at the spine conference as there had never been such a study done before and many of the surgeons expressed praise in reporting these results honestly and with scientific rigor. However, and strangely, when we wrote the study up for publication it was rejected for obscure reasons.

There were many clinical studies that the group embarked on in order to get to some of the nagging answers in the world of spinal care and also to be recognized as a research center. We were assisted by an amount of funding for research from the hospital and had access to the research experts associated with the heart institute. I did a few other specific studies. One included using a specific medication to limit blood loss during surgery which included the modern protocol including: institutional review board approval and being a prospective, randomized and controlled study. This standard was rarely seen in surgical literature at that time. The results did not show an advantage to using that medication and we quickly avoided it and showed the results at the national spine conference so others could be informed.

Another longitudinal study I did included collecting a series of 10 patients that initially presented with severe incapacitating sciatica pain and were found to have a presumed large herniated disc on MRI scanning. This group of patients were strongly considered to need a disc surgery for relief. However, after 8 weeks of treatment all patients were remarkably improved even though a few had signed up for a surgery. All these patients had a follow up MRI scan to see what happened and fascinatingly all were found to have their large herniations completely gone! One of the patients did have a subsequent fusion surgery and no herniation was found. I went over these scans in great detail with the radiologists who were experts in the area of spinal MRI interpretation. It turned out the initial large herniations seen had particular characteristics of being "bright signaled" indicating also possibly being due to inflammation or to blood. It was concluded that the "herniation" was actually an acute blood clot in the spinal canal causing nerve compression and sciatica as its disappearance 2 months later was impossible for a true disc rupture. Blood clots like this can be looked at as a hematoma or bruise from sudden pressure in the spine and like all hematomas resolve over a few weeks. It is true that disc herniations can reduce in size over time as the body begins to shrink and reabsorb the material but this was known to take up to a few years and didn't happen for everyone. I wrote the study up and presented it the following year at the national spine conference. It was greeted with great interest and discussion. One elderly spine surgeon approached me after my presentation and related his experience of operating on a few patients like this and finding "purple herniations" which were blood clots on the way to being absorbed. The likely anatomic explanation for this phenomenon is that there is a network of veins along the spinal canal, the epidural veins, that could rupture and leak with sudden increase in pressure during lifting something heavy or some other similar activity. Blood would seep into the spinal canal and compress the soft nerves surrounded by spinal fluid just like a disc herniation but expansion would be limited by the bony spaces. The confined clot would then form a defined mass in a closed space. The compressive forces in a confined area would stop the bleeding (just like putting pressure on a bleeding skin wound would) and then the clot would eventually be reabsorbed. Such a phenomenon had not been described before in the literature. While theoretically a patient on blood thinners could have this happen as has been reported in the literature, none of these patients were on one and none of patients were found to have a bleeding disorder. Since this study, many individual case reports have appeared in the literature but the series of 10 patients I reported over a 3-year period has not been replicated. Unfortunately, this study was only presented at the yearly spine conference and was not written up for publication.

There were many other research studies done at the spine center during my time there on various technical and biological topics. However, there remained important questions to answer of whether what we were doing was actually helping patients. Namely, what was our center's success rate in performing spine surgery compared to others? Was our paradigm of evaluation valid in selecting patients for surgery? What were the factors that contributed to patients having a poor outcome? These unknowns were a source of growing concern and discussion among the internists and psychiatrists as we were the ones seeing the failed surgical cases on an ongoing basis well after their surgery. The surgeons were largely busy doing what they liked to do: evaluating and doing surgical cases.

It was obvious to me that many of our surgical patients struggled afterward. Certainly, those being treated with a serious deep tissue infection that required a prolonged course of antibiotics, wound care, debridement and healing had a very long recovery time. Many for 6 to 12 months before complete surgical recovery and most of these didn't seem to have the result that was hoped for pre-operatively. Many other patients who had normal recovery also were left with the same pain and disability. As mentioned previously, standardization of measuring outcome of surgery at that time in the 1990s was at its scientific infancy. Led by Jerome, the internists and psychiatrists put together a metric to measure and study a successful outcome of elective spine surgery. Included in this protocol were measurements of physical disability before and after surgery, use of narcotic pain medicine and its reduction after surgery, return to work status, subjective pain relief and patients' overall rating of improvement. Additionally, the psychiatrists who evaluated every patient before surgery were very interested in the influence of early life traumas on the development of chronic pain and difficulty with surgery improving their condition. The developmental or early life traumas they documented in each patient included: substance abuse in a primary caretaker, abandonment by a primary caretaker, and physical, sexual or emotional abuse by a primary caretaker. They had seen these early traumas over the years having an important factor in patients' continued suffering. We included these data points in our collection along with other life factors such as divorce of parents and patients' divorce as potential psychological factors. Our first study in outcome was done retrospectively. By that method, we chose all surgical patients in the previous 4 months to collect data on and analyze as a preliminary way to see what we would find. It took several months to collect, sort and analyze all this data. The results turned out to be enlightening but not good news. Jerome was a bit sheepish to share the findings with the famous surgeon and his surgical colleagues. Using this method to evaluate surgical outcomes was unique in that it took away the bias of the surgeons evaluating their own surgeries and gave the data an objective standpoint as compared to historically reported surgical outcomes. Our overall surgical success stood at a measly 43%! Much less than half the patients were truly improved. This did include a mixture of first-time back surgeries as well as reoperations. Additionally, the psychiatric data was extremely revealing and predictive for failed surgery. Patients that had any of the early traumas had increasing risk for failure and the more traumas the more predictive it was. So, for patients that had 3 or greater early traumas 85% had a failed surgery result! Interestingly, factors such as divorce of parents or patients' divorce had no predictive value. These results drove home the message that spine surgery was still a very uncertain and uneven science even in the hands of a multidisciplinary center. The power of the psychiatric component predicting success was astounding and unique. Their observations did reflect the work of George Engel, M.D., who 30 years earlier who published his review on *Psychogenic and Pain Prone Patient* in 1959 in which he described chronic pain patients in the context of the encompassing biopsychosocial model of pain. This model was gaining favor in that it put patients' response to illness beyond just the biologic and included their social and economic environment, their upbringing and their genetic underpinnings.

As unique as these findings were, it was equally unusual to have a psychiatrist work directly with surgeons in this manner of preoperative evaluation and postoperative counseling and treatment. It was an interaction I had not seen previously or since. Psychiatrists typically stand off to the side in medical treatment not alongside or integrated. The nature of treating these complex patients brought out the need to include these important specialists in what traditionally was considered a purely physical issue. These were a fascinating group of psychiatrists that had trained together in New Orleans and migrated to San Francisco and created a group practice in general psychiatry and became interested in chronic pain. They had been sounding the warning bells about many of these patients' fragile and traumatized mental state for a few years already and were offering them counseling and treatment to improve their lives. Still, many of these patients were considered worthy surgical candidates even with their concerns. Now we had a clearer understanding of how much of an impact these early life traumas had on patients' ability to benefit from spine surgery. Of course, we didn't know all the details of the interplay these factors had. We couldn't tell if these were inherited psychological deficiencies as we knew alcohol and drug addiction can be but it was clear that these life events were important to predict what happened later in life.

We did a second study of these childhood trauma risk factors on chronic pain patients who presented to our clinic the following year and found a similar association of multiple childhood traumas and persistent pain especially in patients without a significant spinal abnormality that would be amenable to surgery.

These studies validated the caution the psychiatrists voiced over the surgeons thinking to perform surgery. Did the surgeons listen? Well, yes and no. They did take these warnings to heart but also had the belief that the psychiatrist could "fix" the patients' traumatic upbringing and then permit them to operate on their spine. This led to many patients being referred for psychiatric treatment for a period and then a reevaluation. This led the psychiatrists into the world of chronic pain management and some of them took on the role as primary caregiver. By counseling and prescribing various medications including antidepressants, anti-anxiety medications, nerve pain modulators, and pain medications they began to expand their world of care. However, the assumption that active treatment and counseling could reduce the chance of failed surgery had no proof behind it although it served as a rationalization for more spine surgery.

As time went on, the business component of the new spine center started to have its difficulties. After a couple of years all the initial seed money invested by the hospital had been used up and the practice had to stand on its own financially. The doctors soon realized their hard work was not realizing the financial rewards they were used to or expected and quickly realized that the bloated Mayo Clinic corporate structure was at the core of the issue. There were many weekend meetings and heated discussions. I was still only an employee and not a shareholder had no say in the direction of the business although its problems were obvious.

Over the course of the next year, it was clear that the over-optimistic and opportunistic CEO had to go along with all the middle management and after all the firings the practice settled into a more normal-looking multispecialty practice with still a large amount of overhead. Then other regulations changed the business model, as we could no longer be owners of the imaging center that generated enormous revenue from all the scans that were done. Then, the physical therapy center was sold to an outside company. Reimbursement for surgeries and treatment started to decrease during the early 1990s as the insurance industry was reshaping into a contractual and HMO model. At the end of this period of financial turbulence, the clinic and practice looked and felt much different. Due to the changing professional dynamics the physician relationships underwent significant changes as well. The rehab doctors had decided to leave the group and form their own practice in Silicon Valley. The psychiatrists decided to be completely separate and offer consulting services and two of the internists were fired for odd, personal conflictual issues. One of them was Jerome's brother, Les. As the least paid and more productive employed physician, I kept my position. It was then a much smaller and lean ship I was floating on. I always had the sense that this project's overreaching attempt to be too big and important misled the work instead of focusing on the basics of good business and medical practice.

However, now I was confronting the overreach and pressure to look more towards a surgical solution for these patients. This direction was opposite to what my sense of appropriate care had taken. After several years of being in this world, I saw for myself what the limitations of surgery and other treatments were. I couldn't ignore the results of our own research which told a more accurate story of how difficult it was to cure back pain with surgery. I was compelled to follow a much less aggressive surgical approach in the service of being a physician trying to do the best for my patients. I naturally steered patients towards a path of non-operative care and only in the few clear-cut instances where one could accurately predict a positive outcome could I refer a patient for surgery. The way I was practicing medicine felt correct and responsible.

I was further convinced that spinal surgery had severe limitations by the next surgical outcome surgery study done by the surgeons. As the surgical approach had become more aggressive, more spinal fusions were being done with increasing complexity. This was reflected by spine surgeons around the country as there was a trend to fuse multiple segments of the lumbar and cervical spine using more advanced internal hardware devices. Our surgeons devised a study to determine how well their fusions actually fused and to see if the patients were improved. They devised a very simple outcome measure compared to our previous more detailed and objective one. Their sole criteria for "success" was a patient satisfaction survey. If the patient reported they were pleased enough that they would sign up for the surgery with the result they had they were considered a success. Interestingly, and to the credit of the technical skill of the surgeons, 90% of the fusions were solid after one year. Many of these patients had both anterior and posterior fusions, extremely complex surgeries. However, only a small percentage (13%) reported being "very satisfied" while only an additional third reported being "somewhat satisfied". The majority reported they would not have gone through the procedure knowing their status after recovery. What this told me was that a good "surgical" result (bony fusion) did not correspond to reduction in pain and improvement in one's life. The orthopedic spine surgeons paradigm that fusing the spine eliminates pain in the back was disproved here by their own data. It was not what the surgeons thought or believed and they then manipulated the data to make the outcomes look better than it was. I had no say or input to their study. However, the road was paved for my future.

As time went along, I began to experience covert and then overt pressure to refer more patients for surgery. The last straw came when one of the surgeons sat me down in his office with a list of items that he deemed I needed to improve upon. Last on the list, but first on his mind was his conclusion that I was being delinquent in not referring more patients for surgery and that I needed to improve on that immediately. The following week I submitted my letter of resignation of employment which immediately filled me with enormous relief along with a sense of professional liberation but also disgust and sadness at the path these physicians had taken. Blinded by their false belief in their surgical paradigm and influenced by the economic gain of highly reimbursed surgery to support themselves, they had lost the proper perspective and ethics of what physicians need to keep in their minds in order to honor the profession they chose.

Of course, the clinic continued on after I left but it had further difficulties down the road. Within a couple of years, the famous surgeon faced criminal charges in a sexual assault case and was eventually ousted by his partners for alcohol abuse issues. The local medical community had always been largely skeptical of their work and mostly ignored the spine center as something of an oddball practice. Their reputation of being "knife happy" while doing these bizarre complex surgeries increased their isolation and mistrust among the doctors in the area.

After leaving, I had some regret spending so much time with this group, nearly 7 years, but in the end I realized I learned an enormous amount about this other world of chronic pain, the business of a medical practice, physician group dynamics, ethics and the pitfalls of a start-up organization as well as the politics of hospitals and how much work modern clinical research took. All of this directed me back full circle to the world of primary care internal medicine which would be my work life for the rest of my career.

I would like to end this chapter with a general guideline for dealing with back pain as it's such a common problem. This advice summarizes the current scientific evidence as of 2024. Of course, visit your doctor if your pain is increasing or persistent to get a medical evaluation.

For acute back pain, which previously mentioned is a very common human experience, time alone will be the best remedy. If it is accompanied by pain down the leg, sciatica, or numbness this usually means some irritation or pressure on a nerve. Sciatica pain differs from low back pain (which can also just radiate to the buttocks) in its meaning. Low back pain itself does *not* imply pressure on a nerve. For treatment of the pain of only low back pain one can use simple over-the-counter medications such as ibuprofen or acetaminophen as needed. Although the effect of these medications are variable in that they can help some a lot and not at all in others. Commonly, the pain is accompanied by stiffness or spasm in the back in an acute episode. An ice pack can be your friend (instead of heat which can make inflammation worse) for 20 minutes at a time which also helps relieve pain by its numbing action of pain nerves. The best thing to do is try to keep active. Movement such as simple walking helps blood flow to the back and improve healing and inflammation. It is usually best to avoid prolonged sitting as this puts more pressure and load onto the low back. Changing positions frequently and stretching are also good things to do to return to one's normal state. While many folks visit chiropractors and acupuncturists and even physical therapy there is no good science that any of these help in the case of a typical acute back ache that will resolve within a few weeks.

Sciatica is a different story. Pain down either leg which can be worsened by either bending forward (or occasionally backwards) is the definition of sciatica which technically means compression or irritation of a nerve in the lumbar spine. Sometimes there can be a sensation of tingling or numbness along with the pain. There are a couple of important points here. The first is that if one notices one leg or foot getting weak then a prompt medical evaluation is needed. If that is not the case, the second important thing to know is that sciatica, unlike a back sprain, usually takes much longer to heal. A typical case of sciatica can take at least a few months to recover and often can take 6 months or longer before it resolves but again most cases resolve without getting worse or needing surgery. If the pain or neurologic symptoms are getting worse, it is recommended to get an MRI scan to see what is going on. If the pain is stable and manageable, most would consider a scan at about 6-8 weeks after the onset if not resolved. What to do if you have a herniated disc? The best science on this comes from the only randomized study done in Sweden in the 1970s. It followed patients for 10 years which is an incredibly long study in orthopedics. The study showed two important findings: one, that only about 25% of sciatica patients crossed over to the surgery side after being randomized to non-surgical care. This is about the expected percentage of herniated disc patients needing surgery for management of sciatica pain. The second important finding is that after 10 years *all* the patients were about the same whether they had surgery or not and the vast majority improved significantly from a pain and function standpoint. So having a herniated disc does not doom one to need an operation. However, if your pain and disability is not improving after a couple of months, a modern microscopic disc surgery can help you greatly to get back to a normal life without sciatica. Another important point here: disc surgery in general will *not* help back pain, only sciatica pain. Also, if you have evidence of nerve injury (weakness and numbness), the need for a disc surgery is more urgent and recommended to prevent permanent nerve damage. This is a small percentage of patients with a herniated disc. There is one catastrophic complication of large disc herniation that is worth mentioning and that loss of bowel and bladder function known as the *cauda equina syndrome*. This is due to severe compression of all the nerves below the level of herniation and is due to a large amount of extruded disc material occupying the spinal canal. The nerves to the bladder and bowel are under control of the very lower spinal nerves of the sacrum and are not involved in a usual lumbar disc herniation/sciatica situation. However, the acute occurrence of this problem is a surgical emergency and requires prompt intervention. Fortunately, this is quite rare and I've only seen a couple of these in over 35 years of medical practice.

The next complicated issue of the spine is nerve hole narrowing known as *stenosis*. This can be found in the central spinal canal or in the individual exiting holes on the side of the spine. Symptoms of this problem can be variable from no pain to severe sciatica and then possible muscle weakness due nerve compression and damage. This is usually a dynamic problem in that it is often made worse by a patient *standing up straight* or *bending backwards*. So the symptoms are usually made worse in the opposite way as a herniated disc. This problem can be congenital in those born with narrow spinal canal or more commonly develop over time due to changes with aging and narrowing due to disc degeneration. A very common example is an elderly person who stands bent over while holding on to their shopping cart and when asked to stand straight will say "I don't like doing that" or "that doesn't feel good" indicating that their spinal nerves are getting pinched. Also, the discomfort will go away when the person sits down (also the opposite of a person with a herniated disc) because that position will open up all the nerve canals of the spine relieving the pressure on them. This problem is difficult to improve from a physical therapy standpoint and spinal injections do not help this for any long period of time. Often the elderly just slowly adapt to the nerve narrowing with doing life activities that limit pressure on the nerves. Surgery for this problem can be quite tricky especially in the elderly in that it can involve many levels of the lumbar spine which is more prone to complications and further spinal deterioration. The decision for the elderly should be based on trying to do as limited a surgery as possible in a person who is otherwise healthy enough to get through the surgery and has enough limitation of life activities that a proposed surgery can improve significantly. The usual indication for this would be a healthy elderly person who experiences significant pain and who has progressively lost the ability to walk only a short distance. For healthy younger patients, the question of a surgical intervention often is confounded with the surgeon's opinion of *also* doing a fusion. This is controversial and there is no clear scientific evidence that fusion improves outcome in these situations. However, there is one situation where a fusion surgery and a decompression surgery for stenosis is an accepted standard and that is when a patient has a slipped vertebrae, a *spondylolisthesis,* and spinal stenosis. This is often an issue that develops over a person's life due to the spine not forming properly or from childhood injury and is usually seen at the lowest end of the lumbar spine. In this situation the posterior bony bridge of the spine is not attached to the front allowing the large block of vertebrae to progressively move forward over the one below and then develop symptoms of back pain and sciatica. A fusion and decompression in significantly symptomatic patients has a good rate of success in this instance.

There are still hundreds of thousands of lumbar spine fusion surgeries done in the USA every year mostly for patients with back pain. The science on this paradigm of fusing the vertebrae and eliminating back pain is not established but the world of spine surgeons continues to do them with that belief. There are no clear-cut well-done studies that demonstrate a long-term benefit from fusion over non-surgical treatments. The exact indications for surgery for specific spine abnormalities are not clear from the literature. In comparing decompression for stenosis with or without fusion, one randomized, controlled study has been reported from Sweden in 2016 and the results show that there was *no difference* in the patient outcomes after 2 years and 5-year follow up periods. This showed no advantage to fusion over simple decompression for stenosis. Also, complications rates from fusion surgery in the elderly are quite substantial. So, in general, I advise being very cautious about a recommendation of fusion from a spine surgeon. I suggest at least getting a couple of other opinions and discussing the options of different surgeries but more importantly to maximize non-surgical treatments such as physical rehabilitation and pain management. This is especially true if one has had a previous surgery because the success rate of any subsequent surgery goes down significantly.

My final topic to discuss is chronic back pain. This, of course, is a classification of patients who can be quite diverse from the multiple, failed spine surgery individuals to those with little abnormalities on their MRI scan and all those in between. The basic definition is one who is experiencing daily pain for over 3 months. Of course, the mechanical aspect of pain is dependent can be worse with certain activities but also could be present at most moments. Firstly, let me state that treating chronic pain is one of the most difficult problems in medical care and there is no single treatment, medicine or method that is effective for the majority of patients. I am also speaking of those folks that don't have an obvious structural problem that would be improved with a surgery. It is most important to think of chronic back pain (or any chronic pain) using the *biopsychosocial* model of disease as this reflects real life experience. What this means is that there is an interplay and overlap of the biological or physical component with the psychology of the person and one's socio-economic place in society. All three interact to form the experience of pain. So when one has a back surgery to "fix the problem", it is only addressing one component, a structural aspect. Most back pain patients can walk and do basic activities but have difficulty with bending and lifting and twisting. This can be worsened with less physical strength and flexibility and overall conditioning. Psychologically many possess factors of fear and anxiety, previous experiences of injury and recovery and childhood difficulties which can predispose someone to develop and continue in a chronic pain state. Also, depression is very common in chronic spinal pain patients with something over a 50% incidence. From a social standpoint, chronic pain influences the ability to work and often causes financial hardship. Also, one's relationships change in regards to co-workers, family and friends and the world in general.

The majority of chronic spine pain sufferers have this combination of factors driving their mental and physical being down into a minimally functioning state. So what is there to do and is there a path out and a hope? Well, yes and no. One important point is that chronic pain is a severely life-changing event and it is best to think of it as such. Hanging on to a belief that there is an answer that will allow one to "just go back to the way it was before" is unrealistic and can easily trap one into despair when there is no path back to the past. This realization is itself a painful and mournful event but needs to be accepted in order to build a new life with one's current reality. One may need psychological counseling to obtain this acceptance which may include evaluating the mental aspects of one's coping mechanisms. Depression needs to be treated as an illness that is a common complication of chronic pain. Not all depression needs to be treated with medication but it can play a significant role in improving one's mood and motivation which are important in rebuilding a new life. The medical profession often plays a negative role in continuing chronic pain by prescribing addicting medications such as narcotics, muscle relaxers, tranquilizers and sleep pills. Unfortunately, this has led to an epidemic of prescription drug dependence that has now extended over the past three decades. The physiological and mental problems with these medications is that they all paradoxically *worsen* one's pain tolerance and depression while at the same reduce motivation to change one's habits. This is a terrible side effect that often undermines any other treatments including helpful medications such as antidepressants. So an important aspect to rebuilding is to wean off all those medications and give one's mind and body a fresh chance to handle pain in a normal biological way. For most patients, when I have counseled them that stopping addictive and harmful medications is crucial they reply "but I can't survive without these". While it's true that getting off them is difficult and should be done slowly, *all* my patients who have gone through detoxification and resetting of the natural pain fighting mechanisms their bodies possess have told me they either feel the same pain or less pain off the medications and are clearer and better mentally than being on those addicting medications. That is a truism not often communicated to patients. For those with substance abuse issues such as alcohol or illicit drug abuse this is a particularly crucial aspect of mental and physical recovery.

From the physical aspect of rebuilding one's life there is nothing more important than being active. This can be as simple as increasing one's walking tolerance as most chronic pain patients are very inactive and deconditioned. Increasing physical activity has so many benefits that it is paramount to rebuilding a new life. By improving one's muscle strength and endurance one is literally increasing the support to the back which gives the spine 90% of its strength in standing up! There is an old saying: "Feeling follows action." What this means is that physical activity will increase mood and motivation as well as reduce pain. Yes, physical activity increases the natural pain fighting chemicals our brains and body make such as endorphins. Many patients avoid physical activity because they are convinced "it just makes my pain worse" and are stuck in a downward spiral of a weaker body and a pessimistic mental condition. Starting slowly and daily is the best method by even just 1% more per day. There is no specific type of physical activity that is necessarily better than others although a simple walking and stretching program is the easiest. Of course, there are physical therapists or trainers that can guide one more directly. The scientific studies do not point to one type of exercise for back pain that is best. One personal recommendation which is backed by studies are *pilates* exercises. There are a plethora of simple videos on YouTube on pilates. The benefits of these simple, controlled exercises are that they can be done at home without any equipment and incorporate a variety of different ways of slowly improving strength, flexibility and balance while restoring fluid motion. There are so many different ways of doing these various exercises one could find a different routine for every day of the year! Doing just 10-15 minutes per day can have dramatic effects over several months. A couple of important things to remember are that this is a long-term project and that some days will be good and others not so good. Also, do what you can and take it as a positive that something is being done! Many patients have been deconditioned physically for years so this can often be a lifelong project to improve your body while improving your pain, pain tolerance and mental state.

Socially it is important to have connections in the world. Many patients have lost work connections, are not able to do things with their friends anymore and have strained family relationships. This all contributes to the negative frame of mind about one's life and has been shown to be detrimental to physical and mental health. Rebuilding one's social sphere is also difficult. Humans generally do better in groups than in solitary. Seeking out others in a similar situation has been clearly shown to improve one's quality of life. I strongly recommend joining a group of chronic pain folks online. This can be an important way to see that one is not alone in the world and to get support and feedback from others in a similar state. Connecting to others is important to build a new life.

Did you know that your frame of mind affects your body? Yes, good research has shown that just looking at your life activities in a positive manner improves medical conditions such as blood pressure, diabetes and cholesterol and also pain. Rebuilding a new life is greatly enhanced by looking at one's efforts in a positive way. By reframing any of the efforts you make (reducing harmful medications, slight increases in physical activity, etc.), you will improve your pain level, mood and motivation. If unconvinced, listen to the detailed and extensive scientific research on this topic on the podcast *Hidden Brain* on "Reframing your reality".

CHAPTER 4

Private Practice

Starting out, professional quilting, and building up one step at a time

May 1995, I'm driving back from Las Vegas after a bizarre and unsuccessful trip to try to get a business relationship with the Nevada board of Worker's Compensation where I would do independent medical examinations for injured workers. Having recently obtained a Nevada medical license and set up an appointment to meet with the director of their program, I was brusquely told that there was no such meeting on their calendar and there was no opportunity to provide any services for them after arriving at the appointed time. Driving through Death Valley on the way and stopping to take a nice hike to Zabriskie point, I then stayed in a drab, run-down room at Caesars Palace for a couple of nights contemplating and planning my future as a doctor. The bizarre surrealism of the situation was heightened by the empty, artificial grass surrounded, unshaded pool area (casinos don't want you to spend too much time away from gambling) and more so by visiting a pain specialist anesthesiologist I had contacted. This young doctor had grown his practice in less than a couple of years to over a million-dollar business by doing spinal injections on back pain patients. He was very busy, dedicated and entrepreneurial. However, his life with his new wife working 10-12 hours per day, living in a large, nearly unfurnished, McMansion home on the outskirts of Vegas with essentially no social life, colleagues or activities outside of work struck me as desperately depressing regardless of how much money he was making. He encouraged me to come start a practice with him to help manage all the patients he was seeing. I told him I would think about it and with every mile further from Vegas, the idea seemed more absurd and distant and faded quickly into the desert dust.

I was in the first few weeks of my new life as an unemployed physician, having quit my job working at the spine center. I was convinced and encouraged by my fellow colleagues at Seton Hospital about starting my own practice. Due to the negative experience with the group I had just left, it seemed natural to try to set up a solo practice. But one doesn't just "hang out a shingle" and then have an instant practice! I had a mortgage to cover and therefore needed to set about earning enough income from various sources until things became established. This was the rationale behind the Vegas trip. I was hoping to parlay my experience in evaluating and treating complex back pain patients into helping supplement my income. Many of my long-term patients wished to continue to see me to help manage their spine problems (without surgery, of course) but they would not fill my schedule as my former employer sought to block their access to my new office and many elected to stay at the haughty "spine center". Even having a "new office" meant sharing space on a part time basis with another internist. I had asked around and one of my colleagues who I didn't know very well, Marty Lorber, offered to have me use one of his exam rooms, personnel and billing service a few half days a week for a reasonable fee.

Essentially, I found myself putting together a patchwork professional life in order to build a new, old-fashion, solo private practice. This included being on "ER call" which meant being the primary physician for patients that needed admission to the hospital and who didn't have a doctor on staff. This usually meant a few or many patients per 24 hour period. These could be any sort of patient such as a comatose overdose to an elderly woman with hip fracture or a stroke patient or a GI bleeder or anything else that needed acute hospital care. Basically, I was doing general internal medicine that I was trained to do and was happy to get back to my medical roots after a several year hiatus into the weird world of chronic pain and spinal surgery. It was a true breath of fresh air to see sick people again! I began to get new patient referrals from many of my specialty colleagues I worked with as some of their patients didn't have a primary internist or were unhappy with their current one. Unclear of how much income I could generate, I signed up to work for Kaiser for an afternoon per week in their musculo-skeletal clinic seeing various joint pains and injuries working alongside a couple of other very nice docs who were doing it as their career. As the clinic was in Marin county, I got to escape the city and get out in the country and could go for a pleasant rural bike ride after my work. The patients were upper class, educated and motivated and were fun to treat and help and if they needed something more I could send them to the orthopedists down the hall.

Through the hospital grapevine, I discovered that our hospital's wound care clinic needed doctors to evaluate and treat patients with chronic wounds from diabetes, venous disease or other sources. These were mostly leg wounds that could take months or longer to heal and could often get infected and cause significant complications and even lead to amputation if not treated well. I took their course on protocols for treatment and learned the techniques of debridement and wound care and started in the clinic one morning a week. The director of the wound center was one of the friendliest and upbeat guys on the hospital staff, John Crew. Besides being a vascular surgeon, doing arterial bypass surgery or placing a stent in a blocked leg artery, he was a jolly, large, lumbering fellow who sang in a barbershop quartet on the weekends and was more than happy to help out on any of my cases in the clinic by just asking. The protocol of debridement included scraping off the accumulated debris (pus, fibrin and dead tissue) that the body made on top of these wounds that prevented them from healing and then covering the wound with materials that would keep it moist and clean to enhance healing. One could also use a specially prepared serum from the patient's blood that included platelet factors that promoted healing if the wound was deep and complicated and not healing. On rare occasions, the plastic surgeon needed to do a skin flap to cover a large, non-healing wound. The debridements were done with a scalpel and since most of these were in diabetic patients with neuropathy, it meant that they didn't feel anything during the procedure. It was greatly satisfying to see these awful looking wounds heal and form normal skin over the course of many weeks of treatment. The wound clinic had a wonderful, caring, upbeat staff that welcomed and coddled the patients and were equally helpful and supportive of the doctors. That was coupled with a friendly, low key, interactive relationship with the other doctors working there. I found it so rewarding that I worked there for many years.

By the end of the summer, my subletting experience was beginning to feel a bit stifling. I was appreciative of Marty for giving me a place to work and to be able to use his personnel for my administrative needs. He struck me as more interested in running his business and having free time as he was only in his office a few days a week. He had hired a couple of young internists who were very good and were working super hard. Marty and I even chatted a bit about joining his practice but I was gun shy of the idea. His billing personnel were not as attentive to my practice as I needed, which was crucial to my income, so when my cardiology colleague and friend, Ken Lehrman, offered to share his large office, I decided to hire my first employee and make the move.

Fortunately, my income was sufficient from all these different sources that I could continue to pay my mortgage and live in San Francisco. Slowly my practice was building. After the new year, I became aware of an inexpensive office space in the older office building next to and owned by the hospital and for $700 per month, I happily signed my first lease. The space was huge but had 3 other doctors there, two internists and a cardiologist, Tali Bashour. I now had my own office, 2 exam rooms, an area for medical records and a window at the front office and was ready to hire my first medical assistant. While we shared a large waiting room, I quickly figured out that it was ridiculous and impossible to schedule patients on Tuesday and Thursday afternoons after 2 p.m. The reason was that Tali, who was an extremely busy cardiologist, also did primary care and scheduled about forty patients during each of his only 2 outpatient clinics per week. His patients included a huge cachet of Arab patients as he was from Syria and spoke the language and in a minority community word spreads quickly if there is someone from your part of the world. Daly City and its surroundings were populated with a diverse population of immigrants from the Levant, east Asia, the Pacific Rim as well as Europe, Central and South America. We were all practicing truly international medicine from every corner of the world! Tali was a wonderful, friendly man who was never in a bad mood or stressed out. He always greeted and ended his visits with his patients and their families with a hug and pleasant demeanor. No wonder his patients would begin to line up after lunch on Tuesdays and Thursdays and many would sit out in the hallway waiting for him all afternoon into the evening. Tali was also incredibly busy in the hospital and usually had about 20 patients to take care of both in the ICU and throughout the hospital as well as doing cardiac catheterizations and various complex procedures in the ICU. During his time from the early 1980s into the 2010s there wasn't the specialization of hospitalists and intensivists (ICU docs) as there are today. Tali was one of the specialists that did all this work. He worked seven days a week and rarely took a vacation. He became involved in helping start a new medical school in Beirut and used to fly there to serve on the board and give lectures for a week at a time every few months. Also, in the evenings he would write medical papers to submit to cardiology journals on topics that interested him. The guy did everything and was loved and admired by the staff, nurses and patients! He hosted an enormous annual holiday party at his large home and invited all the hospital employees, nurses and staff and it was the grand ball of the year every December.

It was a big deal to hire my first medical assistant, Michelle, along with getting my own computer system for billing and having my front office assistant, Carmen, learn all the software and hardware functions. I was learning the ropes of the business of medicine on the job and was enjoying the challenge and process of being independent.

Then in June, I was presented with an opportunity to expand my practice significantly. Joe Muscat, M.D., died suddenly while at the Baylands horse racetrack with his friends. Joe was from Malta and had all the local Maltese as patients. He was an internist in his 60s and I knew him a bit and we actually did some weekend call coverage for each other at times. Joe was short and stout with a thick neck which did not allow him to button the top of his shirts but always wore a tie loosened enough to breathe comfortably. Joe was in solo practice and there was no-one to take care of his patients after he died which meant they would scatter around the primary care community. On the urging of many on the medical staff, I contacted his grieving wife and we agreed upon a sale of his practice for a reasonable price of twenty thousand dollars after a review of his finances by my accountant. Suddenly, I had a large influx of patients that needed care and were used to seeing the gruff but friendly Joe for many years. He had been part of the older group of docs at Seton that settled in the area in the early 1970s. Quickly word got around to the patients and I sent letters to them explaining the situation. It was hard to say but I believe most of the patients ended up transferring over to my practice as it was an easy move as my office was just around the corner from his. I considered moving my location to his old office but it was three times the rent so I decided to stay put until I saw how this all shook out. As my schedule began to fill up, I gave up the gig at Kaiser and spent more time in my office. Then at the end of the year, an office upstairs from mine opened up for rent. This was the perfect spot for my growing practice with 3 exam rooms, a decent private back office for myself and sufficient space for the front office and waiting area. I jumped at the opportunity and the hospital negotiated a new lease and included doing all the upgrades that I requested. It was a bit of a whirlwind but in less than two years, I had a nearly full medical practice with my own patients, staff, office, equipment and presence in the medical community. I don't think I could've planned it any better. One important piece that got filled in along the way was the weekend call group. There were 4 other internists close by in solo practice and no-one wanted to work every weekend, so we created a pleasant schedule of every fifth weekend of outpatient calls and hospital rounds for all the patients. While it was a fair amount of work on those on-call weekends with admissions of our sick patients to the hospital, calls from the hospital at night, hospital rounds taking many hours and outpatient calls from patients we didn't know, it was worth it to have those other weekends free. This was the real life of an internist in the 1990s.

The Mess known as the Medical Insurance Industrial Complex

One of the strange, confusing and complicated parts of being in solo practice was dealing with medical insurance companies. The business of medicine went through a major upheaval and transition from the early 1990s. Insurance companies no longer paid doctors what they were billed. By the late 1980s, they limited payments to "usual and customary" compensation. Then the fast advancement of managed care came in the early 1990s to try to limit the explosion of medical costs which were rising nearly 20% per year but also brought in an entirely new business model to medicine. Doctors began to form groups and contract collectively with insurance companies to gain market share. This included the concept of doctors taking "risk" which meant that in exchange for a certain amount monthly (the *capitation payment*) the doctor group would provide all the professional services for that group of patients regardless of how much care they needed. The rationale for this model is that the payments would average out and could be profitable as most patients didn't seek care most of the time. This provided a great accounting and profit benefit to the insurance companies as they could then know exactly what their professional (physician costs) would be every month. This theoretically would benefit the physician group as they would have a steady, calculable stream of income without having to bill the insurance company and then wait for payments. However, the real effect was that this disincentivized the physician groups to authorize expensive care such as seeing specialists and getting expensive tests such as MRI scans in order to keep more revenue. In this model, the insurance companies were successful in offloading *their risk* onto the doctors which added to their profit. As most insurance companies were publicly traded companies (i.e. Aetna, Cigna, United Health Care, etc), their profits and share prices steadily went up. What suddenly developed was this bloated and cumbersome machinery that was put on the individual doctors known as "pre-authorization". What this meant was that if I needed a patient to see a specialist such as a cardiologist for a complex heart issue or to have an advanced test such as a CT scan, my staff had to fill out a form with all the clinical information then fax it to the authorization center of the physician group that held the contract for that patient and we had to await whether it was approved or not. This was in contrast to previous times where I could simply send a patient for a test or specialist because it was clinically indicated. This process slowed down care and made primary care physicians offices an administrative nightmare trying to get patients the proper care they needed. Over the ensuing years in my growing practice, I had to hire two additional staff in order to keep up with this crazy world of trying to get patients the right medical treatment and testing. This nonsense went on for nearly 20 years when it was finally found that it didn't really save any money and just made hassle, waste and expense for the physicians on the front lines!

In a bizarre twist, there developed more physician groups who competed for these contracts with the insurance companies which resulted in each subsequent group bidding for a *lower* reimbursement monthly amount. During this frenzied time in the 1990s and early 2000s, some medical groups took on even more risk by including hospitalization costs (which are always the highest costs in medical care).

The behemoth that the medical world was competing with was Kaiser which was an established HMO (health maintenance organization). Since its start in 1945, Kaiser has grown steadily as a comprehensive model of medical care in California. It is essentially a medical insurance company that owns and employs all aspects of medical care. This includes owning and maintaining its hospitals, clinics and facilities, employing the physicians and staff and providing all aspects of care including medications, testing and ancillary care such as physical therapy all under one umbrella. In turn, patients or more commonly employers can pay a single insurance premium and have complete comprehensive care in one of their many facilities around California. They have expanded to include many other state markets as well. Their business is set up as a "non-profit" entity although the business creates a significant financial surplus that is distributed to the physicians and administrators as well as to maintain and build new facilities and expand programs. It remains immensely popular and has maintained a 40% market share of all insured patients in northern California as of 2024. Their business model worked well in that all medical care and expenses were integrated into one system. Since they owned the hospitals, clinics, pharmacies and testing centers, their costs remained fixed so it didn't matter much if more patients needed a CT scan or another hospitalization for example. Seeing patients who previously had Kaiser as their insurance plan, working for Kaiser as a part-time doc for a year and having physician friends who spent their career there, I got to know the system fairly well. Certainly, the advantages of being able to get all your care at one location was a plus and to not have your doctor bogged down in paperwork or insurance billing issues meant more time for direct patient care. However, many patients I saw after they left Kaiser were on older medications as a cost saving measure which had a direct limitation on optimizing treatment on common problems such as hypertension and diabetes. The biggest issue for patients with Kaiser was when they had very unusual problems that required a specific sub-specialist available only at academic centers such as UCSF or Stanford. The physicians I knew at Kaiser seemed mostly satisfied in that they didn't have too much administrative paperwork although they often expressed their work as being a "job" they clocked into and that they felt like a small cog in a big wheel and had no control over their schedule or say in their individual work life. While their administrative life was much less than mine, they were forced to keep their schedules completely full all the time as the demand for patient visits was very high. The other big plus that Kaiser physicians had over my life was their call schedule was quite minimal. Because they employed so many physicians they enjoyed nearly no obligations after hours in contrast to mine where I was on-call essentially 24-7 during the week and free only on the weekends when my colleagues were covering me. Kaiser has always enjoyed the highest rating of patient satisfaction of any comparable group or system. This is likely due to patients' ability to access care easily and at any time. They implemented an extensive after-hours nursing advice call line and also an easily available Urgent Care clinic that patients can just go and be checked for an acute problem. I actually worked for their urgent care system for a while and discovered that many patients came in on the weekends (when I worked) because they were too busy with their own work during the week. While early on in my private practice life, I looked into the career opportunities of Kaiser, however, it didn't seem to fit what I was looking to do.

The wild west world of contracting with these medical groups known as IPAs or Independent Physician Associations business entities was dizzying. In order to be able to have access to HMO patients (outside of Kaiser), I needed to contract with seven of these groups that were all in my geographic area of the San Francisco Peninsula. Each of them had their own way of paying capitation rates and authorization procedures. Above these IPAs were the big for-profit insurance companies who doled out patients to these entities in an equally obscure way in order for them to maximize their earnings. In the US most working folks obtain insurance through their employer as an untaxed benefit which the employer is able to deduct as a business expense. Usually employees are offered a few different plans often including Kaiser, other private HMOs and the other acronym, PPO, which stands for Preferred Provider Organization. This last one is most similar to old fashioned individual medical insurance where one can go to any doctor or hospital but if that care is not part of their contracted network then the *patient will pay the difference* but it does give one more choice. In an HMO network, there is *only* medical coverage for the doctors, hospitals, labs, etc that are part of that network. This further complicated my life in having to know what specialists, hospitals or laboratories the patient had to go to. Needless to say, the patients were generally entirely clueless about these restrictions. What is well known is that employees pick medical insurance that is the least costly for them, regardless of the restrictions, which is why the HMO market took over in the 1990s. Patients had nearly no out of pocket expenses except for maybe a five dollar co-pay and therefore frequently saw their doctor for any issue as it didn't produce any financial hardship. So, in the late '90s most primary care doctors saw their schedules crammed with HMO patients while trying to figure out (while paying for the support staff) how to logistically care for them and at the same time for many physicians seeing their reimbursement diminish. However, for some clever doctors or groups of primary care physicians who were able to amass a large number of these monthly capitation patients, they saw their income rise substantially as still most patients didn't go to the doctor while they were getting a big monthly check from the IPA. If all this sounds ridiculous and crazy to the reader of this section, you are not alone. Most everyone involved with the system was complaining daily except those able to game the system. The large for-profit insurance companies were seemingly cutting costs (mostly by paying less to specialists, hospitals and for testing) while raking in record profits! Everywhere you read something about medical care, the talk was how the shift to primary care was the best thing in this revolution. However, from the front lines, my practice began to feel more like a factory than a private practice. HMO patients were coming into my office with every minor problem and some had a laundry list of things they wanted done such as seeing many specialists and requesting special tests.

This insane and fragmented system in Northern California broke apart in 2002, interestingly a bit after the *dotcom* bust swept through the Bay Area. There probably was some correlation but it remains unclear if the downsizing caused the numbers of HMO patients to significantly drop. What really happened was many of these smaller IPAs which were run by physicians who thought they could manage a complex business and take on financial risk of which they were not skilled, knowledgeable or prepared for ran into financial insolvency. Overly optimistic over their initial savings of limiting care, these IPAs continued to compete with each other at the insurance companies' benefit for even *lower* monthly capitation. This coincided with the eventuality that patients needed and demanded modern care which continued to become more expensive. So after a flush 10-year period, the cost of medical care again rose significantly and quickly decapitated their capitation of any financial margin these small groups had for being able to pay the doctors what they had contracted. Quickly in a brief 6-month period, we were suddenly notified that many of these smaller IPAs, which had about 20,000 patients each, were out of business! That meant as primary care doctors we were not going to get paid what was owed but we were still legally responsible for caring for all these patients. Only two IPAs were left standing and one was a larger one not associated with our hospital. In response to this the insurance companies who had helped create these bankruptcies by paying the groups less than was necessary had to step back in and take over the administration duties that they had successfully offloaded for a decade. I recall an urgent meeting at the hospital with some of these insurance execs who detailed their plans to return to processing and paying the *future* medical bills of these patients (as was their legal duty) but refused to compensate for the lost revenue of the past many months after all the bankruptcies. This shortfall amounted to at least tens of thousands of dollars for each of the local docs! Did the insurance companies care about this loss? Not at all and justified themselves in a purely legalistic stance. The downfall of the handful of IPAs was actually a benefit to the two remaining ones as they absorbed many of the patients and because the insurance companies took back paying bills directly it did eventually make our lives a bit less complicated. Since that time the number of patients in traditional capitated HMOs has steadily decreased so that now it represents a small percentage of the health care market outside of Kaiser, fortunately. The story of the rise and fall of the HMO health insurance market is one of those that reflects the naivety of the physicians business sense and the ability of very large corporations to take advantage of an opportunity to maximize profit.

The other business contract that remained intact throughout my 23 years in private practice was that in taking care of the poor and underprivileged in California through my acceptance of Medi-Cal patients. Medi-Cal is the state/federal program for insuring the poor and disabled who do not qualify for Medicare. It is known in other states as Medicaid insurance. It doesn't pay well but it does pay regularly and without hassle an amount per month that allows a practitioner to treat these patients. In San Mateo County where I worked and lived, all the Medi-Cal patients were under one umbrella of managed care and by my contract with them, I agreed to treat these patients for a small capitated amount monthly. It seemed to me to be my public duty to help take care of the disabled, unemployed, mentally ill and families in poverty. What kind of patients are these? The same as all the other patients I saw during my career: mothers, teenagers, out of work fathers, people with all the various diseases everyone else gets, some with alcohol and substance abuse problems, some with seriously difficult home lives, some with serious mental health problems not easily treated, many without much education beyond high school, many working minimum wage jobs intermittently, many who were laid off from a good job and couldn't find work again easily, some with a criminal record, and some who were homeless living in their car or on the street. Fortunately, there was no issue with getting these patients the proper tests, medications and hospitalizations they needed. The big issue in their care was getting a specialist to see them and help care for their complicated problems such as gastrointestinal, cardiac, ENT, allergy and several other medical specialties as most specialists refused to sign up for the poor reimbursement from the state/federal system. However, these patients were a great source of satisfaction and the vast majority were very appreciative of having accessible care. They also gave me a chance to see a variety of unusual diseases and problems that are peculiar to the poor and immigrant population.

One example of a very unusual disease was a patient's father who came from Mexico for a visit and had eaten raw milk cheese before his departure. He developed a rare systemic bacterial infection due to the milk being contaminated with Brucellosis in which there are only 100 cases per year in the US. He had symptoms of high fever, severe headache, fatigue and joint pains. The diagnosis was made easier for me because he had gone to an ER recently where they were alerted by his wife's recent diagnosis with the same infection and then did the special cultures needed to grow this bacteria. It was clear he likely had the same infection and while we were awaiting the blood cultures, a compassionate infectious disease specialist was happy to help out, as he had seen only one other case in his whole career of this rare infection. The special cultures were positive and the patient was successfully treated with a complex mixture of antibiotics. Checking around, none of my primary care colleagues had ever seen a case.

Being a general internist meant having a significant number of elderly patients in my practice. The vast majority of these were covered by the federal health insurance system known as Medicare. While there has been a steady increase in managed care/HMO options for seniors under this, most are still covered in the simplified version known as straight Medicare. For me, this always proved to be the easiest system to deal with from a business standpoint. Most doctors sign up to take payment from Medicare based on their fee schedule depending on the level and type of service which is adjusted based on the economic region of the country. While some physicians complain of lower reimbursement on these often more complicated patients, the process of submitting a bill and getting paid by the federal government was always straightforward and timely. There was no questioning or downgrading of payments as with some of the private insurers and most importantly there was no impediment to order tests or consultations or hospitalizations. One could simply treat these patients as they needed according to one's judgment without administrative hassle. What a relief from a business standpoint! Beginning in 2007, Medicare instituted a global payment system for the hospital (not the doctors) based upon the patient's diagnosis. While this caused the hospitals to put pressure on the doctors to discharge patients as quickly as possible, we were under no obligation to do so and many patients with complicated illnesses stayed well beyond the estimated time to ensure their care was complete.

A Day in the Life

So what was a typical day for me in this world of private solo practice as a general internist? Well, as I usually had patients in the hospital to see, I would start there first thing but with a short stop in the doctor's lounge for a cup of coffee, a piece of donut and a chat with whoever was there. This exclusive space was located on the first floor just above the parking lot and was an important informal early gathering of those that did hospital work. There were couches, a TV tuned into the news, the daily newspaper, the San Francisco Chronicle, and of course a coffee machine and some "goodies" delivered early each morning. The goodies were always of the unhealthy kind such as various commercial pastries, greasy but delicious donuts but also some fruit. There were also several computer terminals where one could check various test results and read transcribed consults from the previous day. So a combination of very functional tasks were performed in the lounge. Namely, daily gossip around the hospital, short political and cultural discourse, going over details of complex patients with consultants, not infrequently asking a specialist to see a complex patient, reviewing data of inpatients and checking the latest news and sports. The fluidity, brevity and randomness made this the perfect stepping off point to starting one's day and I literally could not miss a stop here unless I was dealing with a very urgent hospitalized patient. These short medical staff interactions grounded our personal and professional relationships, and it was our "water cooler" moment of the day. Of course, the day's tasks were just ahead which made the calculation of those 5 or 10 minutes a bit pressing but if there was a light load or one had more time, a 15-minute session with the colleagues almost felt like a luxurious social event. So much subtlety was accomplished during these meetups it is hard to underestimate the efficiency and cohesiveness along with important learning tidbits of medical care that were often dispensed. It was a crucial small slice of my life as a doctor.

After a coffee, snack and chat, I really did need to see the sick ones in the various parts of the hospital. Typically, I would start in the ICU as these were the most complicated and in need of in-depth evaluation. It was unusual for me to be the only doctor on one of these cases. These could be patients on a ventilator for severe respiratory issues and would also have a pulmonary specialist managing the details of their lungs. Some could have serious sepsis (blood bacterial infection) with low blood pressure and other organ compromise and be seen by an infectious disease specialist or other specialists. They could be post-surgery and need close observation for recovery purposes. A whole variety of severe and complex medical problems go to the ICU. My job was to review all the various components and to offer any treatments or further testing that might be needed in addition to the management by the specialists. The nurses in the ICU generally are the best and brightest in any hospital and they often can give very important insights into what is going on a minute-by-minute basis and even suggest various therapies that may be very helpful. The ICU is truly a team activity and my role was often as overseer, coordinator and importantly communicator with the patient and family what was happening in understandable language. This included talking honestly about what the medical team was dealing with and the expectations of treatment.

While modern medicine does a decent job with getting very ill patients through difficult times, however, there are many times where it doesn't or can't. Patients who had a severe stroke from an intracranial bleed and then developed increasing brain swelling and damage who were not going to wake up or have a meaningful recovery. Patients with deteriorating heart failure on maximal treatment, those with advancing cancer and severe secondary infections and a whole host of other medical failures were encountered. Here is where crucial conversations with the family were needed to explain the situation and discuss considering letting go of aggressive treatment to allow a natural death to occur. These discussions were always better if I knew the family well. Many times the spouse of the patient was also my patient and so that personal connection helped the family trust and listen to my explanation and permitted us to engage in a more compassionate and realistic plan. I could answer any questions and concerns in a more relaxed way, and we could settle the important end of life issues of shifting to delivering comfort care. Sometimes, there was a difficult display of family dynamics. An example I encountered several times was from a domineering relative (not the spouse) who would take on the role of decision maker for the family (usually an alpha male type), challenging and not accepting the unchangeable medical situation while bullying and embarrassing the other family members. These interactions made it difficult for everyone, taking copious amounts of time to explain and reason with and often prolonged the unfortunate patient's suffering.

After the ICU, I would head up to the general medical floors for rounds on patients in various stages of treatment and recovery. Pneumonia patients needing IV antibiotics, fluids and oxygen but "stable" enough to not need the ICU. Heart attack patients recovering on the monitored floor with all their new medications while starting to get mobilized to walk and do regular activities. GI bleeders that required blood transfusions and getting scoped at either end by the gastroenterologists and observed to assure they were not going to bleed again. Patients with blood clots in their legs or lungs requiring IV blood thinners and oral anticoagulants. Diabetics in ketoacidosis from severely prolonged high blood sugar levels needing intense IV fluid recovery and complete medication regimen adjustment and teaching. And, of course, a whole host of other serious medical problems needing inpatient hospital care.

Hospital care has changed radically over the nearly forty years from the end of my residency in the mid-1980s. Length of hospital stays have decreased significantly and many previously common "hospital requiring illnesses" were able to be treated with minimal time as an inpatient and in many cases became common outpatient care. There are many examples of this. Two weeks in bed after a lumbar surgery where the patient was mostly restricted to bed rest in the early 1980s, to a 3 day stay and out of bed the day after surgery in the '90s, to now where most lumbar microsurgeries are done as an outpatient procedure. Heart attack patients often go right to cardiac catheterization and stenting immediately and if all goes well are discharged in 1-2 days as compared to at least a week or two in the 1990s. Most uncomplicated leg blood clots can be treated with oral medication as an outpatient these days as compared to a week on IV blood thinners and transitioning to oral warfarin. GI bleeders are often stabilized, scoped and sent home within 48 hours now. Pneumonia patients are mostly treated as outpatients unless they show signs of sepsis. Many surgical procedures that required many days or a week post op in the hospital are now done as outpatient procedures such laparoscopic cholecystectomy (done with a tiny incision and operating scope) for gallstones; renal stones are pulverized by ultrasound as an outpatient; appendectomies are also done by a laparoscope with discharging the patient the same day. My 84-year-old mom had hip replacement surgery done at my medical school hospital and spent a total of 30 hours in the hospital before going home! The vast amount of orthopedic surgeries are now done as an outpatient. This reduction of hospital time has been a true revolution for medical care and reflects the advances in skill, knowledge, medicines and technology in our era of modern medicine. However, this shift has changed the typical patient in the hospital to now being quite complicated and more ill. Along with this there has been increasing pressure to discharge patients earlier from both the hospital (particularly Medicare patients where they get a lump sum) and from private insurance companies (looking to save money). This increased pressure began in the 1990s and progressed to the point that hospitals hired many "discharge planners", nurses that oversaw the progress of patients and daily urged the doctors to release their patients. There also developed penalties for patients that came back to the hospital too quickly for the same problem. Medicare instituted a no payment for patients readmitted for heart failure after a short period at home.

The other big development in hospital care was the institution of full-time docs, *hospitalists*, who only took care of patients in the hospital and are literally in the hospital 24/7/365. This trend has swept through the country over the past 20 years and is now in place in nearly every hospital in the US. These docs are hired and paid by the hospital and usually work 12-hour shifts, somewhat similar to ER docs. Since they are there all day and night, patients get more direct and quick care for their problems and patients admitted through the ER get a prompt evaluation and care plan for their hospitalization. This has created a whole new genre and specialty of the physician workforce. Many of these docs come directly out of Internal Medicine residency and can easily do the same type of work they were just doing without needing to do any outpatient care or join a practice while collecting a decent paycheck right away. Because inpatient volumes have decreased and acuity has increased, many community primary care physicians like myself gave up their hospital duties to these physicians so that these days it is rare for an Internist to go to the hospital to directly care for their patients. I saw this developing in my own life over the final 7 years of my private practice. I found myself with only 1 or 2 inpatients most of the time along with no longer having a call group and realizing that the time, energy and also the reimbursement was one of diminishing returns. It became possible to have these eager, available hospital physicians take care of these patients that included all nights and weekends. Hospitals pushed the programs in order to have better statistics over length of stay and to also collect payment for the doctor services. Some doctors' groups contracted directly with the hospital to provide coverage for this service. While there was a convenience to this new system, it was my patients that didn't like it much after I transitioned. "Why didn't you come take care of me while I was in the hospital?" was the guilt inducing question I would get from my elderly, long-term patients after their hospital stay came to see me in the office. I then made a point of doing "social" rounds in the hospital to at least say hello and chat with my long-term patients after they were admitted which helped them feel more secure and safely looked after. Seeing a brand new unfamiliar young doctor when you are at your sickest moments is certainly a bit disconcerting but is the way modern hospital medicine is now practiced. Lack of continuity easily leads to repeating tests and procedures that were previously done as an outpatient. Also, knowing patients over the long term allows one to focus on the most important components of their hospitalization and not chase down every little abnormality. The biggest pain for me after one of my patients came back to my office after being in the hospital was that they were unclear of all that was done and that many of their usual medications were changed or stopped. Treatment that I had often fine tuned and found worked well over a long period of time working with the individual. With the copious repetitive testing and evaluations there were lots of frustrating moments in seeing my patients after a hospital stay! This was also a common experience to my other primary care colleagues who had stopped seeing patients in the hospital. However, the times had changed permanently and there was no going back. Is seeing a Hospitalist better than one's primary care physician when hospitalized? Well, maybe yes if the primary is out of touch with modern medical care. However, in terms of efficiency and money saved it remains to be definitively proven by the data that there is a clear advantage. There are definitely disadvantages in not knowing the patient's medical history well including previous tests, responses and adverse reactions to treatments along with patient preferences and their psychology.

This system of divided inpatient and outpatient care has been in place in most of Europe for a very long time. I recall traveling in Sweden with friends when I was in medical school in 1980 and interacted with docs there who explained their medical care system. It struck me at the time that maybe they were missing out on seeing everything. I was happy I had the experience of "doing it all" for a long period of my career and I wonder what the younger physicians are lacking by not seeing severe acute illness after their training unless they work as hospitalists.

Our hospital for a very long time also had a Skilled Nursing Facility aka SNF on the top floor where patients who needed rehab or treatment after their acute stay such as a few days of IV antibiotics. These sub-acute care facilities are also scattered around in the community as free-standing facilities. These are labeled Nursing Homes and are also for long-term care patients who cannot be at home due to their problems. The SNF facility is for those patients expected to transition back to home at some point. Most of these patients are elderly and Medicare covers this benefit at one hundred days in a SNF per calendar year. For myself and the patients it was quite convenient to continue to care for these patients after their acute hospitalization and complete all their needed care and then transition them to home. Typical patients could be those recovering from a stroke, a complicated orthopedic surgery, a severe infection requiring prolonged antibiotics and many others. This would be my final stop in the hospital and sometimes I would stop by after lunch or in the afternoon as these patients were the least urgent in the hospital setting. There was always a slower pace on the SNF floor as the patients were on a different track of care, one that was measured more in weeks than days. Some patients could not progress well enough to go home and then needed to be transferred to a true Nursing Home facility which would be their final residence. For a period of time, I got privileges at some of the local ones but realized that mostly this setting was for patients who were really there for long term custodial care and not active medical treatment. Some of my internist colleagues built up a large clientele at these places but it never appealed to me and seemed to fit the stereotype of "god's waiting room" too well for me to stay interested in going there once a month for rounds. To be honest, these facilities were simply too depressing to go to and still are. Nursing homes are a "growth industry" in the western world as folks can live for many years with end stage dementia or debilitating strokes that have no hope of improvement neurologically.

After rounds in the hospital it was time to head to the office. As a solo practitioner, it felt good to get to "my place" on the 5th floor of the old office building next to the hospital. Everyone was waiting for me. My staff, my patients and of course all the paperwork and details that needed taking care of such as messages, reports from the lab, radiology and specialists as well as a host of administrative and business tasks to fill up my life. An outsider might ask: "ain't that all a bit much to deal with every day?" Funny though, and this came to me some time after doing this for a few years, is that going to work didn't feel like "going to work" in a typical sense. My work didn't seem like a chore I had to show up and do. My workday flowed naturally through my life. I truly enjoyed interacting with patients as they were so entertaining and often very interesting as medical puzzles and people. I had hired my staff and trained them to do all things that helped me do what I did best, namely see patients. The business stuff was a bit tedious but necessary and it just got done in the least amount of time possible. I couldn't complain as there was really nothing and no-one but myself to complain to as I had mostly devised and configured what my work life was about except for, of course, my patients' problems. There was this distinct sensation that I was somehow in the midst of this course on life, discovering and learning about all the various aspects of the human condition from a physical and psychological standpoint. So, the concept of my job never seemed a trudge but was simply moving along from one thing to the next. I suspect this is the real secret of private practice but was rarely discussed. And, of course, I was able to make a decent living doing it. Not the big bucks of a specialty practice like orthopedics, cardiology or dermatology but fine for my needs which was satisfying enough.

It was always nice to see some patients waiting for me when I arrived back at the office through the back way. After a few pressing questions and issues I needed to discuss with the staff, I was off to the first patient awaiting in one of the examining rooms. The essence of outpatient medicine is one patient and one physician in a private room. It's a simple format of sitting together with the chart, a couple of chairs, an exam table while listening, asking questions, doing an examination followed by discussion and advice. It's astonishing what can be accomplished and the depth of interaction that can occur in a 15-minute appointment. Of course, many times more time is needed to fully unpack a complex situation. The confidentiality and intimacy during an office visit is not to be underestimated. Patients come in and will explain the most profound, important, embarrassing, and difficult parts of what they are experiencing in life. Many times without any plan to do so. It's the perceived safe space that allows an outpouring of directness and honesty not seen in encounters in other parts of life. As their physician and trusted confidant, I needed to be ready and willing to not only to hear anything but to react in a compassionate and humane way to assure the patient that their experience is part of real life. Of course, many times there are no easy answers to complex life situations such as an impending divorce, loss of a loved one, the news of having a terminal illness or an incurable medical condition so just being present, understanding and empathetic can sometimes be the only and best medicine.

Many if not most office visits are for rather straightforward, simple problems like colds, aches, pains and strains and review of stable chronic problems like hypertension. These "easy" visits allowed me to check in on the patient's life and get a broader insight into how they were as people and what their lives were about including their jobs, families, hobbies, travel, relationships and important stuff they wanted to share. While I knew many docs who didn't like to hear about a patient's life and wanted only to focus on the diagnosis and treatment, I really enjoyed getting to know what my patients were up to and thought about in various parts of their lives. This important background gave me a foundation of understanding their life view which could be crucial in choosing a way to approach an important medical treatment that might be needed at a later time.

After a morning of seeing my outpatients the staff and I always took lunch for one hour. This was super important for my staff and also for me to go and have some mediocre food at the doctor's dining room in the hospital. This was a relaxed meal where many docs got together to socialize and chat about whatever was on one's mind. This was a fairly large room with many round tables that sat about eight each. At one time during its peak in the early 2000s one would enter a room with thirty or more colleagues in various combinations at different tables. This was also the height of the cohesiveness of the medical staff. We all knew each other and shared patients, stories, humor and gossip. This was where we got to know each other as plain folks. Having it be exclusive to only doctors meant also that we could "let our hair down" and discuss various things such as vacations, families, hobbies, political and religious views as well as tell interesting and funny stories of patients we encountered. Everyone enjoyed our neurology colleague, Bob Hoffman, who regularly told great jokes loaded with irony and sarcasm. The dining was where all the specialists and primary care physicians were on the same level without any hierarchical importance. One grabbed a tray of food and randomly found an empty seat. This kept the interactions fresh and varied. While the hospital supplied food was just barely acceptable, it was the most efficient way to easily have a meal and not have to go anywhere else as it was a short walk from one's office. Most of the docs at Seton were located in one of the two large professional office buildings adjacent to the hospital and were connected by an enclosed walkway. All the different specialties showed up for lunch: cardiac and general surgeons, gastroenterologists, pulmonologists, allergy specialists, cardiologists, oncologists, orthopedists, ophthalmologists, radiologists, plastic surgeons, dermatologists, ENTs, ER docs, internists, family practitioners and even psychiatrists. It was a complete mélange of the medical professions enjoying a meal and a break from their hectic day. Sometimes I would need to cut my lunch break short to visit a patient in the hospital or to go admit a patient from the ER. I remember getting great recommendations for interesting vacation spots to visit, restaurants, shows, museum exhibits and films to see. Docs, in general, have a great and natural interest in culture and travel. It was fantastically enriching to hear and share experiences outside the world of medicine. One example was my fantastic lunch relationship with Bert, a partially retired general surgeon, who was one of the greatest film buffs I have ever known. Bert had spent nearly all his free time as a young man watching and studying every film made. We would chat at times the whole hour on a particular genre of film after mentioning an interesting one I had recently seen. It was like getting a film appreciation lesson!

Unfortunately for all, the number of doctors going to lunch in the hospital decreased significantly over the last 10 years of my private practice. Hospitalists were being integrated into the care of hospitalized patients and less primary care physicians were coming to the hospital. Shorter more intense hospital stays made hospital-based physicians have tighter schedules. Some of the specialists moved to different hospitals with the changing insurance and contracting landscape. Some docs just retired. Some got ill and died. So in my last few years we were down to a core group of about six docs who met around one table in this large dining room. We all sensed the changing of the times and the end of private practice medicine and lamented the passing of great congenial times together we knew over the past several decades but carried on the tradition of great discussions.

After lunch I was back in the office for a full afternoon of patients. The sight of patients in my waiting room was always an interesting one as it seemed as if the United Nations were in town. The variety of patients from all cultural, geopolitical and religious make-up reminded me of the mid-1980s anthem "We are the World". There sitting next to each other one could find an Israeli and a Palestinian, a Mexican and a Filipina, a Fijian and a Korean, a Bengali and a Pakistani, a Black and a white, or a Maltese, Brit, French, Russian, Italian and German. Literally any combination that the world could throw at you could be found awaiting an appointment in the waiting room. This great mix often gave rise to conversations that demonstrated humans can bridge any cultural gap. There were also the "old guard" of Daly City, South San Francisco and San Bruno that were a significant part of my practice. These were families and often the elderly that had lived in the area since their families settled the area particularly in post WW2 growth of the suburbs south of San Francisco. Many of these knew each other or their families and would chat over shared friends and family. My staff were also from the local area, Carmen, Michelle and Allison all had their families close-by and knew many of long-term locals and could share some "inside" information on their lives that was often helpful in understanding them better. Medicine doesn't discriminate against cultural, racial, geographic or religious lines. Illness and disease are human issues common to all.

Like many primary care docs, my afternoon schedule was usually a combination of long-term patients in for re-evaluation of chronic problems such as diabetes, hypertension, COPD, acid reflux, chronic joint pains as well as follow ups from recent testing and treatments that needed close review together as well as acute problems such as colds and flu, acute abdominal pains, headaches, dizziness and various musculo-skeletal injuries. I kept a rather open policy of trying to fit in patients for acute illnesses the same day as best we could. This kept my calls after hours to a minimum and kept patients out of the ER for minor problems that I could easily handle in the office. Of course, it was always nice to fill the schedule if it had some holes in it as I was going to be there all afternoon anyway. On occasion, some of the old-time locals would just show up in the office and ask to be seen for something or the other and we usually accommodated them telling them they would need to wait. Many simple acute illnesses didn't require much time to evaluate and treat. Some were sent off for an X-ray or a lab and told to come back the next day or that I would call them later with the result if it were urgent.

On a rare occasion, a seriously ill patient would come in and we would need to make arrangements for admission to the hospital or to be sent to the ER for stabilization. This is when having my office next to the hospital came in quite handy as we could simply put the patient in a wheelchair and roll them over to be admitted or to the ER. My patient Curtis was a 50-year-old man who had been having progressive angina (heart pains) for several days and was in the midst of a serious heart attack. I quickly rolled him to the ER where he was greeted by the cardiologist who promptly took him to the catheterization lab where he had four blocked arteries and was then sent for bypass surgery within an hour which saved his heart and his life. He thanked me every time he saw me for the next 15 years. The experience shocked him into quitting smoking and he cleaned up his lifetime habit of a poor diet and no exercise. He was doing well in his retirement the last I saw him. On many occasions, my fragile asthma patients needed admission to the hospital when they deteriorated with their home treatments. Getting them straight to their room with all the orders for their care in their lap got them on the road to recovery quickly. Often, I would stop and see them in the hospital after my afternoon clinic was finished before going home to check on how they were doing and order any additional treatments.

I always enjoyed the urgency and drama of treating asthma patients and seeing them get better. Usually those with asthma have both a sense of an attack coming on and frequently have a sense of denial that "this one will *not* be a severe one". Nearly all asthma patients have inhalers they use for acute situations and also have additional ones for managing their chronic symptoms. An asthma attack can be triggered by a viral respiratory infection, allergies, stress and sometimes for no reason. Usually there is a period where one senses the early constriction of bronchioles (small tubes in the lungs that transport air deep to the lung tissue for gas exchange) and some mild difficulty of breathing and this seems familiar and manageable to the patient. As the process of the disease continues several things are happening at once that can get the patient into a serious situation. From a physics standpoint, as one's breathing tubes in the lungs begin to constrict the openings become drastically smaller with just a slight diminishment of the diameter of the tube because the area of the opening is a function of the square of the radius. So a reduction of 1 mm can reduce the volume of air by half in the small airways! Constriction of bronchioles occurs primarily by the smooth muscles contracting due to various stimuli and nerve activation. Along with this logarithmic narrowing of the bronchioles, the lungs develop a generalized inflammation response so fluid and inflammation cells swell the tissues and the lining of the lungs begin to make more mucus. This cascade of events evolves over several hours or days with the end result that the patient feels like they are trying to breathe in and out of a small straw. This situation becomes quite anxiety provoking especially when the little handheld inhalers one is using are not able to get the medicine deep to the lungs. The worst thing for a physician to hear when examining an asthmatic is not the loud, prolonged wheezes of air moving through narrowed tubes but *less* sound as this indicates air *not* moving well into the lungs. Treating the patient in the hospital can tackle all the components of worsening asthma. Continuously inhaled bronchodilators (usually a combination of two medicines) delivered by a mask over the mouth and nose via a moist mist allows the medicine to begin to penetrate deeper into the lungs to open them up. In addition, intravenous cortisone turns down the inflammation and mucus production allowing the lungs to recover although this component takes several hours to start having a definitive effect. IV fluids help as patients are often dehydrated from a high respiratory rate. Some patients need supplemental oxygen if their level is low or borderline. Seeing patients turn around and begin to literally breathe easier is one of the more satisfying feelings in the world of medicine. An acute progressive asthma attack usually takes about 48 hours to get the patient's bronchioles dilated back up to an acceptable level and reduce the inflammation and mucus production. However, it often takes an additional week of intensive treatment with corticosteroids to assure the attack doesn't return after patients are released from the hospital.

Fortunately, triaging sick patients for immediate care to the ER or the hospital was an occasional significant event in the office. For the majority of patients there was not an obviousness of urgency when analyzing a patient's symptoms but a more nuanced calculation of the *potential* seriousness. What I mean by this is that each symptom has a range of what diseases are possible from life threatening to very benign. Someone with chest pain could be having a heart attack, or a pulmonary embolism, or a dissecting aortic aneurysm all of which are life threatening and very important to consider and to reasonably "rule out" before moving on to less dangerous diagnoses. This is the background mental processing that doctors go through when evaluating patients and the process is a combination of factors. First is how likely the presentation or history of the symptoms and any associated data correspond to a life-threatening condition. Taking chest pain as prime example, a middle aged male patient with a consistent history of pressure in the chest when doing exertional work that lasts for greater than 5 minutes and also has the same pain in the office with an EKG that shows ischemic changes is quite definitive for serious coronary artery disease and needs a prompt cardiology evaluation and treatment to prevent that person from dying from a myocardial infarction (heart attack). In contrast, a 19 year old anxious woman who experiences a fleeting one second sharp discomfort in her right chest that occurred at night a few times over the last 6 months while lying in bed and has a normal EKG has an extremely low likelihood of having any serious heart or lung issue and doesn't need any further evaluation or treatment and can be sent home safely with confident assurance that she is not experiencing anything serious from a medical standpoint.

Medical diagnosis probability calculation is the true "art of medicine". In the office setting, one cannot order a CT scan and a full battery of lab tests on everyone with abdominal pain as is done routinely when the same patient is in the ER. This, of course, means taking *some* risk with all patients seen in the office. Certainty is a mental construct not an absolute in medicine.

The ranking of potentially life-threatening symptoms to the benign and its nuances is the essence of clinical thinking and decision making and it takes time to develop this brain muscle. Its refinement begins in internship and residency where one is fearful that every symptom in the ER or change of status of a patient in the hospital can lead to a rapid death that might be avoidable. Hypervigilance, testing and re-evaluation becomes the way to not let any possible serious problem be addressed. This way actually makes medical care in the ICU or ER "easier" in that one gets to use the bastion of the latest medical technological tests and treatments at one's fingertips so that any-and-all bases can be covered. This is not at all possible or practical or even good medicine in the real world of office-based medical care. The human mind is built to discriminate information from useful to trivial. In the outpatient world of medicine, physicians naturally adopt the Bayesian method for decision making. They begin with a set of "priors" or data from the patient's story of illness, include the background of what is known about the patient, take in any relevant physical findings or recent tests/information and map this onto possible diseases and begin to include or exclude what is most probable. Sometimes more data or testing is needed to get to a comfortable zone of diagnostic decision. Sometimes a trial of treatment is necessary to see the response and recalculate the probabilities. This process continues all the while knowing that the unlikely or highly improbable might be present. If this predictive model starts to favor more serious or more unlikely disease states then more testing or consultation with a specialist may be needed to get at a more certain answer. The common presentation of someone with abdominal pain is a good example. In medical diagnoses, it is taught and well known that a complete history gives 90% of the information to get a correct answer. So the real art in medicine is listening and questioning the patient closely. For abdominal pain these questions need to include the location of the pain (right upper quadrant can mean gallbladder disease, right lower quadrant pain can mean appendicitis); the quality of the pain (sharp, dull, pulsating), the duration of the pain (a few seconds, all night); and associated symptoms (fever, nausea/vomiting, diarrhea, constipation, blood in the stool) all of which are crucial for whittling down the possible etiologies for which in abdominal pain could be in the hundreds! In abdominal pain evaluation the physical exam is actually quite an important component in that if there is no palpable pain, along with normal bowel sounds, no masses and no guarding or referred pain then the probability of serious intestinal or organ problem is lowered significantly (although a rupturing or expanding aortic aneurysm is not). It may not be comforting for the reader, but all physicians' decisions are based on what is most probable. Fortunately, careful history taking, examination and experience brings the level of accuracy to a quite high level. But what about the unusual or unknown that can and does occur? The main safeguard against being incorrect is to retain a sense of incertitude. If any new data should come to light, then adjusting one's "priors" allows an adjustment of probability to entertain other possibilities. This can simply be facilitated by having the patient call back if there is any change in their symptoms or their response to treatment. A patient with epigastric pain who most likely was experiencing excess stomach acidity who then reports dark black stools or vomits "coffee grounds" is then bleeding from an ulcer.

Another good example of trying to figure out the serious from the benign is fainting, or syncope in medical jargon, also known as passing out. Fainting is a fairly common phenomenon and can occur in the context of a serious heart arrhythmia, the common vasovagal reaction causing pulse and blood pressure to go down quickly, hypotension from internal bleeding, medication reaction from various drugs, and several other conditions. A common presentation is "Oh doctor, I fainted last night for a few seconds but I'm fine now" which on first blush seems as if it would be a benign event but doesn't rule out a serious problem. Sorting out the possibilities here include what was going on right before the faint as it is not uncommon for an older person to faint after going to the bathroom caused by vagal nerve stimulation in a case of "post micturition syncope". Were there any other symptoms such as feeling one's heart speed up suddenly (atrial fibrillation or sick sinus syndrome)? Was there pain that occurred at the same time (pain induced syncope)? Was there mental stress that was recently encountered (emotional stress syncope)? What food or alcohol intake was (or was not) involved before the incident? And, of course, what did the patient feel like right after awakening—OK or confused with no memory (indicating a possible seizure)? Rarely, fainting can be caused by a seizure, so having someone there and reporting on the event can give important clues to the etiology. Of course, what medications and when they were taken are crucial in knowing if they played a part in the syncopal episode (blood pressure meds and others can lower blood pressure when one has mild dehydration). After examining the patient and checking various vital signs including any changes in blood pressure from lying to standing, a reasonably good estimate of the cause can be arrived at by taking in all the variables above.

Of course, as with any human mental calculation, one can be wrong. Being wrong is embarrassing and occasionally dangerous for the patient but always makes an important learning point and serves to keep one humble in the profession. One can find out about being wrong from a call from the ER when the patient has some other problem than what was deduced. Or from a specialist who saw the patient with a different lens and found the correct diagnosis. The diagnostic answer from hindsight is sometimes the only thing that is available. Sometimes common problems can present strangely, and strange problems can present like common problems. One never forgets one's mistakes in medicine.

Running a business

Private practice is a small business venture. Everyone who has experience with running one knows the very simple formula for profitability—bring in more money than you spend. As the owner, proprietor, CEO, CFO, administrator, etc. it was on me to make sure all was in place to keep the business running, i.e. supplies, office equipment, competent employees, etc. Behind the scenes there are a whole bunch of important and regulatory things to keep up and maintain. From an insurance standpoint, I needed to have malpractice insurance in case of being sued by a patient (fortunately, this has never happened in forty years!), but also worker's compensation insurance for my employees and business liability insurance in case someone incurred an injury in my office (such as tripping and falling). Many regulations had to be followed in several areas and were subject to intermittent inspections. The various health plans had their own requirements for office practices. These included keeping all medicines in a locked cabinet, a specific emergency kit in case of a cardiac arrest, keeping all medicines up to date and replacing expired ones, keeping a specific plan for medical and environmental emergencies and of course strict billing practices for submission of claims including time limits in order to get paid. We had various scheduled inspections a few times per year from various insurances and were required to make any updates under their rules. My lease was renewed every two years with the hospital. I had to maintain my medical license with the state of California every two years and prove that I completed the required continuing education courses which were twenty-five hours per year. There was health insurance for my employees and I set up a retirement plan. My accountant set up a schedule of paying my employees every two weeks along with electronically submitting payroll taxes to the IRS but how was I to pay myself? Well, based on a conservative estimate of revenue I set up a payroll for myself. Of course, if there was a significant shortfall, I would have to reduce or delay my pay as everything else came first. Fortunately, at the end of most years, I could pay myself a modest "bonus" based on excess revenue which always was a nice sigh of relief and made the new year a happy time. I also always gave my employees a bonus for their hard work throughout the year.

There were various expenses related to maintaining records, initially paper charts but then when we switched to electronic records, the entire office was connected with a private networked computer system. I was incredibly lucky to have one of my patients be my main IT person. Michael C. had a full-time job at the hospital and then at Stanford as a high level IT manager, but agreed to help set up and keep my system running. It was crucial to have someone help when the computer system experienced problems or crashed. On several occasions part or all the system went down which meant that we had no chart or schedule to rely on. Many a weekend were spent with Micheal troubleshooting and then fixing the tech problems. He was worth every penny for his crucial help in keeping the office going.

The important aspect of my business was to oversee and delegate all operations but to try to have the employees do as many logistical tasks as possible so that I could do what I did best, which was seeing patients. Life evolves in a small office setting and the employees did not have one specific job description and there was always a crossover of front office, medical assistant and business tasks that needed to be done. On a rare occasion when someone didn't want to learn a new computer program or do certain tasks that were important they had to be let go in order to keep a fluid, functional office going.

Perspective

Overall, my nearly 25 years in private practice was an extraordinarily rewarding and life expanding experience. I got to be my own boss and make all the mistakes along the way setting up a business. I was immensely rewarded with being the trusted general doctor of my patients which made my motivation and purpose to do what I could for them at the top of the priority list. My patients gave me enormous opportunities for learning about humanity and how disease worked in real-life, real-time circumstances. My colleagues were crucially helpful in evaluating and treating complex patents and generally my employees did an excellent job supporting my work and business.

It's fascinating to me to see that I was part of the last of a generation of private practitioners in my area. Of the 20 or so local primary care docs, they each had a background story. Many joined an existing practice and developed their patient base. Others left a larger practice to start a solo practice. My situation was a bit of a combination in which I left a larger multispecialty organization to start my practice and then had the opportunity to take over a physician's practice who had suddenly "nonvoluntarily" retired (died). Several colleagues started several years before me from taking over from the retiring "old guard" that had set up their practices in the 1960s and '70s. The entrepreneurial and individualistic spirit is part of the personality of most physicians in solo or small practices. So nearly all of my internal medicine and family practice colleagues (who were equally split between men and women) were in either solo private practice like myself or with one other person as a two-person practice. We often joked at lunch that we were the "last of the dinosaurs" of this type of practice as no new primary care docs came into the community over the last half of my private practice. What did happen was that those primary care docs with an increasing workload hired nurse practitioners to help see patients. While this became somewhat common, it never seemed an option for me as my patients only wanted to see a doctor and myself specifically.

While there remain a few colleagues still practicing good old fashion private practice medicine, it is a dwindling minority that hang on. Large organizations have taken over hiring young primary care physicians and it seems no-one has the desire and drive to go into solo practice with its inherent instability and complicated and difficult insurance contracting issues. Also, I have seen the world of primary care medicine as an employed physician take on an entirely different look. These days the vast majority of primary care physicians are women who are able to work part time. It is extremely common now that most work only half or two-thirds time which allows women to have a career, a stable income and a family which I applaud as a great deal! Medical care in the US is heading in this direction for everyone and will not be going back to previous generations such as myself. Of course, there are pros and cons of every situation but I cannot say that I envy the current situation from the perspective of my ability to have been part of the complete world of medical care including hospital, ER and office work. To look back, it feels that I was especially lucky to have been part of this type of work, which never felt like "work". I am forever grateful for the opportunity to participate in such an extensive and enhancing medical community.

PART 2

Unusual, Fascinating and Deeply Moving Patients

CHAPTER 5

Photographic Skin from Russia

It was a long Thursday afternoon, and the waiting room was slowly emptying out after a full schedule of various patients. Going back and forth from the exam rooms to the front office giving Allison, my medical assistant, some instructions on the previous patients, I glanced out to see a group of three people sitting in silence in one corner. The sight of the elder man caused me to take a second look, but I moved onto the next patient ready to be seen. On finishing with that patient and coming back to the front, I stood and stared for a few seconds at this man with seemingly gray skin of his head and hands contrasting white hair. Odd. Was it the fluorescent lighting giving this strange appearance? He was the last patient of the day and was accompanied by his wife and daughter-in-law who translated Russian for the truly gray headed man who was about seventy, Vladimir.

On the intake sheet which included space for describing the main problem as well as a complete medical and social history, there was only the written complaint: "trouble with urine" and no other symptoms, past history, medications, allergies, surgeries, smoking or alcohol. Allison proactively had Vladimir give a urine sample that could be tested in the office for infection or blood. The result was complete when I entered the room and was normal.

Sitting down with the three of them, I began the open-ended questions of what was bothering Vladimir. His daughter-in-law explained that he had been experiencing a mild irritation with urination for some time. "How long?", I asked. "About 20 years or so." "Has he seen another doctor about this?" "No, he hadn't been to a doctor since he was a child." "Did he notice any blood, back pain, fever, or difficulty starting or finishing his urination?" "No," she answered. I told them his urine test was normal but that we could also send it for a culture in case there was an occult infection. He stated he didn't think it was an infection. I mentioned that I should perform a prostate exam and also send him for a blood test to check for any abnormalities. He didn't want me to do that and refused.

After a brief silence, I brought up the color of skin which was clearly a deep uniform gray from the top of the collar of his shirt including his entire neck, face and head. Also, both his hands were of the same hue. Interestingly, his wife's hands were partially gray as well, not as deep as her husband's. Something I've never seen before and began the mental rolodexing of medical conditions that might be the cause. Yes, the daughter-in-law stated, he had this coloring since she has known him for over 10 years. Bluntly I asked, "Any idea how this happened? I've never seen such a skin color." She explained that he has been taking "silver treatments" nearly his whole life. "What do you mean by 'silver treatments'"? She clarified that a few times a week Vladimir put a plate of pure silver with two attached electrodes into a glass of water and plugged it into a standard wall socket. She described how the silver plate exudes bubbles at the edges which reminded her of champagne. She went on stating that after several minutes, Vladimir unplugs the electrodes and lets the water sit for a short bit and then drinks it down. He usually gives some to his wife and to the rest of his family. The daughter-in-law states she has tried it but rarely takes it. Vladimir encourages his son and grandchildren to drink some but doesn't force them to. She says most everyone has taken some sips at various times. She was told that the silver water is to keep infections away and to keep one healthy according to Vladimir.

OK, so now it pops in my head what's going on here and the word for condition somehow makes its way from the reaches of first year medical school pathology class to my consciousness. *Argyria!* The medical term for silver poisoning. The condition is just as described.

This old practice of using electrolysis to bring silver ions into solution and then ingesting them for "health" purposes. What happens is that the silver in solution is an ion that is absorbed easily in the intestines. Then it is distributed throughout the body via the bloodstream to all organs in the body. In the skin it is taken up and trapped by a type of immune scavenger cell, the macrophage, and stays embedded in the layer below the dermis. There it undergoes a reaction when sunlight "exposes" the organic silver complex very similar to a photographic plate which then eventually creates this peculiar and somewhat ghastly, ghostly skin appearance. At this point I am intently listening to her explanation while also reviewing my medical database of the condition to get more details. Vladimir and his wife sit there stoically and occasionally answer a question for clarification from the daughter-in-law. She explains sheepishly that their appearance creates a bit of disturbance when he is out in public. People give them odd glances and avoid sitting or standing near them.

The medicinal uses of silver goes back many thousands of years. It was observed in ancient Greece that using containers made of silver kept water and food from spoiling and it was reported by the Macedonians that using silver plates on wounds prevented infections. Hippocrates used silver preparations to help heal skin ulcers. Through the ages it was tried as a treatment for various problems including epilepsy but there was a consistent use for purification and as treatment for infections. In the pioneer days, the antiseptic use of silver coins for transporting water and milk was well known. The use of silver utensils by the upper class in the pre-colonial era grew out of this notion of making food safer and that silver interacted the least with food as well as showing a level of status. Many cases of *argyria* reported in the aristocratic class of Europe denoted a significant silver ingestion inducing the distinguished bluish-gray coloring of the skin. This led to the infamous coining of the phrase "blue blood" for the rich. The grayish coloring of Vladimir occurred because of the changes that occur after significant sun exposure. In the mid-19th century, a physician, J. Marion Sims, (a fellow alum of my medical school, Thomas Jefferson Medical School in Philadelphia) became known as the founder of modern gynecology by using silver sutures to sew up pelvic complications from childbirth, fistulas, that before no one was able to treat because of continued infections preventing healing. It was discovered in the late 19ᵗʰ century that applying a solution of silver nitrate to the conjunctiva of newborns prevented neonatal conjunctivitis caused by bacterial infections. This practice was adopted by western medicine and was used until recently being replaced with antibiotics drops. Currently, silver-based creams are used commonly for wound healing for patients with burns and ulcers.

In the first part of the 20ᵗʰ century prior to the availability of antibiotics in the 1940s (penicillin was discovered in 1928 by Arthur Fleming but was not developed for use until WWII), ingesting silver colloid solution became a very popular remedy for just about any type of infection. There were even silver colloid intravenous injections given in medical settings and there were medical reports of successful treatment of bacterial sepsis. Of course, chronic ingestion led to many cases of argyria and doctors knew of this condition in the first half of the 20ᵗʰ century. It has been estimated that skin coloring changes would be noticeable after 1 gram (1/30ᵗʰ of an ounce) of elemental silver had been ingested or injected.

Our Vladimir, who was born in rural Russia in the early 1930s, likely had very little contact with doctors or medicine and learned and relied on local folk remedies for treating various ailments. In fact, on questioning, he couldn't actually remember visiting a medical doctor in his life. The use of colloid silver ingestion was a widespread and accepted practice during this time and he learned this simple way of making a home brew of silver colloid which he used throughout his life for both prevention and treatment of any symptom that might be attributable to an infection.

So there was the answer to his skin, but what about his urination issue and the rest of his health. I performed a general examination. The mucous membranes of his mouth and nose also had a bluish hue, however, the rest of his skin not exposed to sunlight was nearly normal colored. There was a dramatic demarcation of the deep gray exposed skin of his neck, face and hands with that of the rest of his body. Then I listened to his lungs and then heart. Uh-oh! His heart rate was quite irregular and his pulse was only 30! On asking if he noticed that he got dizzy or felt like he ever was going to pass out, he said no. His blood pressure was 100/60, low but acceptable. I next had Allison do an EKG. It revealed a complete heart block indicating his heart's electrical system was severely damaged. Big trouble here. This is a problem that can result in sudden death if not treated with a pacemaker right away. Our heart rate is normally regulated by the nerve fibers that pass through the heart starting in the upper chambers, the atria, and moving in a coordinated wave down to the main pumping lower chambers, the ventricles. With complete heart block, only the intrinsic beating system of the ventricles is working and results in very low heart rate as the electric system is short circuited. The result of this untreated condition is often cardiac arrest, arrhythmia, syncope (blacking out due to lack of blood flow to the brain) and death. In Vladimir, this was due to his silver ingestion damaging the pacemaker electrical system of his heart causing it to be short circuited. There is no known treatment to remove silver from the body once it has built up.

So at this point, I urgently counsel Vladimir that he needs to be admitted to the hospital and have a pacemaker inserted in order that he will not die of this condition. He refuses. I tried several times through his daughter-in-law to explain the extreme gravity of this situation. He was steadfast and adamant about not going to the hospital even after another 15 minutes of serious warning. Defeated in convincing him, I then explain what can happen and that they need to call 911 if he passes out or feels any chest pain or trouble breathing or anything strange! I also make a plea to not take any more silver treatments. In addressing his main complaint, I tell them that he likely has silver deposits in his lower urinary system causing his urinary irritation, hoping that might work to get him to stop.

Over the next few weeks, thinking about the danger Vladimir is in and how easily treatable his heart problem is, I call his home every day to see how he is doing to try to convince him to get a pacemaker. Most of the time no-one answers and there is no answering machine. Occasionally, he or his wife answers and can't understand me, a couple of times his daughter-in-law is there and I try to get her to convince him to get to the ER or I can arrange a cardiology evaluation ASAP. She tells me he feels fine and still refuses. Silly stoicism!

I didn't hear from him or his family in the following months and was never notified from the ER or the coroner's office of his death at home. However, about a year later, I got a call from his daughter-in-law. They had all relocated to the Seattle area. She told me he had begun to pass out and went to the ER there and finally agreed to a pacemaker but that he still was taking silver treatments.

Since I encountered Vladimir over 10 years ago, I've told nearly every colleague this story. No one had ever had a case of *argyria* or even heard of another case from someone they knew. So this was not just a case of once in a career but once in a hundred careers for modern American medicine at the turn of the 21st century. Vladimir's case is a throwback to time in rural Russia over 50 years ago where there were few doctors, no antibiotics and folk medicine was practiced. In this case of silver use, the practice came from centuries of observation. In the literature on *argyria*, it was generally thought that outside the skin color changes there was not much toxicity. In this case it may have been only coincidence that he developed heart block as this can occur without any specific cause. However, it is known that silver ingestion causes deposits in all organs of the body except the brain and never is eliminated so toxicity is highly likely with higher amounts.

I wonder how many other cases there might still be in remote parts of Russia.

CHAPTER 6

Son of America's Most Wanted

Tim possesses a difficult, complicated and nearly incredible life history. His complex medical issues are only part of his whole story. After many office visits going over his medical situation and reviewing a bunch of his old records, I found myself sitting across from him sighing and shaking my head saying: "Jeez Tim, if you didn't have bad luck, you'd have no luck at all!"

The full story of his life of tragedies took a few years to fully unpack. In fact, in order to fully comprehend the details, we spoke together several times after I retired from private practice. In order to fully understand where he was coming from, I had to read, discuss and compare what was presented in the book written in 1975 by his father, John "Jack" Clouser, in *The Most Wanted Man in America*. After spending many hours going over his life on Ground Hog Day, 2021, he summed up his life with this simple statement: "I was built for survival not for education." Tim has given me permission to tell his story.

I first saw Tim as a patient when he was in his early 50s and was looking for a new doctor as he had been in the San Mateo County Medi-Cal health system for many years. He had already been disabled for nearly 10 years after several ankle surgeries which didn't go well in helping his pain, improving his ability to get around or allowing him to return to work. He used a cane and walked slowly and gingerly. He had been on chronic narcotic therapy since he injured his ankles and was taking a whopping 240 mg of oxycodone a day. He might have researched that I had some expertise in treating chronic pain patients but he was seeing me as a general primary care doc. Unusual in my experience, he was interested in trying to get off his pain medicines. Desperate to get some improvement for his disabling ankle pain, he sought consultation from a local orthopedic surgeon who recommended removing the metal hardware in his ankles. In addition, Tim suffered from terrible anxiety issues and was taking a good amount of the tranquilizer, clonazepam, several times a day to keep this at bay. To his credit, he had quit smoking and was using nicotine patches to keep himself off cigarettes. His other medical problems included chronic constipation from the narcotics which required medical care and hypertension which was reasonably controlled with medication.

After recovering from the surgery to remove the hardware in his ankles he seemed to get some relief from his pain and we proceeded to slowly reduce the oxycodone down to 180 mg per day. He tolerated the lower doses and was doing "OK" but he was still minimally active, living with his girlfriend and going to church which gave him spiritual grounding.

Over the next 5 years under my care, his life was on a rollercoaster that mimicked his earlier life. He would have periods of feeling a bit better and even went to vocational training to try to go back to work. There was a constant struggle to keep his health insurance. A combination of physical, psychologic, situational and relationship difficulties kept his good times to a minimum. He moved to Sacramento for a year with his girlfriend but then came back when the relationship soured. His ankle worsened when he inadvertently jumped off his truck. His mood and morale were brought down in trying to help his drug addicted son get straight. We tried many different combinations of antidepressants and counseling (which was not covered by insurance) with only minimal benefit. I was called from a local hospital when Tim had run out of his clonazepam and had a devastating panic attack that required psychiatric hospitalization for several days. A short time afterward, he broke a toe by tripping when walking. Desperate for a solution for his pains, he met with various orthopedic surgeons and podiatrists. At Stanford, they gave him the option of either fusing his ankle or a joint replacement. Scared by such big operations, he came back to see me to go over alternative treatments and seek an opinion he trusted. We discussed extensively the pros and cons with him deciding to not go through more surgery. Throughout our time together, he remained disabled but managed his life and pain in an admirable, reasonable way.

Tim was born in Orlando, Florida to parents that were well matched to each other in the sense of both being nightmares in the same dream. His mom, June, a fiery redhead with half Cherokee Indian heritage, who had met Jack, his father, while working together as police officers in Orlando. The marriage and their jobs didn't last very long. Both were heavy drinkers and had explosive personalities that erupted frequently. Jack became a corrupt cop, taking bribes from the Mafia and was eventually caught and put in jail with the help of the testimony of his wife.

John "Jack" Clouser was born in Knoxville to a southern family that had blood connections to Andrew Jackson, the 7th president of the US from 1829-1837. Jack was a restless, wild, misbehaved but intelligent boy and young man who often got into "little jams now and then" as he described them. This included being kicked out of several schools for wild pranks and promiscuity. He was a good athlete playing football in high school and then in college until a knee injury ended his athletic life and studies as his life turned toward womanizing and crime. He married young and had two children but his first marriage ended quickly after they moved to Orlando. He decided to become a cop after being attracted to the status and the pay. Quickly, he was taken in by the culture of corruption in his department and the fiery redhead meter maid. With June, his life took an accelerated path with two sons (one of them, Tim, born in 1960) along with increased stealing on the job and bribe taking. Jack was ironically proud in describing his criminality in the late 1950s. He claimed to have helped Castro's revolution by selling illegal weapons to Cuban gun runners. Jack moved up in the police department to sergeant detective where he saw the position "as where the money was". However, he was forced to resign after being found out in a corruption scheme of running numbers. As a civilian, he became involved in the crime world of Orlando. Jack was charged in a couple of armed robberies and fled the law with his family but was ironically turned into the authorities by his mother while hiding out in Tennessee. He served two years in prison and was then released on an appeal for a retrial.

After Jack's arrest, Tim, age 3, and his brother became too much for his alcoholic, unstable mother who then lost custody. They were left to be cared for by Jack's mother, Lilian Jackson, in Tennessee from the time was 3 to about 5 years old. These were golden times for Tim without his two wayward, deranged parents around creating havoc. For the only time in his life, he had a stable, loving, secure and safe environment with his grandmother who helped send his father to prison. This respite ended when his mom cleaned up long enough to regain custody of her boys. This return to the hell of his childhood started when his drunk mom arrived in the middle of the night and carted off her sons after physically molesting their grandmother.

His bizarre, chaotic, carnival-like life continued into his teen years as his deranged alcoholic mother took up prostitution in order to pay for booze and living expenses. Intermittently, Tim was sent to various foster homes when she lost custody due to her alcoholism. He and his older brother were subjected to his mother's open prostitution at home. June even "shook down" her own sons for their neighborhood chore money to support her drinking. The door was clearly slammed shut on any real mothering. On reflecting on these events, Tim summed his childhood: "I never got a fair shake, and could've been a better person."

One night in this brutal time, Tim developed a serious viral infection that drew him toward a spiritual awakening. Around age 9, he got ill with severe flu causing his temperature to soar to 106 degrees while being nauseous and hallucinating. He thought he was going to die. He recalls crawling to the bathroom in the middle of the night alone, glancing up out the window at the full moon and seeing a white Pegasus stallion riding toward him. Scared to death, he hid under his bed shivering and eventually fell asleep. The next morning, he awoke to bright sun and found himself completely recovered. He has attributed his remarkable recovery to a mystical, heavenly force that looked down and helped him. Years later, attending a Baptist church service, he experienced the congregation speaking in tongues. He was spiritually transformed as the elders of the church took him in to accept Jesus. With their support, for the first time, he was overcome by a state of calm euphoria he had never experienced before. The sensation of his spirit floating out of the church with the congregation stayed with him for weeks. Since that time, Tim has sought refuge and solace from life's difficulties by the community of his church. Affirming to me on many occasions that prayer has helped him emotionally more than anything else.

At around age 13, in 1973, his tortuous mother developed psychotic signs initially by seeing devils while they were living in a condemned house. His tolerance for her crazy abuse ended when she beat him for 10 dollars he had earned. He lashed back by punching her on the nose, leaving the money and fled to find his dad, John Clouser. He didn't see his mother again and she ended up dying at age 52.

In the meantime, his dad had been living quite the life of a fugitive. While awaiting a new trial after he won an appeal in 1963, he was then charged with armed robberies and kidnapping and was back in jail. Facing possible decades in prison if convicted, he smartly schemed up a fictitious insane character based on the mythological character he read about, Wolfeim. He was able to convince the judge of his insanity by his strange foaming mouth behavior in court and was sent to the Chattahoochee mental institution in Florida. Not believing his ruse for a second, the district attorney fought to have his insanity plea reversed. Knowing his crazy persona was suspect, Jack escaped from the insane hospital with a few others and spent almost 10 years on the run. His escapades while being on the lam are colorfully documented in his book. It's actually a fun first person account written with an author about all the details of staying away from the law but it is impossible to know how precise they are. The book has an obvious air of narcissism and hyperbole of his abilities and proclaimed intelligence in evading capture by the FBI. It includes a minimization of his guilt of the crimes he was accused of and likely excludes some of the more nefarious aspects of his behavior. He portrays himself as a man wrongly accused, looking to live a free life and find honest work. He finds day laborer jobs in various parts of North America while occasionally interjecting his regret of not seeing his two sons although he makes no attempt to contact them during his 10 years on the run. His ability to create different identities was quite inventive as he journeyed from the east coast to Canada to the Midwest then to California, Mexico, Hawaii and back to the Bay Area. His story does make entertaining reading even with a skepticism of accuracy. Along the way he names himself "The Florida Fox" and puts this nickname on the cover of his book. Culturally, his exploits of life on the run in America during the 1960s are telling of that time period. Particularly how he was able to adopt different identities stolen or made up which included procuring various social security numbers, driver's licenses and other forms of identification fairly easily obtained during a time which had no easy access to computer databases and when people were believed at government offices without any documentation.

John Clouser was placed on the FBI's 10 most wanted fugitives list after it was known he had crossed state lines. In an example of life imitating art, his life mirrored popular TV in the '60s as two of the most popular TV shows on during that time were *The Fugitive* about a doctor, Richard Kimble played by David Janssen, on the run after being wrongly accused of killing his wife which ran for 4 years in mid-'60s. The other show that Jack watched religiously was *The FBI*, starring Efrem Zimbalist Jr., which portrayed real stories of catching federal fugitives and was supervised by the director of the FBI, J. Edgar Hoover. At the end of the episodes which aired Sunday nights, the latest list of the most wanted were portrayed. Jack frequently describes his cringing and defiant reaction to his poster shown on the show. He engages in a one-sided personnel feud against J. Edgar Hoover and tries to portray himself as a victim while also being smarter than the authorities. The poster Jack saw in post offices around the country during his time on the run was placed on the back cover of his book. On several occasions, he writes letters directly to Hoover that proclaim his innocence while other letters taunt him over his ability to stay free. There are no documented responses from the infamous FBI director. Jack gets a huge boost emotionally when he finds out Hoover has died in May 1972. By this time, Jack has settled into "family" life in San Francisco for a couple of years and actually had a steady job and even got married, all with a fake identity. He truly had been able to outwit the law for nearly 10 years. In early 1973, he discovered that he was no longer on the 10 most wanted list after scouring the posters in the post office. The FBI website today still lists all previous "most wanted". John Clouser is listed as former 10 most wanted *#203* where it simply states that his "federal process was dismissed in 1972". Historically, there have been 506 fugitives on the list where their cases have been settled which does not include the current 10 most wanted criminals.

While living a comfortable, secret life Jack managed to bring it all crashing down by being charged for rape in San Francisco. He describes the incident after a night of drinking and pot smoking as being entirely fabricated by a "crazy woman". However, he is charged and finger-printed and knows they would eventually be matched with his federal fingerprints. Fearful his true identity will be revealed, Jack is forced to go on the run once again and abandons his wife and stable life. In a fateful twist of mimicking popular culture, while awaiting a flight from Reno to Minneapolis, he buys the recent bestseller by a famous hit man and his co-author named *Killer* and begins for the first time to think about surrendering and getting something out of his story. Exploring the idea, he contacts the same co-writer about writing his memoirs. He decides to surrender after his book concept is accepted by a publisher. In a well scripted and planned media event, John Clouser surrenders in the midst of cameramen and reporters in August 1974. He is held on bail but then many of his previous charges are dropped or reduced for unclear reasons. However, he goes on to give many interviews on TV and radio and develops a minor celebrity status as "The Florida Fox" and publishes his book. Jack's book includes a group of photos of himself with his various identities and of his fake IDs. Seeing these pictures immediately struck me of the resemblance of Jack and my patient, Tim. They have eerily very similar facial and bodily features.

Tim contacts his dad while Jack's legal issues are settling out and he is back living in San Francisco. After 10 years, he had only a few short telephone calls with Jack after his surrender and was well aware of his father's fame and minor fortune from his book sales. Pleading his desperate situation, Jack agrees to take him in and buys him a plane ticket. Arriving at SFO, Tim looks like a homeless kid wearing a torn T-shirt, holes in his pants and sneakers worn through. Jack takes him back to his rented cottage in the Diamond Heights neighborhood of San Francisco and is given the attic to live in. Finally, Tim has somewhat of a normal life. His father had taken up with a new woman and was doing odd jobs. Tim attended the local public high school where he got good grades and, similar to his dad, played varsity football. He graduated from McIntyre High School in 1979 and did all the typical stuff like the prom, backpacking, high school dances. As Tim's life blossomed, he thought about going to college. Unfortunately, Jack squashed this idea and had him start working in order to pay rent. Tim found various jobs over the next few years including at a printing company and then a union job working with his dad. That ended when they both were fired after Jack started a fight. Tim was subjected to his dad's ongoing forays into criminal behavior. He was continually lured into various schemes including buying Jack guns as he was ineligible as a former felon. In a drug deal, Jack wanted to kill someone and take their portion of the deal. Refusing, Tim was done with this parent as well and left to find an acceptable legal life.

Initially, Tim went to bartending school. Working in various bars in San Francisco, he found himself making a lot of money while also being exposed to and falling into the rampant cocaine culture of the city during the 1980s. Realizing the path his life was taking, he made a crucial pivot. Finding himself emotionally exhausted and empty, Tim decided to move back to Orlando where his brother was located and found a job as garage door installer.

Here is where I find one of the great contrasts of how life works out for different folks and speaks to the differences of individual psychological makeup having a big effect on one's life as compared to events. On the one hand, Tim's father, Jack, had a stable, loving upbringing in Tennessee but from an early age and throughout his life leads a life of cheating, crime and self-deception while having many opportunities to "go straight". Tim, on the other hand, had some of the worst experiences one can have growing up with his mother's alcoholism, abandonment and abuse and his father's never-ending criminality. Somehow, he realized the danger of falling down the rabbit hole of drug and alcohol addiction and avoided the life of crime he was tempted into and had the resilience to leave that situation behind and look for a stable life! At age 28, he found a career as a heavy equipment operator at an airfield in the Orlando area. During this time, Tim got married and had two boys. Tim worked there for 18 years until his bad luck found him again.

July 4th, 2000, Tim and his family are at home enjoying the holiday. Fireworks are legal in Florida and Tim was safely letting off a few in his backyard and kept the last big one for the end. In a life-changing misfortune, one of his young sons pulls out the fuse while Tim is holding it and it explodes near his face and in the shock Tim falls into a hole in the yard and feels his lower leg and ankle snap. Sustaining a compound fracture, he underwent surgery and returned to his job after a few months even though it continued to bother him with pain. However, this was also the start of his life metaphorically falling into a hole and breaking apart. After his recovery, his wife's low grade depression became more prominent and she began to talk of suicide intermittently. She sought mental health and was eventually diagnosed with bipolar disorder. Their relationship deteriorated and they eventually separated but Tim remained dedicated to helping raise his sons and would do various house chores and repairs for his mentally ill wife.

One weekend he was putting in a needed drainfield at his wife's home, which was a hard, long, labor intensive job that he completed late Sunday afternoon. His wife asked Tim to stay with her but he had to return to Orlando for work on Monday morning. He heard her say to him, "I'm going to die before you" even though she was many years younger. Tim didn't appreciate the meaning of this statement until he was informed the next day that his wife was dead from suicide. Tim was a suspect by the police and wasn't allowed on the property when he returned and could only cry and give a kiss when she was wheeled out in front of him in a body bag. Devastated, he was unable emotionally to care for his two boys and they were sent to live with his wife's mother. They were 9 and 11 at the time.

Death seemed to surround Tim at this time. Before his wife's suicide, Tim experienced the loss of several relatives. One of his aunts in Orlando had died from cancer as he had helped take care of her. Then an uncle and cousin died shortly afterward all preceding the death of his wife. After all this loss, his chronic ankle pain became more prominent and he found himself unable to continue his work the following year.

Hopeful but unsure of his future, he decided to return to California and take his two sons with him. Unfortunately, both his sons did not adapt well to being teenagers and one fell into drug use and the other into petty crime. Tim describes the terrible distress of seeing his sons have so much difficulty while trying to get them help as his physical pain and disability worsened. Unable to work, he successfully applied for disability but required increasing amounts of pain medication and anxiety medicine to keep his life in some sort of tolerable state. I can't help but see a correlation to his mounting physical pain and ongoing mental distress. Metaphorically and literally, he had his life tripped out from underneath him on many occasions.

In talking about his life, Tim is equally perplexed as he is sad about what has happened. Through everything, he remains a pleasant person to sit and chat with. He has a grounded, reality-based perspective on his difficult life, even without answers and he even maintains a sense of humor about all the craziness that has happened. It truly inspires and amazes me that one can actually still have a desire for living, be engaged in relationships and seek minor pleasures with such a life story. I applaud Tim for his bravery and his resilience and I am eternally grateful to him for teaching me important lessons about what humans endure while still being a caring person. A deep thanks for sharing Tim!

CHAPTER 7

Letting Go

The plain fact that everybody dies in their own way either by a mortal disease or accident or the sequelae of such events is a simple truth of life. "Nobody gets out of this life alive" I have said in joking with patients for decades when casually the subject comes up talking about life and death. While the "why we die" question is often easily answered, the "when we die" is often a nebulous but fascinating topic. Doctors are terrible about predicting when someone will die even when someone is close to death. We cautiously skirt the question and give a wide berth for prognosticating the final breath when family members ask. Inside the medical profession, we don't really concern ourselves much with the question of when, as we know the course of someone's illness can vary enormously. We are more concerned with the question of "is there anything left worth doing treatment wise for this person that can have a definitive impact?" After a career of seeing folks get sick and die, the fascinating and entirely unstudied phenomenon of why someone dies when they do can take on the deepest and telling aspects of being human.

Frank and Rosemary had one child, Lucas. In his late teens, Lucas developed a very severe, rare deterioration of his lungs due to pulmonary fibrosis which then damaged his heart. As his health was failing they sought out treatment at one of the preeminent medical centers in the world, Stanford Hospital and Clinics. Near death Lucas was offered a new and complicated treatment, a heart-lung transplant. After a difficult time of hesitancy, he and his family realized this was his only chance, so he went for it. This was in the late 1990s when transplants had become commonplace but this type of transplant was still unusual. While technically feasible and manageable, there was not much long-term outcome information on how these patients did and how long they lived afterwards. Frank and Rosemary owned and worked together at an auto repair shop in South San Francisco. Frank knew cars and trucks and Rosemary knew bookkeeping. Their business did well. Frank started seeing me as a patient a year after Lucas' transplant. Frank had high blood pressure and some back pains but had never been sick a day in his life at the age of 51. We went over his medical issues and I asked how his son was fairing after such a big operation. He couldn't stop talking about Lucas. Particularly since Lucas was having a rough time of it. Lucas had difficulty with pain and a slow recovery after the massive transplant. He had infections and trouble with the immunosuppressants to control the rejection of foreign organs. He showed me a picture. Lucas looked like a concentration camp survivor, so emaciated with sunken cheeks and a scruffy beard. He didn't look happy and Frank kept asking if they should not have gone through such an ordeal. Lucas still struggled with breathing and was not much more physically active from before the transplant. Frank explained how much it aggrieved him to see his son in such a state but he was obviously committed to helping him as much as possible. He monitored his medications and took him to all his doctor appointments at Stanford.

Sometime after Frank's first visit, Rosemary came in to see me as well. She was a pleasant, soft spoken large woman who had type 2 diabetes that needed help. She was not very interested in taking charge of her diabetes from a lifestyle viewpoint but was quite compliant with taking her medications. She was also not interested in getting routine lab tests or any preventative care and seemed to be seeing me at the urgence of her husband. This was a turnaround of the usual wife leading the husband to the doctor ("I'm fine, why do I need to see the doctor" is the usual excuse for men). On asking about her son's issues, she spoke distantly and curtly and obviously was not there to talk about her family.

Over the next year, Frank came several times for checkups and random minor symptoms. Nearly all of the visit time was spent talking about Lucas and his ups and downs. Frank had an extraordinarily busy life. While working full-time at the garage, managing employees and watching over Lucas' medical care he never complained of being tired, conversely, he exhibited frenetic energy. He was mostly worried about his son. He never spoke of his relationship with Rosemary. Frank seemed to have boundless energy for all the tasks of life that required his attention. At some point many months later, Lucas' condition worsened and I didn't see Frank for a while. He came in a few months after Lucas' had died of infection and transplant rejection.

He sat leaned over in a chair in one of my exam rooms, despondent, defeated, fatigued and a bit confused. I did my best to console him over this enormous loss in his life but there is not much one can say to help someone in the grief of losing a child. I was reminded of another patient father of mine who revealed that his teenage son was killed in a car accident and started crying uncontrollably throughout that visit and every other visit as the loss was always hanging close to consciousness. Seeing the doctor triggered his memory and we ended up just sitting together while he cried and all I could do was hand him kleenexes.

Frank sat there, his eyes to the ground, shaking his head sideways, unable to understand the years of pain and sacrifice that he had endured and the emptiness that he had to look forward to. "Frank," I said trying to get some focus back, "your blood pressure is quite high, have you been taking your medicine?" "No, I've been too busy and haven't refilled my prescription for about 6 months." "OK, let's get you back on your medicine and I want to see you every couple of weeks until we get this back on track." "Oh, OK," he mumbled. I gave him a hug and put my arm around his shoulder as we walked to the waiting room. He had come alone, no Rosemary. "That's a bit odd," I thought to myself.

Frank did come back as requested but his blood pressure never got down to a reasonable level. A couple of months later, he looked a bit odd and puffy in my office. "What's happening with you, Frank?", I asked. "Don't feel too good, my feet are getting puffy and I get short of breath going up the stairs." I examined him and he did have some pitting edema at his ankles and his heart sounds were a bit faint. An EKG looked like he could have had a heart attack in the past but not currently. I immediately set up an appointment for an echocardiogram and a consultation with a cardiologist downstairs from me. They saw him right away. The results were awful. He had developed a very severe cardiomyopathy and congestive heart failure. His heart was pumping at only the force of 10% of normal! I was surprised he could work or do anything physical. He said he was still working but having his employees do everything. He underwent coronary catheterization which did not show any blockages. The cardiologist started a regimen of medications to relieve his weakened heart muscle and recommended an implanted defibrillator to prevent sudden death from arrhythmia. Frank refused it. A week later, I got a call from the coroner's office that Frank died at home in his sleep and he was requesting that I fill out the death certificate without needing an autopsy. I tried calling Rosemary but no one answered the phone. I saw her one more time about 6 months later when she asked me for prescription refills and told me she was moving out of the area and had sold the business. She didn't say much when I asked how she was getting along after her losses, choosing to keep our interaction purely professional.

This wasn't the first time someone's health rapidly deteriorated before dying, but the timing of Frank's rapid decline and complete loss of energy from a literally broken heart was due to the death of his son. It struck me as an obvious connection, that he was only held together by trying to support his son. Without the need to continue to help his son, his life force quickly drained out.

Cases of the "broken heart syndrome" have been written about in the medical literature for over 30 years. First described in Japan, it has been nicknamed "takotsubo" meaning an octopus trap which has the shape of an expanding balloon similar to what is seen in the damaged hearts of these individuals. Most research points to an excess of catecholamines (e.g. adrenaline) released during a period of stress as the cause of the heart muscle damage. Like Frank, these patients do not have blockages of the coronary arteries. Certainly, it could have been that Frank's heart had been on the decline for some time and was just able to compensate and ignore his symptoms. However, this doesn't seem to be the case as his rapid decline and death, in my view, fits this recognized scenario.

Laverne and Hugo Keller had been married for 40 years before they started seeing me as patients after they and their former physician retired in 1997. Hugo had been a butcher and Laverne had done administrative work while they raised 2 sons. They were quite energetic to start their retired life together. Hugo was more laid back, but they were both quick to smile and laugh and joke and talk about their travel plans. Laverne had developed a significant case of Guillain-Barre syndrome after a flu shot about 10 years earlier. This left her with a partial paralysis of both legs. She used two canes to help her walk steady but it was obvious from the get-go that nothing slowed Laverne down. She was on a daily exercise program of walking, stretching and weights to keep her physically fit. She never got assistance from anybody for anything related to her residual leg weakness. "I can do it just fine!" she would quickly say if I offered any help. This was an extremely rare side effect of getting the influenza vaccine which can many times afflict someone for months or longer but can also improve back to normal or near normal in most cases but her disability was permanent.

Hugo was reasonably healthy when I first saw him but developed some chest discomfort with walking that he casually mentioned to me on his third visit. He ended up having a coronary blockage that was improved with angioplasty for a couple of years. They always came in together and shared their travel stories and helped correct each other on the medical issues that they wanted to review. They developed a plan of travel to all the places in the US and abroad that they always wanted to see and went somewhere every few months. Hugo eventually developed more angina and his catheterization revealed several coronary arteries with blockages. He needed a 4-vessel bypass operation. While recovering in the hospital about a week or so after the operation he developed shortness of breath and was found to have a large pleural effusion which is a collection of fluid between the lung and chest wall. A not unusual complication that required draining of the fluid with a tube and checking the lung afterward with a CT scan. The fluid was checked and found to be inflammation related to his surgery. However, the CT scan which showed the lung and chest to be OK but surprisingly revealed a tumor of the left kidney that looked like kidney cancer, a renal cell carcinoma.

This was a bit of a shock to all of us. Fortunately, the cancer looked contained to the kidney and no surrounding structures. Actually, this is a common scenario for discovering kidney cancer. While the textbook cases talk about symptoms of blood in the urine, flank pain and fever, these symptoms and findings occur in a small percentage of patients (less than a third) when this cancer is found. Most usually, it is found as an *incidental* finding on a CT scan of the chest or abdomen looking for something else. In Hugo's case the pleural fluid did not seem to have any relation to his kidney cancer although this is possible in a cancer that has spread. We checked the fluid for cancer and did not find any. After he fully recovered from his bypass surgery, he underwent another detailed scan to look for any spread of the cancer and it all looked good. Kidney cancer is odd in that we don't really know the course of it over time. It is likely some people harbor kidney cancer for years before symptoms or a scan leads to its discovery. Spread of kidney cancer is also difficult to predict to know its precise course. One thing about renal cell cancer that still holds today is that one's best chance is surgical removal before it has spread as other treatments such as radiation and chemotherapy still do not have any significant degree of effectiveness. Hugo underwent arterial ablation to cut off the blood supply to the cancer and then had it removed surgically without any complication. The surgery requires removing the entire kidney and attached blood vessels and nearby lymph glands. His cancer was confined to the kidney only, a good prognosis and no other treatment was needed.

After his swift recovery from his surgery, he and Laverne were even more earnest in their pursuit of traveling to the places on their list and they did just that. I saw Hugo intermittently for checkups with Laverne, of course, and I reveled in their recounting of their adventures. They were not going to let medical problems prevent them from living life to the fullest!

Nearly 10 years later, Hugo slipped and fell on his left side injuring his chest and came in to see me the next day. There was no bruise but the area was tender when I pressed on it and he could feel it when he took a deep breath. "You could have cracked a rib, so I'll send you for an X-ray," I explained while telling him there is nothing we can do for cracked ribs except for time and pain pills. The radiologist called me about his X-ray right after he saw it. "There's no evidence of a fracture, but he has a section of a rib in that area that looks like it was eaten away from a metastatic cancer." Uh-oh. Hugo came back to my office and we discussed this finding. I ordered scans, lab tests and referred him to an oncologist. After all the tests and a biopsy were done, Hugo developed a recurrence of his renal cell carcinoma that had spread to his ribs. Fortunately, there was no other area in his body where any cancer was detected. While radiation treatment normally does not help kidney cancer, spread to a bone can be improved by it. Hugo underwent treatment for several weeks and his rib pain went away. He was referred to a kidney cancer specialist in San Francisco for possible new experimental chemotherapy and tried a couple of rounds but it made him sick and he understood that it was not yet proven to have life prolonging effects so he quit it. He came to see me several times during this time seeking advice on what he should do. I explained to him that medicine still does not have great treatment for this cancer when it has spread. I also honestly told him that we don't know what metastatic kidney cancer is going to do. He could have had this for several years and it was fortunately causing him no discomfort and had not spread elsewhere. "So nobody knows what will happen," I told him honestly. Since there is no cure or even treatment, I recommended we keep track of his pain or other symptoms and see what happens. He was fine with this, Laverne too. So they went on with their lives and they knew what was what. Mostly, Hugo had minimal pain and annoyance from this metastasis and occasionally took a Tylenol or Vicodin I had prescribed. Meanwhile they went to the Grand Canyon, the Grand Tetons and Mount Rushmore to complete their visits to all the national parks. They went to Florence, Rome and Venice to bask in the wonderful culture and food of Italy. Because his pain had not significantly changed or worsened and there was no promise of effective treatment, he didn't undergo any other scans or X-rays. This good time lasted for nearly five years. Eventually, the cancer in his ribs spread to his chest, lungs and other areas and he was facing death. He simply and honestly told me: "Well, it's been a good ride but the worst thing for me is to leave

Laverne." Hugo was referred to hospice and died within a few weeks. Laverne was strong and philosophical, "we had such a long and great life together, but nothing lasts forever," she told me.

I didn't see Laverne for about 5 months after Hugo died. When she came in, she had a stack of records from a hospital in Lake Tahoe where she had been visiting with her sons. She had developed a very unusual fungal infection of her lungs called aspergillosis which is often seen in those with an immunosuppressed condition. She was doing OK for about a week but then called me and needed admission for worsening shortness of breath. There was a large collection of fluid in her left lung that required draining and analysis. My friend and pulmonary colleague, Tom Bowstead, evaluated her in the ICU. Adenocarcinoma cells were found in the fluid and a scan found swollen lymph glands in her chest and masses in her liver indicating the cancer had spread. With stage 4 cancer there was no hope for treatment and after hearing this, Laverne stanchly decided to have her final days assisted by hospice at home. "It's my time to go," I remember her telling me in the hospital. Her son called me a couple of weeks later telling me she died in her sleep.

The time course of Laverne going from healthy to rapidly dying a few months after her lifelong partner's death seems obviously tied together. It is quite possible that she may have harbored her cancer for some time, but it is known that the stress of loss can weaken one's immune system which allowed her cancer to flourish quickly.

The third example in this series is not a patient but a colleague. Michael Roy was a psychiatrist I worked with in the late 1980s dealing with complicated chronic spinal pain patients at a multi-disciplinary clinic in San Francisco. He was in his late 30s, smart, sardonically funny, acutely analytically of the way the mind works and gay. Actually, he was part of an interesting group of psychiatrists that had trained together in New Orleans at the now defunct but famous Charity Hospital. Charity, a public hospital, was well known to have a full spectrum of the most unusual cases of medical and psychiatric pathology that existed. After Hurricane Katrina flooded it, it closed for good. Michael and a small band of psychiatrists that trained together there migrated to the Bay Area for their professional work. The AIDS epidemic was raging in late 1980s and it got Michael as well and thousands of other young professional men. At that time the prognosis was invariably an early death after battling opportunistic infections and strange cancers. I knew Michael and his partner Glen socially as well as professionally. He revealed to me after about a year of knowing him that he had the "radiation" as he called it. There was only one medication available back then for treatment, AZT, and it only helped for a short time as the virus became increasingly resistant. This was before the revolution of antiretrovirals that were developed in the mid-1990s that allowed those with AIDS to live a near normal life for many decades after. Michael continued to work through his illness and it was a joy to go over his insightful and often humorous consults of these very difficult patients we were treating. Michael and Glen were well connected in the gay community and as result they and their friends saw many of their friends succumb to the "radiation". It was not unusual that gay men endured over a hundred or more of their friends die. It was a tough time, but the gay community responded with a strong safe-sex campaign which helped reduce the spread. However, the visibility of the AIDS epidemic was clearly on view on the streets of San Francisco with emaciated, skin cancer ridden young and middle-aged men hobbling with canes or wheelchairs.

As Michael's health began to seriously deteriorate, I saw less of him but kept in contact especially with Glen. He was hospitalized a couple of times but recovered from pneumonia and blood infections. He had a large circle of friends and family that wanted to visit him which could be fatiguing in itself. I had a short visit with him at his gorgeous, perfectly appointed condo on Nob Hill a few months before he died. He was cheerful, acerbic and funny, as usual. He had lost some weight but looked OK. I checked in with Glen on his progress on a regular basis. His family and close friends were vigilant of his condition. I got a call from Glen a few days after Michael had died and he told me the story of his last days. Michael had a conflictual relationship with some of his family who stayed in town who tried to be with him constantly. He also had close colleagues and friends that visited regularly. Many times Glen thought he was going to die on the spot over a few weeks period when various folks were visiting. However, in the style of his protected vanity, Michael hung in there through the visits of family and friends looking like he was on death's door with intermittent gasping, winching and confusion. After having seen everyone for the last time, he died one evening with only Glen and his rottweiler by his side gripping a hand and a paw, smiling and saying "thanks" as his final muttering. Glen knew he didn't want anyone else by his side when he took his final breath and was able to muster the will to accomplish his goal.

There are many other examples of one letting go of life at the opportune time of their choosing but I think these three are representative of what health care providers have seen over time. All of my primary care colleagues, when asked, can easily relate similar cases. To me, it's a fascinating aspect to our humanity of both our will to live and then to die when it is time.

CHAPTER 8

Gerry C. Cole

At the end of my last office with Gerry C. Cole after enjoying rehashing the prior 20 years of medical adventures and life, we shook hands and hugged (even during pre-vaccination Covid times) and we welled up with watery eyes and as we nearly said our final goodbyes I looked down at his chart I noticed something new. "What does this 'C' stand for as your middle name?" "Cool," he replied coolly with a straight face. We then both laughed and slapped each on the back. "No really," I persisted, "I thought it might mean 'Cat', as you love them so much." "No, it's Cool." "OK then." And that is how we left it.

Mr. G. Cool was born in Nashville during WW2 to a Marine dad and a mom whose heritage stretched back to slave owning plantations in Tennessee. This may have inspired his Elvis look in later life being a big guy with long, sharped edged sideburns which grew white as he aged. While an infant, he was taken to San Francisco by his mom who had family there to help for the duration of the war and after which his family stayed on.

Gerry grew up in the growing middle-class post-war Excelsior district in San Francisco and graduated from the famous Riordan high school. He promptly married at age 17 and went to work at a gas station like his dad did after returning from the war. He changed to a better paying job at the supermarket chain, Safeway, and bought his first house for $16,000 a year later. Showing his early ability to be financially pragmatic, he sold that house 3 years later for $21,000 and promptly bought his current house in the newly developed suburban Westborough district for $28,000 against all the advice of friends and family who believed he would go bankrupt due to the high mortgage payments. Demonstrating his frugality and determination he paid off the mortgage in 15 years in the late '70s and still lives there now.

His work life brought him to progressively better paying jobs. At one point he owned a liquor store which he didn't like but made a big profit when he sold the license. He wisely invested in the 1970s in "deeds of trust" which netted him 25% interest payments. He inherited a rental property and at age 39 determined he had enough money and decided to retire! He had never taken a true vacation and had put his 3 kids through college.

However, early retirement brought a huge stress issue to his marriage. Being an organizational freak and a newly minted empty nester, he drove his wife crazy by gradually taking over many of the household chores including emptying the dishwasher. Fed up after less than a year the two were home together, she issued the ultimate ultimatum: "You either get a job or I will divorce you." Gerry was a bit shocked but didn't want his marriage to end over cleaning up around the house.

Not looking for anything serious, full time or even well paying, the cool Gerry went to the Cow Palace, the only and largest indoor event facility on the west coast at the time, located near his home in the southern district of San Francisco where he knew a couple of people who worked there. The Cow Palace, a depression era WPA program project, was finished the year before Gerry was born in 1941. It was originally conceived as a livestock show place but being a six acre indoor facility it quickly became the west coast showcase for nearly every other large gathering including: heavyweight boxing matches (Muhammed Ali), political conventions (1956 and '64 Republican National Conventions), professional sports such as basketball, tennis and ice hockey; circus shows (Ringling Bros), boat shows, and concerts (the first Beatles US concert, Elvis Presley, etc.).

Jerry strolled in on a bright weekday morning in October and explained to the employment office that he needed "any job to make my wife happy" and applied for a job as a popcorn maker. One of the managers walked in and asked him, "Do you know how to bartend?" as he needed help for an upcoming event. After a chat, he finds himself working at the best bar in the arena as a part-timer and astutely signs up for all the busy shows. Within a year, the now *very* cool Gerry becomes the bar manager, a position he kept for the next 20 years! Mr. Cool is now getting paid to witness some of the greatest shows around and has dozens of attractive, young female bartenders under his supervision all to the dismay of his increasingly jealous wife. In order to keep an eye on him, she demanded that he get her a job but it only increased her jealousy even though Gerry was always faithful and never even drank or partied. "I was just doing what I was told," he told me. Conflict continued as she demanded he quit his job. After he refused, she leaves him for a year then returns but after a few months decides to have a "legal separation".

The pragmatic Gerry understands that his marriage is over at this point and decides to make it final by filing for divorce. Being a person somewhat fixated with dates, he made sure the divorce was signed on his 32nd wedding anniversary, July 8, 1990. Along with the 50 pairs of shoes and various furs she left with, our Gerry gave her a brand new 1992 Ford Thunderbird as a divorce gift while continuing to drive his '79 Mercury which was "working fine". On her way out the door to relocate to Chico, California, she emphatically stated, "I'm gonna be remarried within a year, so there!" A statement he gleefully reminded her of over the next 30 years of her still unremarried life. He, on the other hand, openly stated at the time, "I'm never getting married again" and has stuck to his guns.

During the period of time from the early 1980s and over the next 20 years Gerry began a parallel accumulation of houses and cats. He began acquiring houses by purchasing and inheriting. Initially, he acquired one local house after another in order for his extended family to live in and not for rental purposes. He got up to a total of seven. His cat collection developed more circuitously and goes back to his childhood when he continually begged for a puppy that his dad refused to allow him. After his mom clandestinely allowed him to get one, the dog promptly befriended his dad, abandoning poor young Gerry. Twenty plus years later a parallel situation developed when his son brought home a kitten against his orders. This feline fur ball then proceeded to fully attach itself to this next generation of pet refusing dads. While Gerry became quickly smitten with the kitten, he tried to recapture his lost puppy youth by deciding to make his new cat into a dog. "OK, we're going for a walk," he informed the little white kitty and proceeded to do whatever the new master commanded including coming to bed when called.

He described the path to acquiring his next 6 cats as emanating from the initial kitty dispersing its cat smell and then attracting needy felines. "One told another and then they showed up and that's how I got so many," he once explained to me. Two stray ill cats showed up on his doorstep one day and he promptly took them to the vet, paid for their care and took them home. Then a mother with two kittens was in his backyard. An aunt gave him one of her sick ones, and along the way other strays showed up on his property. At his peak, he had nine lucky felines occupying various parts of his home. He and his aunt, who also had a collection of cats, shared a philosophy and stratification of a multi-cat house. Since cats in general and particularly feral cats rarely get along and are often quite unfriendly to humans, he needed to segregate them to an area that fit their personality. So he had "backyard cats" for the most nasty ones, "garage cats" for those that needed to be indoors but were unruly, "downstairs cats" who had a modicum of friendliness and cleanliness, and "upstairs cats" for the most lovable ones. His power of compassion and deep pockets for these felines apparently knew no limit. The first and longest living lasting cat developed significant health issues starting at age 15, including a stroke, diabetes, and kidney failure. That one cost him an estimated $40,000 of veterinary care including hiring a local vet to come over daily for a year to give the cat injections of insulin and fluids. He extended this financial support to his cat collecting cohorts. His aunt, who when one of her 10 cats became ill, came under the wing of Gerry and he paid for all its care. One of his girlfriends, Beverly, was a master cat collector of 26 felines and gladly accepted financial support for her sick cats. Who knows how much Gerry spent on vet bills over the past several decades? He never thought twice about it.

Cats die too. And Gerry wanted the best resting place for his feline friends. He has 21 of them buried near each other in the infamous Pet Cemetary on the hill in San Bruno which sits above human cemeteries in Colma.

Gerry started seeing me as a patient in the mid-1990s when his only other adult doctor retired. Dr Salteri was known around the South San Francisco area as a "good, solid, general practitioner". I barely knew him as I was starting private practice during his last years of his work. He along with a few other hardy "old-timers" took care of nearly all the folks who lived in the area since the early 1960s. Several of these docs continued to work well into their eighties and I knew and greatly respected many of them. Ed Nolan, Jerry Murphy, Steve Wald and the others in that category would be seen early in the morning before hospital rounds in the doctor's lounge. This was a room on the ground floor of the hospital where one could find coffee and donuts supplied by the hospital and colleagues gathered around to chat and complain about the hospital administration and hear the latest gossip. These older docs usually breezed in for about a three minute stay and then were on their way to see their hospitalized patients. On a rare occasion, one could overhear them talking about the old days and one could even ask them to elaborate about what practice was like back in the 1960s. Mostly what I gleaned from these chats was that life as a doc back 30 years ago was much more difficult. These guys were on-call just about all the time—day, night, weekends and holidays. They were so used to that life that they only were free when on vacation which was seldom and they covered for each other for those brief respites. They all saw all their own patients in the hospital 7 days a week. In order to build a medical practice in the 1960s you had to do house calls all the time. These were mostly mildly ill, worried patients calling in the evening. After dinner these guys would drive around checking in on patients at home. When someone was sick in the ER in the middle of the night, they got up and came in to admit them to the hospital. Such a difference from now, where after-hours calls are taken by "advice nurses" and hospitalists (doctors who only work in the hospital) take care of the hospital patients 24 hours a day in shift work fashion.

I actually saw Gerry first when I was helping one of these other older docs who was cutting back to a couple of days a week and asked me to come to his office to see the overflow. This doctor, Dr. Cunha, was in his mid-70s and was a surgeon who stopped doing surgery and was filling his time seeing general medical conditions and had been friends with Salteri during his career and temporarily took over some of his patients when he retired. Gerry knew I wasn't going to retire for some time so he decided to stick with seeing me instead of hanging on for Dr. Cunha's last days of work. He was reasonably healthy and still working and in his mid-fifties and carried a diagnosis of "pre-diabetes" back then.

On our first visit I ordered a battery of updated blood tests to check on his status. Not surprising, his levels of glucose, glycohemoglobin (which gives an estimate of the glucose level over the previous 3 months) and his lipids were elevated. "Do I have diabetes, doc?," he asked bluntly. "Well, it looks like you are on that path, let's repeat your labs in a month and discuss this further then," I explained, trying to soften the blow of giving him a significant diagnosis for the first time in his life. The next results were worse, his sugar level was nearly 300 (normal is 100) and his glycohemoglobin was over 10% (normal <6%). "Sorry to give you the bad news but you definitely have type 2 diabetes, Gerry." "Oh, jeez, how can this be? No-one told me about this before." I explained that this comes on slowly over the course of a year or more until the test re-sults put you in that category. "Let's go over your diet," I asked. "Well," he said and took a big slow breath, "since my wife left several years ago, I just decided to eat what I want. I got in the habit of just having desserts instead of dinner when I got home late from work. Then I just started having donuts and pastries for breakfast, pie for lunch and ice cream and cookies for dinner." "Oh," I said slowly. "How long have you been eating like this?" "Well, probably over 5 years now." "Well, looks like time to change that up." "Do you ever eat vegetables, salad or fruit?" "Never, I hate salad and all vegetables except for potatoes!", he exclaimed. "But, I do eat meat sometimes," he clarified. Well, well, well, I could see this was going to be a major, delicate project of convincing, rearranging priorities and detailed explanations to this middle-aged man clearly stuck in his dietary habits.

And then there was the need for medications. Gerry demonstrated the typical triad of problems known as the "metabolic syndrome" which includes type 2 diabetes, hypertension and elevated cholesterol all of which require treatment. I gave Gerry the choice of either a cataclysmic lifestyle change or medications. He chose medications with significant protestations and only after I informed him of the severe health risks of heart attacks, strokes, loss of limbs due to neuropathy and an early death which were accurate in this context. However, being the excellent negotiator that he is and my need to be prudent to get him on some road to better health, we agreed to start one medication at a time and he began with the most important for diabetes.

Gerry turned out to be an excellent patient. After understanding the need for treatment, he completely took on the task of listening and complying. Of course, with some of his idiosyncratic caveats along the way but after 6 months of slowly adding medications, coaxing him to reduce a fully processed sugar diet and monitoring his lab results he was showing excellent results. His A1C (the 3 month glycohemoglobin test for diabetes) was down to an acceptable range of 7.5% (normal is up to 6%), his blood pressure had improved from 160/100 to 135/85 and his cholesterol level went from 320 to 215. He truly enjoyed sitting down with me at our monthly visits and going over how the medications were doing with him and the lab results. Each time a lab report came in, he demanded a copy and kept a neat file of everything that was done in chronological order. He was able to cut down from a dozen donuts in the morning to only a couple with substituting other healthier items along the way. He went back to his traditional dinners of meat and potatoes with an occasional vegetable but he honestly admitted this was due to large size *TV dinners*. He adamantly and continually refused to consider ever eating a salad, "I just can't!"

He continued to improve so much over the next year with his diet changes, medications, and a small increase in exercise helped him lose 30 pounds that his "numbers" then looked excellent! His A1C was now at 6%, his blood pressure was in the normal range and his cholesterol was under 200 with a very nice reduction of the bad cholesterol component (LDL). When we sat down together to review all this I said,

"You know what, you are my star patient and if I had one of those gold stars from grammar school I would put it on your forehead and have you wear it around town to show everyone." He beamed, "Thanks for that, am I really your star patient?" "Yes, you've earned it!" "Great," he countered, "now can we talk about something very important?" "Of course, Gerry, what is it?" "Can we get rid of some of these medications now that I'm doing so well?" "Well, that's an honest request but at this point since you're doing much better with them and not having any side effects let's not 'mess with success' and keep them going," I replied.

My star patient did well over the next 15 years or so on a combination of medications, improved diet, and reasonable weight control. He would always ask if he was still "a star" and also ask if I could reduce or take away any of his meds after an extensive review every 4-6 months of recent lab tests. The rewarding truism of these metabolic disorders of diabetes, hypertension and hyperlipidemia is that the patient and the doctor can often keep it under control. Gerry admitted during the years after his divorce that he was a "sugarholic" where the more he ate, the more he craved. He was able to return to a meat and potatoes diet with an occasional veggie. He initially lost that 30 pounds but slowly gained weight as he became less active and got older. Unfortunately, diabetes often worsens due the further loosening of the body's metabolic control mechanisms. Gerry's A1C began to creep up to over 8% and reached 9% for the past few years. So he did lose his star status and instead of talking about possibly stopping medications, I tried to cajole better behavior with the threat of adding more medications. He already had a blood thinner ordered by his cardiologist for atrial fibrillation. I then added one of the newer better diabetic pills to get better control which did stabilize his higher sugar levels. He asked about needing insulin but I reassured him that it would be the last resort to start as he was still on the upper limits of control and the current thinking is to avoid insulin as long as possible in type 2 diabetes. Because he was on a couple of newer medications, his "discussions" in the office included discussing the costs of these. One was $400 per month and another was $350 per month and because they were not generic, they had minimal coverage with his insurance. He alertly and honestly asked, "Can I take cheaper ones that do the same thing?" A common issue in today's world where new medications are "better" than the old generics but often only somewhat (and statistically) an improvement. In Gerry's case the newer medications offered better protection of complications from his diabetes and less side effects of bleeding from his blood thinner enough that I recommended he continue on them. I enjoyed his honest layperson's approach in trying to logically figure out what was best. Unlike most patients, he put thought, research and time into his arguments and allowed us to go through all the reasons for his treatments in a spirited and fun discussion. In the end, he agreed to spend his money on his health.

One other medical issue that we bantered around for a long time was his need for a heart valve replacement. His astute cardiologist, Dr. Girolami, had been following this problem for about 10 years as well as his heart rhythm problem, atrial fibrillation. He was on medications to prevent a stroke but his aortic valve continued to worsen by becoming hardened with calcium buildup and narrowing. This is the most common modern heart valve abnormality, *aortic stenosis*, and it causes blood flow from the heart to the body to be restricted as it narrows the main opening from the heart. As it narrows, there is increased risk of low blood pressure and fainting, or a stroke from lack of flow to the brain, or progressive weakening of the heart due to chronic strain and even a heart attack as it worsens. There is an excellent, accurate and non-invasive method of assessing the valve using an echocardiogram (external ultrasound of the heart) which can measure when the reduction in blood flow from the heart becomes dangerous. In Gerry's case, he was close to the critical narrowing when first discovered and then worsened over the years. He was clearly a candidate for surgical replacement of the valve which is the only true treatment available. However, there were two factors that kept him from signing up for those 10 years. One, he felt fine and couldn't accept a risky heart surgery when he had no symptoms. "Why should I do something that might kill me, when I feel good?", he would ask. Hard to argue with this type of logic and Gerry successfully held off the procedure for nearly a dozen years due to his reluctance and also because the surgery itself was in the process of a transformation.

Until recently, to replace a heart valve one needed to open the chest, put the patient on a cardiopulmonary bypass machine and then cut out the old diseased valve and put in a replacement which is either from a pig (bioprosthetic) or mechanical (made of metal). However, from 2010 to 2020 there was a steady increase in doing the procedure via a catheter through an artery and eliminating the risk and difficulty of a big surgery. The safety and experience of this new way of dealing with an old problem became the more common method as of 2019. Gerry waited until 2020 for his, not without a lot of questioning and concern for all the doctors involved. But things went well in his procedure with the exception that he also needed a cardiac pacemaker for an electrical block during it. He got to tell the specific details of his conversations with the interventional cardiologist who did the procedure. "First he wanted to put in one type of valve then I asked him why and then when he was explaining it to me he decided to put in a different one!" I wasn't sure if this was the way it happened but Jerry was emphatic about his role in the decision making.

Since divorcing his wife over 25 years ago, Gerry has had many "girlfriends" although most have been platonic affairs. There may be a minor form of his "collecting" nature in his opposite gender friend-ships as well. At the end of our time, he was down to only one although he informed me "we're not seeing each other much anymore". One of his girlfriends who was 90 had recently died and left him her house and cat, his only cat of this writing. He would commonly report a steady relationship with usually 3 women at the same time over the past 15 years or so. One, 20 years younger, another his age and the other 20 years older seemed to cover all the age ranges. It seemed these were mostly good friends and all knew of each other and had no issues with him having female friends.

Life goes on for Gerry the cool, cat loving, sympathetic, pragmatic, organized one. It was a joy to have him as one of my star patients! He heartily gave his permission for me to write his story as he anxious awaits the publication of this book.

CHAPTER 9

Pink Elephants from the Nursery

John was a widower who kept working at his nursery business mostly because he didn't have much else to do. Over the last 15 years of his life, the business essentially didn't make any profit but he went to work every day and paid his employees, a collection of pleasant hard working Mexican immigrants who tended to the plants and filled orders for his declining customer base. His grandfather emigrated from Italy in the 1880s and bought a plot of land south of San Francisco in the foggy area that would eventually become the city of Daly City. He was part of a new crop of immigrants from Italy that followed the large Irish immigration after the potato blight. Many of the new Italians found a way to grow cool weather crops where others could not including artichokes, broccoli and brussel sprouts in this fog belt near the ocean. John's grandfather started as a pig farmer in the 1880s. His son then changed the land over to become a plant nursery for the area for the growing homes, businesses and cemeteries in nearby Colma. Business was thriving through the 1930s and post-war era. John took over from his dad in the 1950s and kept his dad's business reputation. However, he developed more than a habit for alcohol which didn't have much effect on his ability to manage the nursery. However, larger, more diverse nurseries began to eat into his clientele but he stayed profitable up until the mid-1990s, which also corresponded to his increasing all day drinking habit. The death of his wife cemented his need to get through a day with a bottle of vodka. This is when he started to see me as a patient in 1996.

141

It didn't take long to know that the drinking was beginning to take its toll on him. Over the next dozen years of our relationship most of our interactions were in dealing with his over-imbibing, including many visits to the ER and hospitalizations. Several times after a severe binge, he would then limit his drinking for a period of time. John had other health problems as well. The significant extra calories and lack of movement caused his weight to be over 300 pounds although he didn't look terribly fat being six foot five inches tall. He just looked big and puffy with thick lips and a limp. He suffered from intermittent bouts of asthma that were reasonably handled with various inhalers and medications when it flared up. Being a widower gave him reason for going to work 6 days a week to try to compensate for his loneliness. He frankly told me that he had nothing better to do and kept the business going mostly for that and to keep his employees on a paycheck. He didn't make any profit from the business any longer but didn't care. He had 2 children that he saw on a rare occasion and didn't have many close friends and no other life interests except for the company of a bottle. He bemoaned the changing world and loss of his wife and gradual loss of his business stature. He longed for and spoke of the "old days" often. However, he was not a depressed guy. Actually, he was reasonably upbeat and liked his employees who were from Mexico or El Salvador and kept his customers very happy. He enjoyed discussions about various topics of local and world politics and was well informed. He read the papers and listened to the radio all day long. He'd visit the iconic local restaurant, Westlake Joe's, where he would socialize with the old locals. Many of which were long time functioning alcoholics like himself and some of which were also my patients. That joint was something out of the 1960's Frank Sinatra "Rat Pack" scene with large booths, a long counter and a separate room for music. Some very regular "important" patrons had their "own" spots where they could claim a booth or a certain spot at the bar and could always be found. John would wander around the place and chat with many of them. He fit in well to the social fabric of the Daly City community that evolved from the old days.

I understood his "lifestyle" and even visited his nursery on his insistence after he offered me rose plants for the umpteenth time. As with all things human, seeing the real person in their environment reveals much more than any word description. His nursery was on a backstreet and was about an acre plot of land with unkempt fences and signage. A simple rusted, faded "John's Nursery" sign hung at a slight angle from the high chain linked fence. There were several workers doing various duties while his main assistant, Jose, showed me to his small office piled high with papers. John sat in a large old dark wooden swivel chair that he could lean back to near full reclining position and put his feet up on his old metal desk. A position he could nearly always be found in, sometimes sleeping, reading the paper or just listening to the radio and sometimes reaching for the bottle of vodka hidden under the desk. A few metal file cabinets of various heights lined the walls. "Hey, doc, good to see ya, come on in" he motioned to me after he saw me walking in.

I said, "so this is where everyone gets their plants?" "Oh, not so much anymore after all these big nurseries and Home Depot came into the area." His guys had nearly a dozen potted roses ready for me. "I got you a mix of different colors, hope you like them." We chatted about his business and I met a few of his workers and loaded the roses into my SUV and after thanking him I chatted with Jose, his main worker. He told me he was the one mostly getting John his booze from the liquor store when he ran out at work. I tried to convince him that it was not a good thing for his health and asked him to stop. I then drove home and planted all of those nice roses in the beds in front of my house.

A couple of months later, I got a call from the ER doc that John is in and will need to be admitted. He had drunk himself into a stupor, fell and bashed his eye, had severe electrolyte disturbances and had a large infected pressure ulcer on his sacrum. When I saw him in the ER, he was dazed and slurring his words and barely recognized me mumbling something about his daughter who I called to tell her he was going to be admitted. Fortunately, the CT scan of his head did not show any skull fractures or bleeding. His protime (clotting) level was elevated indicating his liver was ill and not making sufficient coagulation factors. This along with his lowered platelet count made him at high risk for bleeding either into his brain or his gut. He needed close monitoring for this as well as active treatment for his altered metabolic state.

Alcoholics are at risk for permanent brain damage from a deficiency of thiamine. This consequence of heavy chronic alcoholic abuse is known as *Wernicke-Korsakoff syndrome*, described in the 19th century by the German neurologist, Carl Wernicke. He made the association of the confused mental state (encephalopathy), eye twitching (nystagmus) and unsteady walking (ataxia) of alcoholics and associated specific areas of brain damage on autopsy. A few years later the Russian psychiatrist, Sergei Korsakoff, described the chronic amnesia and cognitive deficiencies in alcoholics that became a permanent state. It was a few decades later that these acute and chronic brain changes caused by alcohol were known to be caused by a deficiency of the common vitamin, thiamine (B1). While thiamine deficiency can cause a similar problem, it is fortunately in many food groups: meats, breads, nuts, beans, peas and other vegetables so it's unusual if one eats a reasonably balanced diet. Alcoholics develop the deficiency from a combination of inadequate intake, poor absorption, decreased liver storage and impaired utility. Thiamine works in crucial steps of glucose metabolism throughout the body but is particularly important in the brain as the brain uses glucose nearly exclusively for obtaining energy. The brain uses a lot of energy, at least 20 percent of the entire body's energy goes to the brain and this must be in the form of glucose. So, if there is a shortage of energy, nerve cells (neurons) stop working properly and are easily damaged. Along with the direct damage that alcohol can have on nerve cells, the havoc that thiamine deficiency causes to a glucose hungry brain essentially produces a short circuiting of normal electrical activity which is not conducive to proper thinking or mental alertness or movement. On repeated episodes of these acute injuries, the brain develops literally small holes in certain parts of the brain caused by tiny hemorrhages. While it can take some time, these damages accumulate to cause permanent malfunction of important areas of memory and thinking. Chronic alcoholism can damage nerves outside the brain as well. The most common is toxic permanent injury to long sensory nerves that go from the spine to the feet. Peripheral neuropathy, as it is called, manifests with a combination of loss of feeling and a sensation of burning pain due to damage of sensory nerves and other nerves that transmit pain and is most commonly felt in the feet of affected individuals. The other important medical issue about thiamine is that if one just gives an alcoholic glucose in an IV solution without thiamine first it can make the brain damage and mental function much worse without this crucial vitamin.

John got a nice whopping dose of thiamine in the ER and was set up with an IV of electrolytes and glucose, wound care, neurologic monitoring and medications for sedation in case he became agitated along with oxygen and asthma medication if needed. Around midnight a call came from his nurse. "Mr. O. is having visual hallucinations." "He sees snakes and large spiders in his room and is freaking out." "The good old D.T.s have set in," I told the nurse. Delirium tremens is not related to thiamine at all but is plain old fashion severe alcohol withdrawal. It's actually not that common anymore it seems. This was my first real case in some time and reminded me of my residency days when I moonlighted at a hospital in Boston that was known as an alcoholic detox facility. That was somewhat of a revolving door situation where drunks would show up at any time of the day or night, often after the bars had closed and their wifes didn't let them in, for medically supervised detox. They would get a medication cocktail to keep them calm from the shakes and after a day or 2 leave to go back home. Occasionally, one would come in after their last drink was 24 hours previously and be in full withdrawal mode: shakes, fever, delirious and some even had withdrawal seizures. As alcohol acts as chemical sedative on the brain cells, prolonged drinking the brain becomes used to this effect. After stopping drinking, seizures occur in the electrically "hyper excited" brain. These seizures are not related to underlying brain disorder that requires long-term seizure medication but is managed easily with common sedatives until the detox is completed after another 48 hours or so. Actually, giving alcoholics seizure medication after their detox can be more dangerous, as they often stop their medication along with going back to binge drinking which can easily provoke more seizures. Withdrawal seizures require treatment and observation but not long-term medication.

A century ago, *Delirium Tremens* was fatal about a third of the time. With modern treatment and monitoring it kills less than 5 percent of patients. Still, it is a serious medical condition and John exhibited all the signs of full-blown D.T.s: hallucinations, fever, agitation, altered mental status, tachycardia, hypertension, and diaphoresis (sweating). He was given regular doses of a short acting benzodiazepine intravenously which is safer for someone with liver disease as the drug's metabolites don't continually build up in the bloodstream which can result in oversedation. His IV included a cocktail of electrolytes, glucose and vitamins. He wasn't allowed anything to eat but could have supervised sips of water or ice chips in order to prevent aspiration pneumonia. His vital signs were checked hourly and he was given acetaminophen for fever.

When I revisited him later that day, he was still mumbling and agitated about the "snakes on the ceiling and coming through the window" and was sweating and twitchy all over. It took him another 2 days to be able to recognize me and stop hallucinating. Slowly, his heart rate and respiratory rate returned to normal and his follow-up labs showed improved electrolyte levels and coagulation studies after 3 days. By the 5th day he was back to his normal self, promising that he would never drink again. His sacral ulcer was still in bad shape, looking like raw hamburger above his buttocks but no longer was oozing pus and he was getting topical ointment and regular bandage changes. He was given a large donut shaped pillow to keep pressure off this area and was told to lie sideways or to sit up to allow it a chance to heal. I discharged him home on the 6th day after arranging for home nursing care and follow up with the wound care clinic. After discussing his situation with his daughter but more importantly with Jose, his employee, I strongly instructed him to no longer supply him with an endless amount of booze as it will kill him next time. Hoping that the fear of no longer having a generous boss and a place to work would inspire his cooperation in limiting his drinking.

In the office a couple of weeks later, John seemed back to his jovial self and kept saying "never again" would he touch the stuff. It's tough to quit drinking, so I gave him both supportive encouragement and instilled the fear of death to try to help. Of course, he refused any medication or to go to AA. Sometimes keeping patients on a short leash can help them stay sober so I had him schedule a regular appointment every 2 weeks and kept in contact with Jose. I even stopped by the nursery to see how things were going. While he slowly went back to an "occasional drink with the fellows," he was not going down the rabbit hole again and Jose cooperated with not getting him a bottle at work at least for a while.

That while lasted for nearly a year until his next serious medical downturn. At that time, his daughter assisted him to be enrolled in an inpatient alcohol detox program at a neighboring hospital. One of the barometers of how extensive his drinking had been was how severe his sacral pressure skin ulceration had become. After this episode it took well over a couple of months to heal but finally did.

Sometime later, he developed sudden abdominal pain requiring emergency surgery for an incarcerated umbilical hernia. Surprisingly, he got through the anesthesia and surgery without any complications and did not have significant withdrawal symptoms afterward.

John had previously showed me his small, reducible belly button hernia which caused no pain. I suggested he could have it operated on but he didn't want to bother. Most patients with a small hernia like this do fine their whole life without an operation. It is caused by a slow stretching of the abdominal connective tissue around the area of where the umbilical cord comes out when we are born. There can be a natural stretching of this tiny hole which can get worse with an expanding abdomen from becoming obese. Many patients elect to not undergo a surgery for these hernias, but if painful it is a worrisome indicator of strangulation of the section of intestine that pops into the hernia defect. If not treated, a bowel strangulation can be a serious medical emergency resulting in that portion of the intestine dying and then leaking bacteria and toxins into the bloodstream which can cause sepsis and death. In John's case, he may have fallen asleep drunk as his hernia became compressed and was slowly developing a gangrenous infarction of the bowel loop caught in tight bind.

After he recovered from this surgery, John was back doing his thing at the nursery. Keeping his business running somewhat, and keeping his drinking to a tolerable level and occasionally seeing me for his various other health issues.

On Monday evening years later, I got a call from the ER that John had fallen on his head and suffered a concussion and likely cervical spine fracture due to a recent binge. He was alert when I saw him that evening but was having difficulty with feeling his legs and moving his toes. An urgent call to the neurosurgeon and another scan of his thoracic spine revealed a herniated disc in his upper back pressing on his spinal cord. This was an unusual event and an even more difficult one to treat. Unlike the neck the spinal column in the thoracic area is more difficult to injure, crack or to squeeze one of the intervertebral cartilage discs out into a herniation. This rare occurrence is even more problematic to treat surgically as a disc herniation is in front of the spinal cord and very difficult to approach because of all the important structures in the chest and that there is essentially very little room to work in this area. The other complicating factor is recovery from a spinal cord injury. In general, the more paralyzed someone is before having a surgery to release pressure on the spinal cord, the less likely there will be a decent recovery. Also, the length of time someone is paralyzed is inversely proportional to the prognosis of full function. John needed emergent surgery for significant compression on his spinal cord. The neurosurgeon I called to consult was very experienced. Dr. Leo Cheng who was also a professor at UCSF medical center in San Francisco and was very concerned with the location of the herniation and his leg weakness when he started the operation. In surgery, exploring his T2 spinal cord, he found a ruptured disc attached to a piece of the end of vertebra bone pressing, squeezing and injuring the front of the spinal cord. After he gingerly removed the fragment of bone and cartilage, he noticed the spinal cord had lost its blood supply at that level. Similar to a stroke that is caused by a sudden blockage of the blood vessel to a portion of the brain, this situation resembles a "stroke" of the spinal cord. The problem is that the nerves that pass below this level can be permanently damaged. Unlike the brain, which can recover remarkably from a stroke as different parts of the brain can take over functioning, the spinal cord has no other alternatives. The spinal cord functions as a thick tube of wires (of neurons) going down to the body and back to the brain. There are no alternatives if the nerve paths are broken or damaged.

When John awoke from the surgery he was paralyzed in his legs. The surgery did not help as damage had already occurred to the spinal cord even though the pressure was relieved. His prognosis was not good but some patients do recover some function after time but rarely. I sat with him in his hospital room the next day after all the anesthesia had cleared from his system. He was alert and calm and had no symptoms or agitation indicating alcohol withdrawal. He was not happy he couldn't move his feet or legs. I took my time explaining what had happened in surgery and the concern and the unknown prognosis whether he would recover his ability to move his legs. "This is going to take some time before we know where you'll be," I said and told him he will need to go to the rehabilitation unit after he recovers from the surgery. He looked down, shook his head and said: "Geez, I didn't think I'd end up like this." It was clear he understood the gravity of the situation. I tried to maintain a positive position of giving this time and rehab but he just looked at me directly and repeated the same statement. We shared a silent moment for a bit. I went out to write some orders for the nurses for his care after the operation. As I looked at the chart, I realized he was 80 years old, but he didn't seem that old. He looked so much younger being so overweight, and his spirit was of a much younger man. I shook my head, wrote orders and a note and went off to see another patient.

Two days later he was medically ready to be transferred to a rehab hospital. No improvement in his paralysis had occurred. "What's gonna happen to me, doc?" he asked. I told him he was going to get all the help he needed to get through this but it would definitely take time. I put my hand on leg and then shook his hand and told him that I will see in the office after he gets home.

The day after his transfer, I got a call from the rehab hospital. John had died the night before from a massive pulmonary embolism. I wasn't terribly surprised, just disappointed and sad. While he was put on prophylactic measures to prevent blood clots namely, compression stockings and low dose heparin a deep vein thrombosis can occur quite easily in a paralyzed, obese person. It could have occurred around the time of the surgery in his legs and then broke off going to his lungs, which chokes off the blood supply back to his heart. Small emboli cause chest pain, shortness of breath and lowered oxygen level but patients can usually survive. Large emboli block blood flow and cause the oxygen to drop below a level of survival and quickly cause the heart to go into fibrillation or arrest.

His daughter called me and was very upset and could not understand how this could happen. After several prolonged attempts explaining the medical sequence in plain terms, she remained confused and perplexed and requested an autopsy which I entirely agreed with. The autopsy confirmed the clinical picture: a very large embolus from a clot in the thigh and pelvis had caused his death. After a long day at the office and another consoling conversation with his daughter, I drove home, got the mail and stopped for a long moment looking at the roses blooming in my front yard and thinking of the man who gave them to me. Those roses are still blooming many years later and give me joy and sadness in having known a good man with a tough affliction.

CHAPTER 10

Fakin' It 'til You Make It (Into the Hospital)

"I don't know what's wrong with you," I said to Kirsti as she, her mom and sister sat in my exam room. I had just gone through a long questioning and extensive review of her complex medical history of the past 6 months. She was 30 years old, slightly chubby, pleasant and seemed straightforward in explaining her condition and quite knowledgeable of medical terminology. Her sister sat next to her taking notes and her mom interjected various tidbits of the events of her medical life. I had a fairly large stack of previous medical records from other doctors and hospitals she had visited and was able to view other medical records from my hospital via online access.

Her story was that she had developed at first gradually and then continuously significant gastrointestinal symptoms over the past year. Prior to that she reported she was in decent health and didn't take any medications and was going to school and working part time. At first she developed a mild upper abdominal discomfort and nausea that occurred after eating. This soon progressed to having bouts of vomiting and occasional loose bowel movements. These episodes then became more severe which required her to visit the emergency room of a hospital in San Francisco, California Pacific Medical Center, on several occasions as she was living in the city then. Her progressive symptoms included extreme nausea, abdominal pain and vomiting after eating.

Sometimes she would have diarrhea afterward and described having fevers at times and that these episodes would last several hours. She was given the diagnosis of *gastroparesis* by a prominent gastroenterologist in San Francisco, one of the leading experts of this problem on the west coast. She had been prescribed various medications, none of which really helped.

Gastroparesis is a condition where the stomach doesn't empty its food contents due to its muscles not working and failing to propel food to the small intestine. Normal digestion of food is quite a complex process that includes coordination of the parasympathetic and sympathetic nerves that go from the brain to the stomach and back to the brain which include actual pacemaker cells in the stomach itself. Patients with gastroparesis often feel continuously bloated after a meal for many hours and some become nauseous and vomit. Most have upper abdominal pain that can be mild or severe. The causes of the condition are many but most cases end up being classified as idiopathic. This is a term in medicine that means the cause is not known. In medical school it was joked that this word was formed as a portmanteau from "a pathetic idiot's explanation" or a more scientific breakdown—"I don't know the pathology" (i-dio-pathic). Regardless, it's an unfortunate, common "etiology" for many diseases even to this day. However, there are real causes for gastroparesis including prior surgery that damages nerves going to the stomach or the most common etiology, diabetic neuropathy. Diabetes can affect nearly everything in the body adversely and commonly the peripheral nervous system. Diabetic neuropathy to the long visceral nerves that go to the intestinal tract causes these nerves that control muscle contractions and digestion to malfunction is fairly common in a patient with longstanding diabetes. Simply, if the longest nerve in the body, the vagus nerve, which goes to various organs and the intestines, controls much of the autonomic functions of digestion is not working properly then conditions such as gastroparesis occur.

Kirsti had an incredibly extensive workup for this problem over the past six months. Evaluations were spread over 2 hospitals and about 10 doctors and multiple ER visits. Her testing included 3 CT scans of her entire abdomen, an ultrasound, every blood test that one could think of in regard to abdominal pain, an endoscopy of the stomach (looking directly using a camera) and a special test that is used to diagnose this condition—a gastric emptying study. In this study a tracing radioisotope is mixed in small amounts of egg whites cooked together and then swallowed by the patient. A special nuclear medicine camera records how much of the food travels from the stomach to the intestines in a time lapse fashion. The typical time for a meal to completely pass out of the stomach is less than 4 hours and usually only an hour or two. So in this test, if a significant portion of radioisotope laden food is still found in the stomach after 4 hours then the diagnosis is given as gastroparesis. Essentially, this means a very slow emptying of food from the stomach.

In Kirsti's case this test showed only a mild slowdown of her gastric emptying with 25% retention after 4 hours. However, it was unclear if she had taken a narcotic pain medication in the previous 24 hours that would have had an effect of slowing her entire GI tract. Narcotics are notorious for shutting down the normal peristalsis of our intestines which is why serious constipation is a common side effect.

As a primary care physician contracted with the program that covered poor patients in San Mateo County, Kristi came under my care being assigned to my list of patients after her legal address was changed. Under this arrangement, I am paid under a program known as capitation. This means that the health plan pays a certain amount to the primary care physician each month in lieu of billing for each visit and rewards the doctor for overall care no matter how much an individual is seen. This payment method makes it easier for the program and sometimes easier for the doctor who doesn't wait to get paid but however in this case gets about ten dollars per month.

Over the next several months, Kirsti was admitted to our hospital about 10 times for similar complaints of severe abdominal pain, nausea, vomiting and presumed dehydration along with very high blood pressure readings. She was given a cocktail of IV fluids, anti-nausea meds, pain meds and underwent various lab and radiologic testing in the ER. Rarely were any of her studies out of the normal range. I would frequently get calls from the evening or night nurses about a very high reading of her pulse and blood pressure that remained unexplained even after an extensive search for a cause. Having exhausted all possible testing and treatments during one of her admissions I was able to have her transferred to Stanford medical center for an evaluation at a tertiary care center. However, after 24 hours of GI and psychiatric evaluation she was sent back to our hospital via ambulance. No specific GI diagnosis was offered other than "functional gastroparesis". The word functional here implies "occurring without a specific cause".

Frustration was building from all involved with her care: the ER staff, the hospital nurses, the hospital administration and myself. Because of the limited reimbursement from the county health system, her care was costing our hospital directly hundreds of thousands of dollars already. These sudden episodes were occurring with an alarming regularity and her seemingly serious condition to the ER docs had often met the criteria for an acute care hospital admission.

Then one evening, I got a call from her nurse from the hospital at 1 a.m. She found the patient eating takeout Chinese food with her mother and sister and also found an asthma inhaler by her bedside. The nurse had come in to check the patient's vital signs as a routine. Apparently, coming in unannounced caused a bit of a scramble of Kirsti putting her food bowl in her sister's lap. The nurse then witnessed her using the inhaler taking a half a dozen puffs all at once. The nurse asked her about this and Kirsti said she had nighttime asthma. However, this was not on her problem list or medication list and she had never discussed this medical issue with me in any of the many encounters I had with her. Kristi then said that it was her sister's and that she used it when she felt short of breath. The vital signs recorded at the time were alarmingly high with her pulse being 150 and her blood pressure reading 180/110! All due to near overdosing on the inhaler medicine. I instructed the nurse to take the inhaler from her and that no treatment for the elevated vitals were prescribed as I was certain this was from the excessive inhaler use. Cautiously, she was counseled on the dangers of using such medications that could potentially be very dangerous.

This weirdness triggered my need to have her consulted by a psychiatrist. My colleague, Frank, who did hospital visits saw her the next day. We met at lunch in the hospital to go over his assessment. Kristi's story was a constantly changing bizarre tale with one twist after another, he explained. She apparently didn't understand how she had gotten so sick but was skilled in describing all the various medical tests and diagnosis in medical terminology. His evaluation coincided and agreed with her psychiatric consultation when she was at Stanford. He explained the "Folie a Deux" situation with her sister as she was always by her side and often spoke for the patient. However, Frank was initially unable to have the sister leave during his interview and only under threat of being removed by hospital security and a phone call to the mother did she comply. Initially, Kirsti claimed to be employed by Aristotle Onassis as an accountant even though he had died 7 years before she was born. He noted how increasingly more anxious she became after the sister left the room and resulted in her speech pattern becoming quite rapid with her mental state scampering around trying to explain her answers in a nearly incoherent manner. Frank noted the many times Kirsti changed her account of past events or attempted to connect impossible occurrences. For example, when she initially mentioned her grandparents were from El Salvador but then later stated they were from Israel and she couldn't answer the question whether they were Israelis or Arabs. In a tangential explanation, she mentioned her mother had converted to Mormonism. Her account of her schooling and work was equally scattered claiming she went to law school and then became an accountant and then denied she worked for Aristotle Onassis but that her father was related to him but later in an anxious outburst stated he was probably not related to him.

What to make of all this from the medical side? Her history with its lack of hard evidence for a specific disease with overt behavior creating false medical crises using asthma inhalers confirmed the suspicion for something very odd going here. The results of the tests and consults resulted in no definable intestinal malady. This in context with someone who actually gained weight while claiming to not be able to keep any food in her stomach along with her shifting, untenable life report gave only one plausible diagnostic entity for Frank and I to entertain: *Munchausen's Syndrome.*

This term was first coined by a British physician, Richard Asher, in an article that appeared in the medical journal, *Lancet*, in 1951 about a group of patients that fabricate wildly dramatic stories about their symptoms and health. He referenced the very popular 18th century book, *Baron Munchausen*, which told the story of a fictionalized German nobleman who was famous for telling great tales that were fantastic and impossible. The name then became a synonym for someone who was a great liar. While Asher's terminology was controversial at first, it brought to light a group of psychiatric conditions called *"factitious disorders"*. Munchausen's syndrome is understood in the context of the most extreme where fabrications form the central focus of the person's life. The disease is medically classified and named officially as a *"factitious disorder imposed on self"*.

Because it is unusual and difficult to identify, the actual incidence in the population is unknown but has been reported to occur more frequently in males. Because patients with this disorder seek medical care in a hospital, they often go to different places and hone their stories over time in order to tell and create a credible history that gains them admission to the hospital for variable periods of time. In this case, her hospital stays were prolonged with her clandestine drug taking causing alarm about her heart rate and blood pressure. The underlying motivation is unclear as most of these patients are not just seeking narcotic medications or tranquilizers. These fakers can remain "under the radar" for a very long period of time due to medical evaluations assuming patients are being truthful. From a psychodynamic standpoint, it is thought that these patients are not psychotic (crazy) or masochistic. The psychiatric explanation remains unknown to the causation and maintenance of this odd behavior, although a developmental history of unmet needs is generally assumed. Scientific studies are lacking due to the evasiveness of the condition and it is possible some patients go through a phase of using these fake symptoms for a period of time and then stop.

In this instance, the care team was confronted with a strange variant of the condition in that the patient's sister and mother were essentially "in on the scam" as they seemed to substantiate that Kristi was actually sick. This *folie a deux* with a family is even less studied or understood as to the family dynamics. The participation of her family seems also quite odd as did they not pick up on her faking her illnesses too? How could they bring food for her late at night in the hospital and see her eat and not suspect something odd?

Ultimately, I needed to confront the patient with her diagnosis and expose her scam in an honest, open and caring way without trying to sound judgmental. I suspected Kristi was aware of what she was doing and so I wasn't concerned about surprising her. I went to her room after lunch the following day and requested her family members not be present but her sister and the patient protested. I informed Kristi that she was allowing her family to hear confidential medical information about her condition and health. I took a deep breath and a pause for several seconds and began with: "Well, I have something very important to tell you. You have a very serious and potentially dangerous condition. Please listen to all I have to say and then I can answer any questions you have…" I took my time giving the details of the medical evidence for giving her this diagnosis and carefully explaining that she does not require any further medication treatment and hospitalization for this condition. I emphasized the enormous risk she was taking by using medications not prescribed for her such as the inhalers. Finally, I recommended psychological counseling for this condition as the most important advice. She and her sister sat there during my explanation without any expression, her sister taking notes. Afterward, I paused for a good 30 seconds giving Kirsti a chance to speak and ask questions. There were none and in the end she softly said "OK". I informed her that she was discharged from the hospital at that point and could leave at any time.

My next duty was to inform all who might come in contact with her in the near future, as I was certain this open confrontation would have no effect on her behavior. I dictated an extensive discharge note for the hospital medical record with the diagnosis of her factitious disorder. It was strange documenting a patient faking illness. Not something commonly done. We are not used to calling out patients as liars and cheats and telling them to "cut it out" in a direct way. Although it felt odd, it also seemed appropriate in the sense of providing accurate medical assessment and counseling. Afterward, I went to the ER and spoke with the director and all the docs in the department about this case. They were all very familiar with her and were quite relieved to hear her diagnosis. She had been to the ER over 20 times in the past few months and it was confusing and stressful when she had shown up for all the staff. We came up with a plan to evaluate her complaints and to perform any needed testing such as labs and monitoring but in the context of her Munchausen's diagnosis, there would be severe restraint in admitting her to the hospital unless there was clear cut medical evidence to do so. So, we were hoping to "cut her off at the pass" by not admitting her each time she appeared in the ER department.

Over the next several months, Kristi did come into the ER frequently with basically the same complaints of nausea, vomiting and high blood pressure. With the medical team on the same page, the ER staff was able to appropriately evaluate her and did not admit her once! I discussed with them frequently along the way and applauded their great fortitude in giving proper care. Then suddenly, Kristi disappeared from the scene for about a year! I knew this because I had an interest in following her ER visits and would often check how many times she had come in. Of course, I never saw her again in my office as she likely found a different primary care physician. Although I never got a request for records or a call from her new provider, she surely had one assigned by the Medi-Cal managed care system. I suspected she may have moved or was going to different hospitals but had no way of finding out. I could only monitor her activity in the hospital where I practiced, which I did for a couple of years. Like a bad penny, Kristi returned to our ER after a year's absence. The ER staff were still tuned in to her diagnosis and only treated her in the ER and limited her care by not giving her any narcotic pain medicines while she was there. Her visits became more intermittent in the following years. It is unknown what eventually happened with her.

The underlying motivation and psychological trigger for this behavioral problem is unknown. It is thought that this conscious deception fills some unmet need possibly related to early childhood trauma or abuse. Other than her immediate family no other person, friend or family ever visited her when she was hospitalized. I had the sense that she was a lonely and isolated person.

Everyone still likes to use the term *Munchausen's* for this odd disease. This entity is distinct from the other deceptive behavioral disorders. For example, *malingering* is defined as illness falsification to obtain obvious *external* benefits such as money, medications (e.g., narcotics, tranquilizers), time off work, child custody, or avoiding criminal prosecution, whereas the deception observed in *factitious disorder* is not accounted for by external rewards. There are other psychiatric disorders that appear similar such as those with *borderline personality disorder* which can involve self-harm but does not use deception. *Somatic symptom disorder* patients, aka "hypochondriacs", are excessively preoccupied with minor symptoms convinced they are something more ominous. *Delusional* patients can have symptoms that have no medical basis but are not deceptive in attempting to convince health care workers to believe them. There is one condition that appears similar but is unconsciously driven and well known, namely, *Conversion Disorder*. Here patients also express symptoms of a serious illness without a conscious intent that convinces the medical system and often leads to hospitalization. My patient, Lulu, clarifies the distinction with her story.

Lulu came to the ER on Christmas eve. She was a distressed 40-year-old Black woman who was in good health until about 2 weeks prior. She had been ill with a flu like illness causing high fevers, cough and general malaise. While recovering, she began to notice her legs going numb and she had trouble walking. When she arrived at the hospital via ambulance she could not stand or move either leg and lost feeling up to her waist. The ER physician was spot-on to suspect a case of *Guillain-Barre syndrome*. This unusual neurologic condition has been associated to occur after a bout of influenza or even after influenza vaccine more rarely. The mechanism is caused by an overstimulated immune system attacking the nerves of the spinal cord and sometimes the entire nervous system. Paralysis and sensation loss often starts in the feet and then to legs in an ascending pattern. In severe progressive cases it can affect the nerves to the diaphragm and chest muscles causing breathing difficulties and then possibly swallowing and eye muscle disorders. In about a quarter of the afflicted respiratory paralysis occurs. In suspected cases patients are always hospitalized, monitored and treated even before the full diagnostic tests are completed to prevent such a dangerous complication of respiratory arrest and death. The standard treatment is plasmapheresis. A complex procedure blood is filtered of harmful antibodies that the body is making and then reinfusing back the purified blood. It is a difficult, costly and lengthy process requiring special equipment. I was on call for the ER that day and admitted Lulu to the hospital. I immediately called Bob, who was on-call for the neurology service. Since delaying care could allow the paralysis to progress, all patients who fit the clinical criteria are started on treatment. Also a spinal tap is done to evaluate the cerebrospinal fluid (CSF) to check for possible meningitis or tumor or any other abnormality. Lulu's CSF was normal which is found in about a third of the cases. Bob mentioned it seemed likely she had the diagnosis but he wanted to make sure by doing the EMG (electromyography) test after one week as that would definitively correspond to finding the changes in the nerves. An EMG tests if nerves are working properly by directly measuring electrical impulses across a section of nerve. It's very accurate and specific for Guillain-Barre syndrome and for other nerve injuries from diabetes, toxins or other causes. Of course, we presumed the worst and didn't want to delay treatment. Most patients with Guillain-Barre syndrome can and do recover and early treatment directed at removing the damaging antibodies can improve their overall prognosis.

Lulu showed slight improvement over the week of treatment. She always seemed quite anxious when I visited her in hospital each day. I attempted to reassure her that the doctors were hopeful she would recover and I attempted to take my time explaining the disease and what she could expect. She never lost bladder or bowel control (a dangerous sign of progression) and there were no symptoms other than her legs.

Bob had his associate do the EMG test in the hospital on a Friday after about 10 days of onset of weakness. We should be able to get a good estimate of the type of nerve injury and therefore a better way of knowing her prognosis. Bob called me right after it was done. "It's all normal," he said with a bit of worry in voice. "Does that mean she doesn't have Guillain-Barre?" I asked, thinking that maybe we did the test too early. "No, she doesn't have it, and there is definitely nothing wrong with her!" he replied. "Uh-oh," I said, "so she's faking this?" Bob, like most, didn't like confronting patients about these sorts of things. I suggested we go up together and that "you can give her the good news from the specialist standpoint and then I will spend some time with her to try to figure out what is going on". When we arrived she was sitting up in bed staring off out the window. "Well Lulu the test of your nerves is completely normal and you will be fine." "Oh, OK," she muttered and turned and slowly swung her legs over the side of the bed to sit up. "Wow, you are getting better," I said. "Yes, I was able to stand up this morning," she said. Bob said a few encouraging words and said he needed to go see another patient and left. "I'm glad you don't have that bad problem," I said. "What's been happening with you and your life lately?" "Have you had any stressful events?" She then looked down and said her son had been shot and killed last month and her mother has terminal colon cancer. "Oh, Lulu, I'm so sorry, this must be just an awful time for you and I can understand your sense of being paralyzed emotionally and physically during this time." I told her frankly, "you will be able to walk normally in a short time but this difficult time of grieving will take however long it takes." I then asked her about her support system and other family members who she can seek guidance with and then requested the social worker and chaplain service to see her and give support. I mentioned that she could go home whenever she felt well enough to walk. The nurse taking care of her called me in the early evening and told me of Louise walking out of the hospital on her own with her pastor after her thanking every nurse and worker on the floor for the wonderful care she received. Lulu's *conversion reaction* to extremely stressful life events was typical for this entity. Her mind literally caused her legs to stop working, for a while.

I would note that the names used above Kirsti and Lulu are pseudonyms for privacy protection purposes.

There is one other extremely strange form of *factitious disorder* seen in the condition known as *"Munchausen's by proxy"*. This rare, bizarre and sadistic behavior is manifested when a parent presents their child as acutely and chronically ill by inducing various dangerous toxins in their child, lying about symptoms and occasionally drugging them into a submissive state. This provides the parent with reinforcing sympathy from caregivers who are unbeknownst to what is happening and often feeding the strange narcissism of the parent by praising them for being so "strong and caring". Even more odd is that the individuals who create this hoax are frequently mothers that work in the medical profession, i.e. nurses. Through their knowledge, they are able to successfully induce serious symptoms and illness in their child and present them to the emergency department in dire medical circumstances. These can include such criminal acts as injecting bacteria to create a serious blood infection, giving medications to simulate coma and various other forms of medical abuse.

While in my career, I have heard of a few of these cases from the emergency room docs I have worked with but there is not a other more dramatic example than the story of Dee Dee Blancharde and her daughter, Gypsy Rose Blancharde, which came to light in the 2015 murder of Dee Dee by her daughter. The details of this fascinating story are available online but a synopsis is as follows. Gypsy was born sometime in 1991 to Dee Dee who became pregnant from her 17-year-old boyfriend who left before her birth. Early in Gypsy's life her mother began claiming her infant daughter had sleep apnea (which tests confirmed she did not) and then a chromosomal abnormality causing poor development and susceptibility to illness (also never documented). Dee Dee had a background of being a medical assistant and there was a suspicion (never proven) that she may have poisoned her own mother. Gypsy was essentially starved to a malnourished state as a child and her head was shaved to claim to her neighbors she had cancer treatment. Gypsy was chained to her bed when Dee Dee worried she might run away. There was some suspicion by one of Gypsy's neurologists that this was a case of *Munchausen by proxy* after all testing was normal for Muscular Dystrophy. Dee Dee also falsely claimed Gypsy had a host of other neurologic conditions while keeping malnourished Gypsy in a wheelchair well into her later teens. Child protective services were never notified by any of her providers. Dee Dee successfully convinced all the neighbors and family members that her daughter was severely disabled and sick and was constantly praised for being such a great, caring parent. However, by the time Gypsy turned 20 she had started using the internet and was becoming also obviously aware of her physical abilities to walk. She began to attract young men over her Facebook account. Secretly from her mother, Gypsy was developing the motivation and tools to escape the torture of her mother and enlisted a mentally ill boy from Wisconsin. Gypsy convinced this young man to come to Springfield, Missouri and to kill her mother by stabbing with a knife. In an ironic twist, Gypsy essentially induced a "murder by proxy". Her trial was a complicated affair in light of her life of abuse but she was convicted and served time in a Missouri prison. Interestingly while in prison, Gypsy researched her mom's diagnosis and confirmed every symptom. In interviews in prison, she states when she was young she believed her mom's claim of having cancer for many years. The gruesome and extensive details of her life are revealed in the 2017 documentary *Mommy Dead and Dearest*. Gypsy served 7 of her 10-year sentence and was released in December 2023 to the husband she met while in prison.

CHAPTER 11

Babs Divine

Babs was in for a follow-up appointment to go over her many medical issues. "So, how's it going?" I asked. "Not so good." "What's goin' on?" "Well, I'm getting divorced," she replied. I looked down at her chart again to confirm her age of 82. "Huh? What happened? Uh… wait, how long have you been married?" "62 years," she answered. "He just pulled the last straw," she stated, somewhat matter of factly.

Her explanation surprised me and was certainly novel in my history of hearing many variations for breakups. She had recently seen a mortgage statement from her bank documenting the amount of loan and repayment schedule which perplexed her because her house had been paid off years ago. The statement had her husband's name on it. Because of her mistrust of her husband's previous handling of their finances she went to the bank herself to find out what was going on. She was furious and then anxious to learn that her husband had refinanced her home and took several hundred thousands of dollars of equity and did something with it. She was very concerned because of his past habit of compulsive gambling. She still didn't understand how this could happen without her knowing about it as both their names were on the deed. She was flabbergasted to find out from the bank that her husband had told them she was *dead* and he was entitled to refinance himself. A sinking, morbid feeling came over her as she heard this from the bank official. "But I'm here and obviously *NOT* dead" she declared. The bank official told her what was done was done and they could do nothing to change the refinance.

This was in 2004. She went home and told her daughter and son-in-law the awful news and to try to find out what he did with the money. They discovered that her husband had given the money to his illegitimate daughter for a down payment on a house. Babs had known about this other daughter for about 20 years. She knew her husband had carried on a "double life" with another woman but decided to not break up their marriage then and to just go on with him. She had never met this other child and didn't want to.

"But, obviously, the bank has made a serious error here" I interjected. "They are culpable for their mistake and you need to pursue this legally and get a lawyer to help resolve this" I offered. Yes, she said she was looking for one with her daughter's help. "And he refuses to leave the house, because he has nowhere to go and legally I can't kick him out" she sighed. Ouch, I thought. This was a nightmare from so many angles I couldn't imagine having to deal with it. Yet, Babs in her simple, direct style told this story with a shaking head of disappointment and with a wry, comic smile. We sat in silence for a few moments looking at each other, me soaking in these bizarre details. During the quiet, I began to get an insight into the long, deep connection to this event and her entire life.

However, there was also the medical side of this visit to deal with. Babs was not in great health. She suffered from long standing back pain which had been treated with Vicodin for decades, she still smoked although only a handful of cigarettes per day, she had high blood pressure, chronic obstructive pulmonary disease (COPD), a kyphotic upper back from severe osteoporosis and physically was quite frail with about 100 pounds to her five-foot-four frame. We went over her meds and how she was doing with her pains and I pleaded with her again to try to stop smoking and scheduled a follow up appointment.

She returned a few months later with a sudden new back pain from bending which started from below her shoulder blades. She had used up all her pain medicines to quell the unrelinquishing ache in her upper back. An X-ray showed a new thoracic spine compression fracture at the 4th vertebrae. "Your vertebrae are like Styrofoam back there" I informed her. "This will heal up but will take several months." "Oh, I really need more pain medicine, doc" she asked. I upped her usual prescription for the next few months and also gave her a stronger narcotic to use "when it was really bad" which for her was at night trying to lie down. "And oh, how are things at home?" "Not good," she deadpanned, "the lawyer doesn't think there is anything I can do to get the money back, but I don't know if he knows what he's doing as he's an old friend of the family." Uh-oh, I thought.

Over the subsequent years, I saw Babs on a regular basis for various other medical issues. She subsequently broke both hips in separate falls each requiring long stays in a rehab center. I was quite proud of her quitting smoking at the ripe age of 85.

The fraud complaint against her bank was never resolved and her then-husband, as she never completed the divorce, died of a heart attack suddenly one day leaving everything as it was. In his will, he left half of his estate to the illegitimate daughter. She took all this stride and then sold the house and moved into a nice assisted living space, the Magnolia, where I made house calls until the end of her life.

Later, as her daughter and son-in-law were also my patients, I was curious as to the life Babs had before I knew of all the difficulties she endured at the end and was filled in with the entire story. She was born in San Francisco in 1922 to immigrant parents. Her mom was from Liverpool, England and her dad from Genoa, Italy. She had an impoverished and difficult childhood. Her mother took to heavy drinking when she started school. As a teenager, she read in horror from the local daily newspaper that her father was a bigamist. The social ridicule of her mother's divorce worsened their financial and social life. However, she was showered with love from her mother's parents, her English grandparents, who doted on her calling her "queen" while enhancing her life with opera and singing lessons. During the depression of the late 1930s and into the early years of WW2, she struggled working menial jobs. It was at this time that physical symptoms began to manifest including back pain and ulcer symptoms. These would haunt her all her life. From a reactive standpoint they could easily have been the somatic expression of her sorrow of being abandoned by her father and living with an alcoholic mother.

She met a local boy her age and became pregnant and married him at age nineteen in 1941. He was a shipyard worker who was drafted into the Navy. Babs and her infant daughter were, fortunately, taken in by her in-laws in the Italian section of San Francisco, the North Beach area. However, trouble reached across the ocean when she learned of her husband's gambling compulsion and requests for money to pay his debts. Nothing changed in his behavior after the war and she struggled with the idea of divorcing him. However, haunted by her mother's regret of divorcing her father she decided against it.

Life never really improved with her decision. While her husband's liquor store business thrived, all the profits fed his gambling addiction. Eventually, he was even barred from the casinos in Reno for bad debts. She endured years of fending off collectors, while his business ventures tanked. Somehow, they had managed to pay off their house during all this. He was forced to take odd jobs but never lasted very long at any of them. Unbeknownst to her, in their mid-life years, her husband had an affair and a child with another woman. Sometimes he spent weeks with them without Babs knowing where he was. Somehow, she tolerated this and life went on. She eventually found out about this other family after about 20 years. She remained resigned to her situation, remembering the anguished alcoholic cry of her mother's lament divorcing an equally terrible man. However, she found great joy, interest and involvement in her own daughter, granddaughter and family. She was the one always trying to help others while she never sought any.

I recall Babs often smiling and laughing about the absurdities of her life. She maintained an upbeat attitude and always had something nice to say about her family or others. She was one who, obviously, could get through a lot of tough times.

At the age of eighty-eight, she ended up having a stroke that required extensive care. At discharge from the hospital, her neurologist placed her in hospice. The doctors did not think she would live long. But tough ol' Babs outlasted her allotted six months and was released. I continued to do home visits to check up on her. She could do most things for herself and had her dedicated daughter help her daily. When I saw her during this period, always with her family, at her assisted living facility, she actually was in much less pain, but was becoming extremely frail. It was decided to not bring her back to the hospital if she became sick again and she died peacefully with her family close by at the age of ninety-two.

Fortunately, Babs did not pass on the pattern of recurrent bigamy, addiction and abandonment to her daughter who has remained in a stable loving marriage herself now for over 50 years. Babs' life of chronic pain, anxiety and difficulty also included an enormous capacity for love, compassion and resiliency that was incredibly admirable to hear about and witness. Babs is not her real name but her family has given permission to tell her story here which I greatly appreciate.

CHAPTER 12

President of the South San Francisco Historical Society

Can you imagine being born in the same house living there for the next 103 years? This is the story of the remarkable life of Eleonore "Ellie" Fourie. She was the 3rd of five children of Pierre and Annette who both hailed from the lower slopes of the French Pyrenees emigrating at the turn of the 20th century and was born at their home on Baden Avenue in South San Francisco on August 26, 1915. Baden was the name given to the area by one of the landowners in the mid-19th century where he built his country estate amid the grazing cattle.

The development of "South City", as it is called, followed the fates of its northern more famous neighbor, San Francisco. Situated just below San Bruno Mountain a few miles to the south, it grew from a pastoral grazing and farming community to become a magnet of big industry and then shipbuilding along its eastern shore, the San Francisco Bay. Lured by its proximity and large tracts of undeveloped land it incorporated in 1908 amid much local bickering over land use. It then saw a progressive increase in industry to rebuild and expand San Francisco after its devastating earthquake in 1906 and then found more manufacturing in building the world expo of 1915 in San Francisco. Attracting big industry, meat packing and manufacturing through the first half of the 20th century, South City saw many diverse immigrant groups coming to the area including a large contingent of Greeks and Italians.

Quickly, it became a fast-growing hub of housing development as well. The town, proud of its growth, erected a large "Hollywood" like sign on its eastern hill. A sixty-foot-high concrete sign of white letters spelling out "South San Francisco The Industrial City" was erected in 1928. Today, it is obvious landmark from the freeways passing to and from San Francisco. When the Giants baseball team won the world series on three recent occasions, the "S" and the "F" were painted orange in their honor for an entire year and a huge Christmas tree is lit up next to it every holiday season. As big manufacturing and small industries declined in the second half of the 20th century, South City remade itself into a biotech center starting with Genentech locating in the area of the old shipyards on the eastside in 1976. Now with over 200 biotech companies it is home to the largest concentration of that genre in the world. The demographic shift in the past 50 years has seen a large influx of Hispanics and a full complement of pacific rim immigrants settling into one of the more affordable areas of the Bay Area. Today, South City is a modern dichotomy. The western older part of the town retains the look of post war expansion with tracts of houses nestled along the flat land to the foot of San Bruno Mountain. The shabby downtown is marked by various small ethnic restaurants and convenient stores. The eastern side, east of route 101, glistens with modern offices, large laboratory buildings and biotech campuses that bus in their employees to discover and create cutting edge new medications and devices. A town of two worlds discordant and disconnected by a freeway and a different era.

Ellie went to the local public schools and after graduating from South S.F. high in the early 1930s found a job as an administrative aide for the growing Reichhold Chemical Company in town. Henry Reichold, the founder, was developing his resin and paint empire with many plants around the US after emigrating from Germany in 1927 having previously worked for Ford for $4.80 per day. Demonstrating her stay puttedness, Ellie worked for that company for over 40 years retiring in 1978. As commonly happened in businesses then, she became in charge of the financials and ordering as she worked her way up, and at times when her boss was away or when specific important tasks needed to be done she was able to even run the company for short periods. Of course, being a woman in a man's world in those days, she was never promoted to a supervisory position.

While her siblings grew up, got married, had families and moved away, Ellie stayed at home. She never married and when I asked her why in her later years she simply smiled and shrugged "it never happened to me".

Instead of married life, Ellie immersed herself in her community and extended family. She remained active at her local church including being the organist, choir member, religious educator and lay minister. She was a founding member of the South San Francisco Historical Society in 1981 and became its president for many years. Collecting artifacts, stories and mementos of her town and helping to obtain an historical building to put everything and give tours. Two of the other founders were also my patients but they were several years younger. I got to hear from all three of them the fun details and the "good dirt" as their town evolved and grew over the 20th century.

Even though Ellie lived with and took care of her parents into their old age, her mother dying in 1975 at age 93 and her father in 1981 at age 97, she also explored the world. With her wide circle of friends and with her extensive family of 15 nieces and nephews, 27 grandnieces and nephews and 19 great grand nieces and nephews she traveled extensively around North America and Europe both before and after WWII. As I enjoyed traveling to France, she told me of her trip to her parents' birth town at the base of the Pyrenees which is geographically similar to where they settled in the US in the early 20th century. Ellie was also famous for never forgetting anyone's birthday! Everyone thought of "Aunt Ellie" as ageless even well into her 90s retaining her memory, wit and friendly nature.

Ellie became my patient in the late 1990s after her doctor retired. She was in generally excellent health except for some blood pressure issues. She had developed atrial fibrillation which is the most common cardiac arrhythmia (electric disturbance). In this condition, the upper part of the heart's electrical system goes haywire and instead of regular beating starting at the upper chambers (the atria) they just quiver and don't push blood down to the lower chambers (the ventricles) which is where blood is pumped into the body. One can visualize normal heart pumping by putting your hands into open fists on top of each other. The top fist pumps first and the bottom fist pumps just afterwards every second or so. A normal heart rate is between 55 and 90 beats per minute also known as the pulse rate. While this disturbance would seem to be a very serious life-threatening problem it can be often unnoticed by the patient. Problems can occur if there is too much electrical activity passing down to the ventricles causing them to speed up to dangerous levels of 150 to 220 times a minute. At this rate many patients experience a racing in their chest and can pass out due lack of blood being pumped properly to the brain. However, if one's ventricular beating rate is within a reasonable range, say 50-100 beats per minute, one could feel "normal" as sufficient blood is being pumped around the body. On occasion, the electrical pumping of the ventricles can slow to dangerous levels below 30 or so and the patient can pass out. In this case a pacemaker is needed to maintain a normal heart rate. In Ellie's case, she didn't notice anything different in her daily life as her heart rate remained in the normal range. However, as it became increasingly proven that this heart condition is a major risk for future strokes where blood clots can slowly form in the quivering non beating atria and then can break off and go to the brain. Over the past 25 years this risk has been well quantified and guidelines for treatment of this condition now strongly recommend lifelong blood thinners to prevent a stroke. The estimate of risk being about 3% per year for stroke. However, anticoagulation also can have severe side effects, namely bleeding into the gut or into the brain. The risk for this is about 1% per year. So, in the overall risk benefit ratio, many more strokes can be prevented with blood thinners taken indefinitely than problems from the treatment. However, there can be confounding factors. Ellie had been prescribed an aspirin by her previous doctor as a way to somewhat thin the blood without giving full anticoagulation. On our first few visits, I began to discuss the importance of this condition and the emerging scientific data on its treatment. She would sit and listen to me very attentively, and after I finished, she would sit there thinking for a minute or so and then ask the important questions: "Well, what if I don't take the blood thinners and see how it goes? I've gotten along without them so far." "Isn't the aspirin good enough?" Unfortunately, it turned out in studies aspirin does not have any protective effect on stroke prevention in this condition.

A few months later the answer to whether to anticoagulate came to light. Ellie was taken to the ER after vomiting up coffee grounds material and then fresh blood. When blood in the stomach is mixed with acid it gets oxidized and turns brown and forms small clumps and when vomited looks just like coffee grounds. Ellie lost 4 pints of blood that night. When the GI consultant did an endoscopy the next day, he found a bunch of small bleeding areas in her stomach caused by taking aspirin. The bleeding fortunately stopped. She was given a couple of units of blood and powerful acid suppressant medication and recovered. However, in the scenario of a life-threatening GI bleed future use of aspirin and other anti-inflammatories was strictly prohibited. Full anticoagulation with warfarin, the only available drug at that time, posed to me an unacceptable risk. While some experts in this area might still consider warfarin a potential benefit, for me it was like tempting the devil of death too many times. Ellie was relieved with my judgment and was happy to go on living with whatever future risks might come.

A few years later, walking across her front yard in the evening she caught her foot on an uneven patch of sod and fell abruptly forward landing squarely on her nose and face, being unable to outstretch her hands in time. The ambulance took her to the closest hospital which was Kaiser a mile away. She had broken her nose and contused her face but also cracked a small crucial bone in her neck, the odontoid process. This was an unusual and dangerous fracture of an obscure part of the upper spine. The odontoid, which has its name from the Latin root meaning tooth, projects up from the front of the second cervical vertebrae. It works as a pivot around which the top two spinal vertebrae rotate enabling us to turn our head and neck. These are indeed very special vertebrae and unlike any other in our spine. The top one is called the atlas and one below with the odontoid process is called the axis. Both of these are round with large areas on the sides where they can slide and rotate over each other. The connections of these two vertebrae to the skull allow over half of the movement for turning our heads. They also surround and protect the upper spinal cord as it comes out of the lower skull. The odontoid is crucial for motion and maintaining proper alignment of those upper vertebrae. When cracked there is loss of stability of the head and neck to maintain alignment and literally the spinal cord can be squeezed, crushed or damaged by the vertebrae moving too much forward or backward over each other. Ellie was lucky in that there was no injury to her spinal cord with her fall. The worse outcome of this injury would be to be paralyzed from the head down.

When the doctors at Kaiser found this important fracture, they debated about what to do. Like with any fracture, the goal is to immobilize the area to allow it to heal properly over the following few months. They reasoned that since the odontoid was merely broken and not misplaced and with her age that they could place a screw through the front part of the second vertebrae and then into the broken odontoid to hold it in place. The other option would be to do a major spinal fusion procedure with various metal plates and bone grafts to fuse the upper spine which is more complicated and a much longer recovery. Ellie got through the simpler surgery just fine. She was sent home with a neck brace and I saw her in the office about a week or so later. Her face and nose were still quite puffy and bruised but she felt OK with no pain in her neck. I sent her to Leo Chang, my favorite neurosurgeon who also worked at UCSF, for follow-up. He checked her neurologically and regularly X-rayed the area to see how it was healing. After six months, he called me to say her odontoid fracture had healed radiologically. The screw was still in the same position. He contemplated her undergoing the complex fusion surgery to make sure she would not be paralyzed in the future. She came to see me to discuss this in detail. Since she felt no pain and was able to do whatever she wanted and needed she was seriously questioning this recommendation. "If I'm OK at this point, what is the real risk this will cause a problem?" I was thinking how relieved I was that she was not on a powerful blood thinner at the time of the accident as bleeding around the spinal cord would have been likely.

"Well," I said, "the future is hard to predict, I would assume if you don't fall on your face or have a major injury to your neck this shouldn't be a problem." As she was approaching 90, she decided to live with it and let me know if she had difficulty in any way and I supported her decision. I always enjoyed discussing various options with patients and coming to a shared agreement.

Over the next 10 years she would be accompanied by her nephew and her live-in caretaker to my office. She was always a delight to see with a smile and story to tell me. Her medical issues were quite stable and we were able to minimize the medications she was taking. She suffered a small stroke affecting her speech at age 97 but recovered completely in a few months. When her 100th birthday approached I told her what I say to all my centenarians. "There are two important things I need from you: one is that I get invited to the party and two is that you tell all your family and friends that I am the reason you have lived so long!" This is always said with the utmost seriousness followed by a good laugh. The huge outdoor party included all her relatives from all over the country who descended onto "South City". The 200 plus who went had a great celebration and I was given a photo of the big crowd.

Afterward, she became less able to walk and get to the office, and I did house calls at her home. What a joy to see where she lived as she showed me her memorabilia and family photos while sharing stories. Her sharp wit and mind seemed quite well intact. She was still doing daily crossword puzzles at the age of 102! I was so glad I scheduled the visit at the end of the day so we could have a relaxing and pleasant meeting. After over 15 years of not taking any anticoagulation, Ellie had a large stroke and passed away peacefully a couple of weeks after my last home visit.

In 2018 Ellie's heirs sold the house her parents had built in 1913 for exactly one million dollars. An increase in value of one thousand times over its original cost of one thousand dollars. The value of such a life lived so well, continuously and completely in one house goes infinitely beyond any price. Ellie and her family gladly and enthusiastically granted permission to write this story.

CHAPTER 13

Woody Brooks

After 100 years and 10 days on this earth Woody Brooks stood up from his kitchen table turned toward his wife and died while falling into her outstretched arms. So ended a remarkably expansive, interesting and long life that captured me from the first time he came into my office 20 years earlier.

When I heard of his passing from his wife, Dorothy, I felt a sharp pang of regret for not attending his grand gala 100th birthday party. Having been invited but committed to a different event out of town, I heard all about this from the other doctors who also cared for him and attended. His cardiologist gave me a complete rundown in the doctor's lounge the next week. There were over 100 guests for his 100th and there was food, drink and music that lasted deep into the night. Woody stayed for all of it and enjoyed every second which he did with everything in life.

It was not unusual to have elderly Black men come to see me in my office, but I was impressed when I met this relaxed, elegant, engaging man. I recall distinctly entering the exam room for our first visit to see Woody sitting upright in perfect posture in a striking three-piece silk suit with matching tie and handkerchief, gorgeous dress shoes glistening with shine and his hair perfectly combed and oiled. He put his hand out while standing and greeted me with a "Hello, so very glad to meet your acquaintance, doctor." His voice had a smooth lilt with a slight smile of reassurance. "I hope I can depend on you to take care of me," he offered.

"I'll do my best, thanks for coming in today," I replied. So we started a long and complex relationship for the last fifth of his life.

While Woody didn't have acute problems that day, he did have his medical problems and need for medications. However, what remained quite a constant with my interactions over the years, is that he never had a look of being sick even though at times he would see me with severe flare-ups of asthma, quietly gasping as he told me, "I'm having a little trouble breathing today." I found I needed to spend extra time examining him thoroughly to get an accurate picture of his clinical state. One could be fooled because he always looked well. He was also very compliant. He followed the treatments and recommendations I made for him and fortunately he mostly responded well, making us both pleased with our interactions. It was a great relief seeing him in follow-up and him telling me in his slow slight southern drawl, "oh, I'm much better now, thanks to you, doc" sitting serenely across from me, hands on his knees impeccably dressed in a different suit, tie and hanky looking a bit like Abe Lincoln.

Most of the time Woody came to see me he was with his wife of forty-seven years, Dorothy (who also was my patient). They struck an interesting contrast. He, petite at 5'5" and quite reserved, she, tall, large and very vocal. Often Dorothy would do all the talking and Woody would sit there and nod slowly in agreement. She would diverge into various topics of life's difficulties and give me a hard time for not calling back soon enough or taking care of various details of his medical care like ordering more X-rays or labs or consultants that she thought he needed. While her tone was strong and loud, after I explained every-thing to her in my practiced calm, caring doctor voice she would go silent and look at me and say softly "Ohhhhhh, OK, thanks then." She was also always dressed to kill as well, in a nice dress, pumps, stockings, hat and jewelry, it seemed like they were always coming back from a ball or going out to a fancy jazz club. However, they were just in my office at eleven am, visiting the doctor.

Born in 1916, after growing up in Texas, Woody joined the navy during WW2 and ended up in San Francisco afterward having been decommissioned at the Oakland naval base. An eye for making money, having a good time, and a hard-working, determined spirit with a steady, unwavering nature drove him along the path to a full life. After learning how to cut hair, he opened several barber shops around San Francisco. Working and employing others, he built up a steady clientele of Black men seeking the latest styles to look their best. He continued this for the next 50 years. But that was not all. He found a pleasant, part time and secure job at the post office doing inside processing until he finally retired in 2009! Due to his connections in the navy and his barbershop, he befriended a captain of one of the merchant marine ships stationed in Oakland. He was hired as the "captain's assistant" which meant he would go on various trips, often to Asia and other parts of the world, helping with anything the captain would need including, of course, haircuts. These trips would be of variable periods and Woody was not committed to the entire voyage and was paid a modest salary but got to travel and visit the world for free and have his wife accompany him. This is where the connection to all those fabulous clothes came in. One of his favorite places to visit was Hong Kong because one could get custom made suits in just a couple of days. Their stops were often for several days in the various ports which was perfect for him and her to go shopping for the highest quality silk and wool dress clothes for a fraction of the price in S.F. I suspect through the '70s, '80s and '90s they likely amassed one of the best wardrobes in the world. Custom suits, dress shirts, shoes, ties and everything else to make one feel and look good were easily bought by them from foreign ports. After he died, Dorothy told me he had over two hundred suits and countless ties and shoes in his closet. She wouldn't, however, reveal to me her count of dresses. She donated his clothes to friends and charity after his death.

Dorothy and Woody met while they were working in the San Francisco post office together in the 1960s. Woody had been married a couple of times already and didn't have any children. Dorothy had never been married. She grew up in Alabama and came west first to Illinois and then to California in 1960 living with a cousin who was in the army at Fort Ord near Monterey. Fort Ord was a large army base next to the Pacific Ocean which closed in 1994 due to the post-Cold War downsizing. Currently, it's an open space for outdoor activities and a state university. After getting a job at Letterman Hospital in San Francisco (also a former army base) in 1963, she then found work at the post office. They were married in 1969 and lived the life of bon vivants in S.F. Dorothy was thirty-five at the time while Woody was fifty-three. They never planned to or had children.

Woody always worked three jobs, shuffling between the post office, his barbershops and captain's assistant work. He finally retired from part time work at the post office in 2009 after nearly fifty years! He and Dorothy bought and lived in their San Francisco home where they entertained and could go out for the nightlife until the 1970s when they moved south to San Bruno and established the first integrated neighborhood in that town. They stayed there to live out their time together. Woody also had great taste in automobiles buying a new one every three years. A Cadillac Coupe de Ville or Mercedes were his typical choices.

Woody would often come in for a visit wearing a merchant marine cap that the captain had given him. His various medical problems over the years included needing a pacemaker, asthma flare-ups, high blood pressure and a stroke that he recovered from completely and unfortunately and finally that "old timer's disease", Alzheimer's, which crept in slowly like the fog in San Francisco over the last half dozen years of life. Dorothy was aware of it first and told me it didn't cause her any trouble, just like everything about his life. It didn't change his disposition or polite manner one bit. His name on my schedule always gave me a bit of joy. He will be missed and not forgotten as one of my very cherished patients. Dorothy gave me a wonderful portrait of the two of them along with permission to tell his story.

CHAPTER 14

Serious Sometimes Seems Simple

Wegener's granulomatosis is one awful disease. Medical students learn about its gruesome graphic details in first year pathology class. Untreated, it is one of the scariest maladies that the body can be afflicted with. Older textbooks seemed to have taken a particular sadistic enjoyment of showing pictures of its natural progression as an autoimmune disease that begins to attack the body both internally and externally. The disease was also known as "lethal midline granuloma", as one's face turns into a cavitating ulcer while internal organs progressively collapse ending in death. Even though rare, its clinical features were known for some time and were described as individual cases in the early 20th century. However, it was a German pathologist, Friedrich Wegener, in the 1930s and '40s that completed a full characterization of the disease and for which it was named. Later, after discovering his association with the Nazi party, the disease was renamed to a more descriptive term—"Granulomatosis with polyangiitis". There is no known cause for this rare condition, and it occurs mostly in the elderly. Something gets triggered in the body that causes the immune system to start making antibodies that attack, destroy and clog the small arterial blood vessels throughout the body, a vasculitis. This causes those tissues to begin to die from lack of nutrients and oxygen and is seen initially in the skin and structures of the face but can be noticed as patches of ulcers on any section of skin. Without treatment, the progression of damage causes the cartilage of the nose to collapse along with pronounced organ damage to the lungs and kidneys. Without treatment, patients die of renal failure, infection and respiratory failure. Before the modern era of immunosuppressive drugs and high dose corticosteroid therapy, the prognosis for patients was about 6 months of terrible suffering before death. With current regimens, patients can have a prolonged remission and more than 80% of patients are alive after 5 years with many having a normal lifespan. This rare disease is found predominantly "only in textbooks," so its awareness and experience as a potential possibility falls way down in the mind's rolodex list when evaluating patients in a busy office.

Louisa was a no-nonsense widow of Italian heritage. Her parents emigrated from the town of Lucca, Italy to South San Francisco in the early 1920s and she was born soon after they arrived. One of six children, her father grew artichokes and broccoli in the cool foggy areas near Funston beach. As the Bay Area rushed to become a modern suburb in the 1950s, all that farmland area eventually became housing. However, established immigrant communities directly south of San Francisco from Italy, Germany, Ireland and France continued the agrarian and tradesman life with small town markets and stores serving the locals. Louise married a man she went to high school with, had 3 children and led a life that included brothers that went off to World War II and Korea, her husband started a local clothing store that was fairly successful until the development of suburban shopping malls in the mid-1960s caused the business to flounder. She became a widow at age fifty-nine when her husband died suddenly of a heart attack on one Easter Sunday. She had been generally quite healthy all of her life but got used to a style of doctoring that was starting to vanish as doctors became more office based. When her or a family member became ill in the late 1950s and '60s she would call her doctor to come to the house for a good old fashioned "house call". Most of these calls were for various minor infections or aches and pains. The doctor would arrive, check the patient out and give an antibiotic or pain medicine usually from their black bag. This type of attention was somewhat driven by the competitive nature of the doctors looking to make patients happy and build their practices. There were many young physicians starting up who also had families to feed, cloth, and educate. This was also at the time of essentially no health insurance, so all visits were paid in cash, usually dispensed to the wives of the physicians who ran the business side of the practice. Many physicians had their offices in an in-law type space attached to their houses. After the new Seton Hospital and office building was completed in Daly City in 1962 many docs found that they could easily see more patients and attend to sicker patients in the hospital in a much more efficient way and began to phase out the evening trudges around town to see patients with colds.

Louisa's former physician, Dr. Bacigalupi, was an icon in the area. Dapper, thin, and high-strung, he was always on the move and always working. I remember him when I started at Seton in the late 1980s but never really got to know him well. He was part of the old guard of general practitioners that did everything—house calls, hospital visits in the middle of the night, seeing patients in the ER on weekends and doing a variety of procedures including delivering babies in his younger days. He never planned on retiring. When I met him, he was in his mid-70s and going strong. A seemingly nice guy who never said much more than a few words as he grabbed a cup of coffee in the doctor's lounge and dashed out to see his patients, always with a stethoscope dangling from his neck and wearing a finely tailored Italian suit. When "ol' Bacigalupe" died suddenly, it probably surprised him as much as everyone else. His funeral at the local Catholic cemetery in nearby Colma was an enormous event in all black. Most Italians in the area came to pay their respects including a large portion of his patients and their families. His passing seemed to be symbolic of a drastically changing world as well. All the local farmland was now covered in tract housing and a growing wave of Pacific Rim immigrants from the Philippines, Samoa, Tonga, Fuji as well as the rest of Asia had become a significant portion of the local population. This along with the influx of Mexicans, El Salvadorans and Nicaraguans, the nature of this community looked entirely different at the beginning of the 21st century. Of course, Louisa was there at Holy Cross Cemetery dressed in black and quietly crying with all her long-standing neighbors at his funeral.

Later that year she sought out another doctor and found my name to be plain and straightforward enough but suspiciously not Italian enough for her liking. The other local Italian physician had retired a couple of years earlier so this search also marked the end of her grounding in her cultural heritage. At the age of 79, she had not had any major illnesses or cancer or heart disease and lived a simple life in the same house for the past 50 years. A standard home of 3 bedrooms and 2 baths with a backyard and front porch that faced the foggy ridgeline looking west.

When I first met her in my waiting room, she eyed me up and down suspiciously as I introduced myself and asked her how she came to see me as her new doctor. "A family friend knows you. Are you a good doctor? I want someone who knows what they are doing and who can help me when I need it. I hope you can make house calls." I took a breath and sat down across from her in the exam room. "Thanks for coming in and giving me a chance to help you. I know you were seeing Dr. Bacigalupi and he was such a great and beloved doctor around here. Hopefully, I can be nearly as good as him. Yes, I do occasionally make house calls but not every day." I stated truthfully. In my early private practice, I decided it would be interesting and helpful to see an occasional patient that was housebound. Most of my patients lived close to my office and I could schedule a home visit either at the beginning or end of my day. The patients and family greatly appreciated it although it was inefficient from a time standpoint. I wouldn't see patients for minor issues like colds or sprains but there was a benefit in seeing a patient with their family in the cases of severe Alzheimer's, lung or heart disease where mobility and equipment tied the patient to the home. One could get a better understanding of their real-life environment and the family dynamics which helped me plan treatment and communicate directly.

"OK," Louisa responded. "We'll see." After reviewing her medical history, I asked if there was anything bothering her that day. "Well, my neck and knee are hurting all the time." "Does the pain keep you from doing anything you need to do?" I asked. "No, I'm too busy for that to stop me." I examined her and recommended some simple treatment like heat and over the counter anti-inflammatory medicine. "Is that it?", she asked. "Let's give that a try," I suggested. "Humpf." I talked about considering X-rays, physical therapy or seeing an orthopedist but she said, "No, I'll live with it." I finished examining her and talked about a few preventative issues but could sense her frustration and told her to let me know if things got worse and if anything was troubling her she could let me know. She left swiftly after that and I thought she probably would go and find someone else.

A few months later she came back in for a check-up of her blood pressure which was reasonably controlled with an older diuretic. I asked her about her aches and pains to see how they were doing. "The same, I'm living with it." "Do you want to try a prescription arthritis medicine to see if it helps?" I asked. "Well, if you insist." I gave a prescription and a flu shot as it was the fall and scheduled her to have a blood test to check her electrolytes as she was on a diuretic.

A few days before Christmas, she called my office and told my medical assistant that she was "sick" and needed the doctor to come over and treat her. After getting a few details, she reluctantly explained that she had gotten a bad cold and was coughing a lot and had a fever. I thought I could get her on better side by accommodating her and was a bit worried that sometimes stoic older patients are actually a lot sicker than they let on over the phone. I headed over to her house off Grand Ave during my lunch break and rang the bell of her mission style home. She looked through the curtain before unlocking the inner door and then the grated screen door and let me into her living room with a "come in" only. Scanning her living room, there was an immediate sense of old comfort and neatness. Pictures of her family were aligned on the mantel, hanging ceramic flowers on either side, an upholstered couch and chairs with a metal bordered coffee table. I was motioned to sit down. There were small biscottis and a fresh pot of coffee in an insulated container in place. "Sit down, thanks for coming," she motioned to the couch and I could tell she had lost some of her normal voice and had a loose cough. "How are you feeling and when did this start?" I began my questioning while sitting down and putting my black doctor's bag on the floor. Her home had a similar feel to my own grandmother's house in South Philly that I recall visiting as a child, a bit dark and old but well-kept furniture, doilies on the tables, various bric-a-brac items, area rugs and all immaculately clean. I kinda felt I had gone back in time and having my doctor's bag seemed to complete the experience. It was something I got years ago as a reward from answering a bunch of survey questions from a medical supply company. I only used it for my occasional house calls, so it looked all shiny and new, not like the traditional worn ones that previous generations of doctors had who actually did this type of work for a living. Inside it were the basic tools of the trade—stethoscope, blood pressure cuff, otoscope, light, reflex hammer, thermometer, a small container of bandages and a prescription pad. Louisa saw my bag as well and I imagined it may have put her at ease a bit but its newness likely indicated how inexperienced or "new" I was at this type of thing. She explained that she had been developing this cough for over a week and didn't feel well with a slight fever, runny nose and mild stomachache. She wasn't bringing up much phlegm and was able to sleep OK. She only took a couple of Tylenol. I went about examining her in her living room, leaving all her clothes on and did not find anything of concern. Her throat, ears, neck and lungs were all normal as well as her abdomen. I mentioned that she could have a mild flu or other virus but possibly the start of a bacterial bronchitis or even a case of whooping cough. It seemed best to give her a prescription of an antibiotic that would cover the treatable infectious possibilities. I set the prescription for the antibiotic and non-narcotic cough syrup down and recommended that she could also take an over-the-counter decongestant for her runny nose. I tried to reassure her that she should be better in a week but that if she wasn't or got worse that she should call me. "OK," she answered. I complimented her on how nice her house was and she encouraged me to have a cookie which I did and then was off back to the office.

I got a call from her about 10 days later. "I'm still coughing and don't feel that great." She said there wasn't much phlegm and no fever that she felt. I ordered a chest X-ray and told her to come to my office that day so I could listen to her lungs. "My friend thinks I have walking pneumonia" she told me. She didn't look like she was having trouble breathing and her oxygen level via a finger pulse oximeter was normal. Her temperature was 99.9. Her lungs had a few scattered crackles and an occasional mild expiratory wheeze. "This bronchitis could have inflamed your lungs" I told her and gave her a sample of a combination inhaler that had a long-acting bronchodilator and corticosteroid and showed her how to use it. "I never had one of these before. Am I dying?" I told her I didn't think so but wanted her to get the X-ray today and that I will call her when I got the result. I contemplated giving her oral steroids, like prednisone, which can help for any lung inflammation but she wasn't wheezing that much. Also, I thought of a different antibiotic but the azithromycin works in the body for about 2 weeks after finishing the last dose and this could all be the result of a viral infection so I held off until getting the X-ray report. Later that afternoon the radiologist called me. "There are some small areas of consolidation of both lungs, which looks like a small pneumonia bilaterally." OK, so there was a reason to prescribe a different antibiotic. I called her, "your friend may be a decent doctor, it looks like you have a mild walking pneumonia." "Humpf," she grumbled. I called her pharmacy and told her to call me in 48 hours to see how she was doing or if she was getting worse.

"Walking pneumonia" is one of those persisting lay terms that is not part of medical classification of a disease entity. It is used mostly by older generations and implies a serious, but not life-threatening lung infection. It seems to have come about by discovering that some people have pneumonia and are still just walking around instead of being in the hospital. Although in my experience of asking folks about their past history of walking pneumonia most of them have never had a confirmatory X-ray when the diagnosis was given to them. I suppose it was a way to have patients rest and stay at home and see the doctor on follow-up. The word pneumonia certainly has a fearful connotation in the elderly of possibly leading to death. The medical definition of pneumonia is largely restricted to patients that have an infiltrate (an area filled with fluid) seen as a discrete shadow on chest X-ray. These infiltrates are often able to be distinguished from cancer.

Putting a note on my desk, I called Louisa a couple of days later to see how she was doing. "Not great, still very tired but not worse," she reported. "OK, let's give it a bit more time for the medication to help.

I'll need to have you get another X-ray to make sure it's cleared up in a week."

I didn't hear from her for a couple of weeks. One morning, while doing rounds in the hospital I saw Phil, a nephrologist colleague, who stopped me in the hall. "Oh, I saw that patient of yours, Louise, in the ER over the weekend." She had come in because she was exhausted but her labs showed acute renal failure with a creatinine of 4.2 (normal is about 1), elevated white blood count and worsening of the infiltrates on her chest film even though her oxygen level was normal. She had requested that the ER not call me and referred her to a different doctor. Phil was on-call over the weekend and because of her serious kidney disease was called in. He said he debated about whether to admit her but finally did for a couple of days of evaluation and further testing. Her kidney ultrasound showed no blockages. Phil astutely tested for a variety infectious or inflammatory causes of her renal disease. Her ANCA test, (antineutrophil cytoplasmic autoantibody) test was positive. "She has Wegener's," he stated plainly. "Oh, wow" I said in blinking disbelief. "What a diagnostic coup, fantastic Phil." She didn't seem that ill and it looked like just a mild community acquired pneumonia. "Yeah, the combination of lung infiltrates and renal failure led to the possibility," he explained. "How is she doing?" I asked. "Oh, not bad." He had started her on high dose corticosteroids and stopped the antibiotics and was planning on the next phase of treatment with Cytoxan, a chemotherapy drug that quells the overactive immune system that induces this disease. "She should do OK." "Have you seen any other cases?" I had to ask as this was my only real-life interaction with this disease. "Yeah, a few over my 30 plus years in nephrology but this case is one of the simplest and least advanced" he told me. "Well, I guess she's not very happy with me not getting the diagnosis correct." He told me gently that she wanted him to take care of her from now on. I understood well that I was fired as her doctor and not surprised. Shaking my head at this subtle presentation of a really bad disease, I was relieved that she went to the ER and got all the blood and X-ray testing and diagnosis promptly. Better than a long delay with likely more complications. She sure didn't look anything like those god-awful patients in the old textbooks.

It's not terribly unusual that a rare disease can look like a typical problem. Medical practice is not a set of diseases with straightforward treatment but an individual patient with a set of symptoms and abnormalities that can be as variable as the weather. Collectively, we doctors take these presentations as a statistical issue. The way we think is in a priority of what could be the most common along with the possible worst case scenario. We can't assume every symptom indicates a life-threatening disease. Judgements and decisions are based on knowledge, experience and occasionally a hunch but there always is the possibility to change or include other possibilities as things unfold. Medical decision making is quite a complex process. There is an old saying in medicine: "When you hear hoofbeats think of horses not zebras." Naturally, as a younger physician those "zebra" diseases are much fresher in the mind and sit alongside the "horses" much closer in the thought process. After many years of seeing problems hundreds of times with variation, a sense develops to sort through the nuances of symptoms and test results. However, there is never an end to variation and also the possibility of a very rare disease showing up unnoticed.

A few months later, I got an update from Phil. She had responded well to the intensive medical therapy. Her kidneys were nearly back to baseline, the lung infiltrates had gone and she was feeling more chipper on all the steroids. Her treatment was going to last at least a year. Phil never did house calls and so she moved on to another primary care physician who didn't either. Her case did raise my awareness of this strange group of *vasculitic diseases*, so I got an important teaching point with Louisa and was relieved it worked out for her. Thankfully, she has remained my only case of this disease after 35 years of practice! Maybe, I can put it back in the textbook where it belongs!

CHAPTER 15

Stop Bugging Me!

Dot lived a colorful life. She grew up in San Francisco and came of age in the wild post WWII era where the expansive nightlife prior to the 1960s was dominated by cabaret and jazz clubs. In the Fillmore district, Black jazz club owners helped the careers of Ella Fitzgerald, Billie Holiday, Etta James, Miles Davis, Dizzy Gillespie where also a host of other jazz greats flourished. In Chinatown, burlesque clubs like the famous Forbidden City displayed an entertainment mix of singers, chorus girls and magic acts to a full house of white and Asian audiences. Dot was swept up in this revelry and found work as a chorus girl in a variety of clubs around the city. She danced, drank, smoked and generally had a great time as a young woman in one of the most diverse, progressive and open cities in the world. However, in the 1960s as the bohemian culture grew and redevelopment projects changed the landscape of the Fillmore and Western addition districts, nightlife and entertainment shifted in the city. Black jazz club owners moved to Oakland, the city's jazz scene shifted to North Beach along with the mostly white pot smoking poetry coffeehouses, nightclubs closed and were replaced with strip clubs and a few comedy clubs such as the Enrico's and the Hungry I. Work as a chorus girl dried up. Dot found herself working downtown in various office jobs and found a man who she thought acceptable to marry. She had a daughter and a more subdued life as the counterculture exploded in the mid-'60s when she turned 30. On weekends, she got together with her old friends and reminisced about the fun times. The hippy, drug culture never appealed to her as she liked the more glamorous, traditional style of the '40s. Her marriage fell apart in the early '70s due to her husband's alcohol abuse and she found herself a single working mom with a boring job and eventually moved out of the city to the much less expensive, foggy South San Francisco. She was not a big drinker herself and only socially. She eventually quit smoking in her 50s. She had "man friends" but decided that another marriage was not for her and even living with a man "who are all slobs" was untenable.

Dot became my patient in the late 1990s after her previous physician retired. She didn't have many health problems except for hypertension and acid reflux problems which were well controlled with a simple medication regimen. She didn't need much doctoring but came in when she was ill or worried about a symptom. Usually, she was able to be treated and reassured without a significant amount of extended testing or explanation. She was what most physicians would describe as a typical middle-aged patient—not too sick, not too demanding. I enjoyed her spirited, direct, no-nonsense personality and got a kick out of her talking about her wild youth adventures when prodded to do so.

I saw her a few times a year for checkups and incidental illnesses. One time after several years she came in complaining of a "rash" that was itching her all over. On examining her skin, I only noticed a few small areas of scratched skin and prescribed a generic cortisone cream. It didn't seem like either an allergic reaction, eczema or infection. Could this be some bug bites? Bed bugs? It really looked fairly tame whatever it was so I told her to contact me if it continued to bother her. It did. She came back in a few weeks later with the itching getting worse. She was worried something was biting her. This time I only saw more areas of mostly her arms and legs with scratch marks. Could this be scabies? I gave her a prescription for treating scabies and gave her instructions on washing bed sheets and pillows. Two weeks later she was back again without any benefit and she was more worried there was some kind of dangerous condition or infestation. I then sent her to see a local dermatologist who could do a skin scraping for possible resistant scabies or a biopsy and to consider a different treatment if he thought it was something else. The consult report merely stated "no rash, no treatment indicated". Hmmm. On follow-up, she began to insist that there were bugs crawling on her and driving her a bit crazy, especially at night. "Did you see these bugs?", I asked. "Yes, but they crawl away quickly when I turn on the light." Tiny cockroaches? "Can you bring some of these in so I can look at them and get them analyzed?", I asked. "Of course!", she replied. I began to think of conditions that can merely cause itching of skin and not a rash, the medical term is called pruritus. There are many, including mild contact allergic reactions to various soaps, lotions, certain fabrics, heat exposure, even cold exposure. Also, various medications, supplements and foods can elicit a generalized histamine response causing overall pruritus often with a minimal rash or skin redness. Dot's pruritus was generalized but more bothersome on her neck, arms, face and head. Like all problems that cause itching, they are always worse at night. This can be due to simply being unable to focus on anything else but also at night the body cools down a bit making anything inflamed or irritated more noticeable. I went through a detailed questioning of any of these possibilities and instructed her to not use any lotions, creams and certain foods. Also as a possibility, I had her stop her blood pressure medication to see if that was the cause. She wasn't taking any supplements. I prescribed her a moderate strength antihistamine by prescription to be used mostly at night and scheduled another follow up appointment for a couple of weeks.

When she returned, there was no significant improvement, and she had a small plastic food container which she said were the "bugs" that were driving her crazy. "OK, let's see," and I opened the container. Inside were various tiny specs of different sizes and colors, some dark, some white. "Hmmm," I said as I brought out my magnifying glass to examine these on a glass background. There were clearly no insects in this bunch of samples. Mostly, it was a collection of small lint, dirt specs and dandruff. "I don't see anything that looks like a bug here," I told her honestly. "Well, they must have crawled out or dried up so you can't recognize them!" She clambered. I examined her skin again, as well, and only saw some scattered marks where she had scratched so hard from the itching that her skin surface was excoriated with scabs. "You have to give me something to get rid of these scabies or whatever it is!" She demanded. I acquiesced and gave her another prescription for Elimite, the topical treatment for scabies with instructions on how to put it on her whole body at night and leave it on for 12 hours before washing off and repeating the process 2 weeks later. This second treatment for real scabies is recommended because if they lay eggs under skin they will hatch and reinfect a couple of days later. No one wants scabies to come back. Unfortunately, one of the side effects of this treatment is itching! So I informed Dot to be patient and complete the treatment and scheduled an appointment in 3 weeks.

At the next visit, she began by saying how disgusting it was that these bugs were crawling in her mouth, ears and even her eyes at night. She could feel them and see them and that they went away during the day. She had used the Elimite as directed and had thrown out all her underwear and bedsheets and got new ones. She had sprayed her mattress and had the exterminator come in and "bomb" her house for "anything" that might be there. She was on full attack mode to kill the "creepy crawlers" and was talking in a fast pressurized speech of someone under significant stress. I listened patiently to her woes and examined her again and gave encouragement that hopefully all this problem will go away but was becoming more convinced with each visit that this was a delusional infestation and no external treatment was going to help. I was struggling with when to confront her with this very difficult and touchy situation. Conversely, in all other matters of her life she harbored no other delusions and functioned normally. She shopped, cooked, took care of financial matters, occasionally saw and spoke with her daughter and even had a man friend she saw on occasion. I gently asked about any stress issues in life, thinking this could be the trigger. None were apparent. No major new problems had surfaced. She had a decent relationship with her daughter who lived across the bay with her family. The man in her life was OK but "a slob" so she would never live with him "or any other man". She had always been a meticulous cleaner. I decided to not confront her delusional thoughts at that meeting. Instead, I began to research this topic which has a medical diagnosis—*delusional parasitosis*. I talked with the dermatologist I had referred her to who suspected this could be the case and after filling in the details of the events he was convinced that was the diagnosis. He didn't see any benefit or need to see her again as in his experience these patients are nearly impossible to "cure" or to convince that they are imagining their infestations. Research on the topic revealed Dot's case to be quite typical in presentation but because of the rarity of the problem, no great research has been performed. There were expert recommendations for a specific old antipsychotic medication, pimozide, that was thought to help this disorder although not studied very thoroughly. Here is where medical research is often fuzzy and limited. While this condition has been documented for a long period of time, it's rarity and treatment recommendations have fallen to a small number of "experts" who describe some benefit from a form of treatment. In this case, a rarely used antipsychotic medication that became available in the 1950s when Dot was a chorus girl. Antipsychotic medications when discovered and began use in the '50s started a revolution that ended the awful practice of frontal lobotomy for psychotic patients by the early 1960s. These new medications allowed many patients to end their lifelong institutionalization as depicted in the movie *One Flew Over the Cuckoo's Nest*. Patients were able to live reasonably functional lives in community settings with these new medications. Of course, all was and is not perfect in treatment. Some patients don't respond as well as others, there can be significant side effects such as the dreaded tardive dyskinesia which causes a person to have involuntary regular tic movements such as lip smacking and tremors which are not very socially acceptable. Also, getting a crazy patient to remember to take one's pill every day is not that easy either, so formulations of monthly intramuscular injections have been devised but require a monthly visit to a clinic to administer the dose.

Since Dot was otherwise doing OK in life, I was cautious in confronting her and recommending such a potentially complex treatment of her evolving psychiatric disorder. I privately consulted with psychiatric colleagues on her case to get their thoughts on how to approach her problem and responses were mixed as well as this condition is not seen by general psychiatrists either and the ones I knew never really had a case that they actively treated. Only the dermatologists I spoke with had tried to treat this with the recommended antipsychotic on the few cases they had seen. Unfortunately, none of them had a success story in helping or even having the patient being compliant enough to truly tell if it was helpful. Not good, I thought.

Dot didn't come back for a couple of months and the scene was a bit scary and humorous. "Doc, you gotta help me with these bugs!" She declared. "They crawl into my mouth and nose and ears and even my eyes and are driving me crazy! Look what I had to do to try to get rid of them" as she pulled off her head scarf and showed me her freshly shaved head. "Oh, this is serious all right," I replied. My memory flashed back to the character in the TV show *The Addams Family*, Uncle Fester. He had a shaved head and did a funny gag of putting a light bulb in his mouth and making it light up with teeth pressure.

"Did shaving help get rid of them?" "No, not really but they have less places to hide." "I had to shave all over to keep them from going you-know-where!" "You gotta give me more of that scabies cream, I've been using the over-the-counter stuff but it barely does anything." She was referring to lower strength permethrin cream available at drug stores known as Nix. I examined her skin and scalp again and found no rash, just a few scratch marks. "Wow," I said, "you're really being tortured with this, aren't you?" "Yeah, I can't get rid of them. They seem to go away for a short time but then come right back." "OK," I said, "I need to have you see the experts in this problem" and then proceeded to arrange a consultation at UCSF in San Francisco for her. "You need to see some of the world experts in this problem as it is driving you batty." Asking about her life situation, she stated that she got rid of her man friend but otherwise was OK. She didn't look otherwise any different and had been taking care of herself.

Delusions are obvious to those outside them but for one experiencing them, they are relentless and real. They take various forms in the human mind. In the extreme case of schizophrenia, patients hear voices and can have visual hallucinations directing all their thoughts and behavior. One could think of these as being quite external to the person. In this case, delusional parasitosis is more intimate and has a boundary that stops at the external level of the skin. Dot didn't believe someone else was infesting her or that these creatures existed anywhere else except for maybe her bed. This private experience allowed her to see the rest of the world as it actually was. In some way, this is a more manageable psychosis as it does not completely take over one's consciousness.

The call from the dermatologist who saw Dot at the University clinic offered no further options for treatment other than the old antipsychotic medication which is oddly branded as Orap. She was given a prescription and tried one pill but it made her feel "weird" so threw it away.

I sat down with her for a talk after this and tried to gently bring up that this was something she felt but that the doctors couldn't find any of these bugs she thought were bugging her. "But I can see them and feel them crawl into my eyes to hide!" She exclaimed. I told her I didn't know what to do to make these go away but at her request gave another prescription for scabies treatment. Fortunately, there was little harm in doing that.

Dot came back only occasionally over the next 5 years. Each time the "bugs" were still there but she was just doing various home remedies and living with them. I listened and nodded knowing there was little else to be done.

One winter she had a bad bronchitis, wheezing, shortness of breath, productive cough and needed a significant combination of antibiotics, inhalers, prednisone and several visits. After not improving and having a chest X-ray that showed a combination of pneumonia and fluid in the chest cavity next to her lungs, I admitted her to the hospital and called a pulmonary consult to evaluate her. We discovered that her lung and heart were functioning at a very low and dangerous level. Years of smoking had caused significant permanent damage including moderate emphysema. Along with that, she had developed heart failure which was exacerbated and brought to forefront when she got a lung infection. This is a common scenario of one condition bringing out another. She struggled with this combination and we struggled to get her better. As her condition didn't improve, she required care in the ICU (intensive care unit) and when she could no longer maintain a basic oxygen level, she was intubated and put on a ventilator. I was hopeful we could pull her through this severe illness as she had not been this sick before and these problems of pneumonia, emphysema and heart failure while being life threatening were treatable problems. However, she was unable to wean off the ventilator after a week or so as she couldn't maintain an oxygen level that was safe without the machine. We then discovered that the right side of her heart was enlarging. Something unexpected was going on and an echocardiogram (heart ultrasound) examination answered our worry. She had a hole in the septum of her heart which separated the right and left sides and as pressure built up on the right side it pushed *deoxygenated* blood to her left ventricle which made her overall level of oxygen lower than expected and needed. She was not a candidate for heart surgery at 76 years old and with serious lung disease. The struggle we faced had no endpoint as we had tried all the medical and mechanical support we had available and after 2 weeks she was no better. She had developed the serious complication of significant inflammation in her lungs which caused fluid to accumulate and worsened her condition. I had a long talk with her daughter. We discussed a previous conversation Dot and I had about end of life issues. She had told me she didn't want to be kept alive if there was no hope. Her daughter knew this was her mom's wishes as well and made the decision to withdraw life support appropriate and humane. Interesting and unusual in the modern era of medical care, Dot's daughter wanted an autopsy which I fully supported. It showed pneumonia, moderate heart failure, lung edema and a fairly large intra-ventricular septal defect that she had been born with, but which did not cause problems until she became so sick late in life.

The heart is basically a pump. The right side of the heart is the low-pressure side and draws blood back from all the veins from all over the body after it has delivered oxygen and nutrients and then pumps blood to the lungs so that oxygen can again be transported back to the body after it enters the left side of the heart which has the bigger muscular pump action. A hole between the chambers occurs as a birth defect and can be inconsequential and even repair itself if small enough. Most of the time even if it is of moderate size it may not be detectable or even cause health issues as the high pressure left side of the heart is able to pump plenty of oxygenated blood to the body even if a small amount leaks through to the right side. However, in Dot's case where lung damage caused high pressure and dilation in the right ventricle the pressure difference was overcome and then unoxygenated blood went to the left ventricle to then be pumped out to the body. The brain and other organs don't function well in a low oxygen state for any significant length of time and led to her terminable state.

Her pulmonologist on the case, Dale, worked hard to get her through her ordeal but it was not to be this time. He knew of her delusional parasitosis as I had filled him in on all the details of her past medical history. After the autopsy we were chatting about her case in the doctor's lounge of the hospital over a coffee. He mused that "maybe those bugs did crawl into her heart and ate a large hole." Hmmm… I thought about that for a minute, then said…… "Nah."

PART 3

Observations, Opinions and Occasional Rants on the Medical Profession

CHAPTER 16

Healthcare is a Misnomer!

Complaining rant here: it bugs me to be referred to as a "healthcare provider" or a "provider" or a "primary care provider" or a "PCP". I am and have been a physician or a doctor or a trained, licensed, professional who takes care of the sick. I provide *medical* care. This euphemistic appropriation of the field of medicine has been going on for the past 30 years and I'm sick and tired of it and disgusted by it. While this has crept in and now most don't even give the nomenclature a second thought, it *is* an important distinction that deserves a scrutinized re-evaluation and desperately needs to be revised to the original classification. The act of combining these two words together to form a pleasant and misrepresented connotation is at the heart of this matter and is wrong. Although a nice trick by some marketing folks to somehow equate "health" with "sick" to make the concept more palatable does not make it correct. Illness is the opposite of health. When one is in a state of health, one doesn't need so-called *healthcare*. When one is sick and in need of medical care the misnomer, healthcare, is a powerful misrepresentation of what the reality of the situation portends.

I don't provide health, I evaluate and treat folks that are not healthy, namely the ill. Being ill means the absence of health in some manner. The hope of all medical care is to allow the person to return to health at some point but medical treatment with all its complexity is to determine what is wrong and what can be done to right the unhealthy ship. Healthy is the state we are in when not sick or injured. If you're healthy you don't need a doctor, you need to just go on with life as usual. Sometimes folks go to the doctor for "preventative" care, that is, to have something done to keep from getting sick sometime in the future. While this concept sounds fantastic, the real ability of modern medicine to do this has serious limitations that I discuss in detail in a different chapter.

Somehow over the last 30 years there has been a systematic white-washing of illness with this word. This has been quite successful to replace the concept of illness with health and along with it to de-doc-torize and reclassify those providing medical care. How and why did this happen?

It is not exactly clear when this alteration of nomenclature began. Certainly, not in the time of the greatest change in American medical care in the 1960s. LBJ's great social programs, Medicare and Medicaid, were accurately labeled to anoint a new system of medical care and insurance for the elderly and the poor respectively. Nowhere was the use of the word "health" attributed to the practice of medicine in the wording of these two monumental legislative acts.

We can start with the rise in the early 1990s with the then estab-lished insurance product called the "Health Maintenance Organiza-tion" aka "HMO". Most people know this as an option when they pick medical insurance coverage either through their employer or individ-ually. These insurance plans exploded then as a business model to try to reduce the cost of medical care by limiting access to testing and spe-cialists by forcing patients to see their "PCP" first to evaluate and treat them. In this model, HMOs put enforceable restraints and incentives in place to limit referrals and costs that were growing exponentially. The concept included paying doctors and hospitals a set amount of money for taking care of the patients enrolled under each plan. HMOs were and are also a misnomer in that it actually means *managed care* in the sense of a comprehensive subscription service for all medical care. This is opposite to the "fee for service" model where each interaction with the medical system has a value and can be billed separately. His-torically, the first HMO is thought to be when a lumber mill company in Washington state paid a medical group $0.50 per month to provide medical care to its employees. The comprehensive model formed by the Kaiser Health Plan grew in the post WW2 era which included paying physicians a salary while owning and operating hospitals, clinics and services as a closed nonprofit entity. Patients are unable to go outside this system for care. The term Health Maintenance Organization was first coined by Paul Ellwood, M.D., a Nixon policy advisor and pediatric neurologist who was deeply involved with the polio epidemic of the 1950s. He helped develop the 1973 law guiding the formation of this model as a way to limit the growing costs of medical care which at that time were 9% of GDP. He believed that reducing costs for medical care could be accomplished by: 1) "keeping people healthy" (an unproven but popular supposition then and now), 2) having medical groups compete for lower prices, and 3) measuring health outcomes in order to accurately and scientifically recommend proper treatment and thereby reduce costs by reducing unnecessary treatments. He believed in the free market system and the "report card" concept for health plans. However, 40 years later, his assessment was that this movement was a complete failure citing: 1) for-profit plans controlling the market, 2) independent physician organizations competing for better contracts, and 3) the lack of accountability as health outcomes were never truly measured in a broad meaningful way. While Dr. Ellwood was responsible for the word "Health" in HMO's, it came from his unrealistic and unproven expectations that "keeping people healthy would result in lower costs" and of course it sounded better with the word Health at the front of the acronym.

Kaiser Health Plans, one of the largest HMO insurers, especially in California, promote themselves in this healthy light all the time. By their simple slogan "Thrive" seen on buses, billboards and TV, they greatly minimize the actuality of being sick and needing extensive, specific, complicated medical treatment. By simply equating the pleasant concept of "good healthcare" and being more healthy, it fulfills everyone's fantasy of never being sick.

However, as an insurance product, HMO's became synonymous with the phrase "managed care" and not "health maintenance". By relabeling medical care to "gatekeepers" and "primary care providers" insurances quickly relegated doctors as cogs in their rising corporate empires. As a business model this was quickly adopted by contracting medical groups and hospital organizations because payments were in subscription format that sent money monthly to these contracting entities based on the number of enrollees. The less number of patients you saw, the more money you made. The exact opposite incentive is the prevalent fee-for-service system. Managed care insurance companies were able to offload "risk" to the contracting medical groups and hospitals by payment of set monthly amounts. Therefore, very sick patients that require significant care and hospitalizations were looked at as cost "losers", while healthy young enrollees were bottom line "positive". Unfortunately, doctors signed onto this profit and loss game and actively competed with each other, sometimes to disastrous financial ruin as patients still got sick and required medical care, regardless of the lowered reimbursement. The business method of cost containment of keeping premiums steady and lowering the payments to doctors and hospitals while various professional organizations compete for contracts kept the profits high in this model. This led to the famous "networking" of physicians and patients into one closed entity and not allowing very complex patients to be treated by the best specialists or centers in an area. Well, this model did work to contain costs during the 1990s. However, this increasingly became unworkable as costs and usage naturally increased and professional groups began to realize the inefficiency of processing administrative review of everything as patients began to complain more of limited care and choices. Essentially, this adaptation of medical capitalism worked opposite to its intention and the concurrent system of fee-for-service.

The word "Healthcare" flourished and expanded during this era and for excellent marketing and image reasons completely replaced the phrase "Medical Care". Healthcare centers, healthcare providers, healthcare products, *healththis* and *healththat* became the norm. In a psychological sense, this was a most pleasant substitution for the treatment of the sick. Words matter, however, words have meanings and connotations and vernacular that influence, create images and feelings. The word "health" is the opposite of "sick" or "ill" or "in need of medical attention, care and treatment". "What is the prognosis for getting better?" "Can I beat this?" "Will she survive this?" "What can be done?" What am I looking at here in survival time?" are all important and appropriate questions when one is facing a serious illness. There is no health care in the answers. There is medical care and if one is lucky a complete and speedy recovery follows afterwards. A return to health is the hope after receiving medical care is the accurate way of speaking.

When I adopted electronic records in the late 1990s, I first researched the available software for over a year before deciding on a decent and functional EMR to purchase. EMR at that time stood for "electronic medical record" and the one I used for 18 years was well designed by a group of family practitioners in Texas. While there were regular updates to the software, approximately 2 per year, around 2009 the label of software changed to EHR, electronic *health* record. With little notice this became the acronym put forward by those myriad of experts, consults and companies vying for business during the early Obamacare era. Just to be clear, nowhere in the records is there anything about the patient being healthy. There is data on their various medical conditions, medications, surgeries, allergies, complications of treatment, bad habits such as smoking or drinking, results of diagnostic testing and even death if that has occurred. Nothing in the record speaks or documents any healthy aspects. It's all about the patient's experience with medical evaluation and treatment and its results.

Over this time period there has also been a lot of doctor bashing for not being "health" advisors. Somehow with the increase enrollment of HMO's, along with the rise of the concept of preventive medicine and the rise of the supplement industry starting in the mid-1990s, there became an outcry that doctors were not doing enough to advise their patients on stuff like diet, exercise, relaxation techniques, proper yoga form, the right vitamins to take, stress management, marital discord, sleep hygiene, sexual performance, proper use of alternative medicine herbs and techniques, etc. All this was supposed to fit into a standard 20-minute office visit amidst a schedule with 20 other patients. Well, while all doctors felt this onslaught of questions ("What vitamins do I need to take to be healthier, doc?), in all honesty that is not our focus or our main concern. The problem with all this is the true paucity of scientific data to guide people in these important but minimally scientifically researched areas of healthy living. Honestly, doctors are not well trained in these areas. It doesn't mean we all don't do our fair share of counseling on difficult life events. I reviewed some of this elsewhere in this book, but our motivation is clearly to determine the proper diagnosis and be aware of the proper treatment for medical conditions, not to improve one's already present health.

OK, I will end this rant by saying that illness and medical care is messy, complicated, often not pleasant and sometimes not successful but it is the means we have to become healthy again. We need to return to an honest use of the vocabulary to describe what is what and *medical care* is not *healthcare*. And with that, this doctor will go back to evaluating and treating the sick with current evidence-based medical care.

CHAPTER 17

Nocebos = Placebos

Everyone has heard of placebos or the "placebo effect". The term comes from the Latin and translates as "I shall please". For most it means giving a sugar pill to someone who doesn't know it is not a drug and then having the beneficial effect of the drug the person thinks it is. Many would think this a form of trickery, a deception and even unethical to get someone to believe in something inert and then "feel" it is working for them without it actually doing much. Additionally, people believe that if the truth is revealed then a placebo would not work at all. Fascinatingly, this view is opposite from the scientific and physiologic reality of some of the most potent effects in medicine and life.

Placebos occupy an important place in medical science in that they are part of the four components for valid, proper, modern scientific studies of medical treatments. The emergence of *prospective* (done in advance of data collection), *randomized* (participants chosen by chance), *double-blind* (the researchers and participants don't know who is in what group), *placebo-controlled* (half the patients get the treatment and half get the placebo) medical studies developed over the last 30+ years have revolutionized and helped secure our knowledge of what works in treatment and what doesn't. The use of placebo is important to determine what is the true effect of treatment in comparison to no treatment. Even though the placebo effect in most studies is that somewhere around 25% that respond favorably, placebos are generally seen as an annoyance to the data one is researching, not a potential treatment in itself. Many medications can have only a marginal benefit over the placebo group which can mess up the long process of drug approval if the difference does not reach a decent statistical effect. The real problem with the placebo effect is that you can't separate it from the drug or intervention. For example, in a drug study for hypertension, drug X causes an averaging lowering of blood pressure by 20 points which is an excellent effect. However, the placebo group had an averaging lowering of 10 points which does show drug X is doing something beyond the sugar pill. However, one cannot just give the drug blind to see the effect because the drug *itself* has its own placebo effect. For medications the placebo effect continues as long as the person is taking the medication. There is not a reduction of the effect with time for long-term medications. So the placebo effect is always present and cannot be separated out and is looked at as "noise" in the science of studying medications.

Well, what about just giving placebos to patients and having all those beneficial effects for free? Doctors actually used to do that fairly frequently. Various "tonics" for colds, sugar pills for pain or anxiety or an irritable bowel were not uncommon in the past and they worked. For physicians, they were looked at as a tool to help a distressed, worried, medication seeking patient in conditions that did not have a specific treatment and that alternative treatments e.g. narcotics and tranquilizers were potentially dangerous and addictive. However, in the modern era of legal informed consent, the American Medical Association in 2007 issued a report and recommendation that placebos only be used "for diagnosis or treatment only if the patient is informed or and agrees to its use." This dictum shut the door on the cooperation of pharmacists and physicians to issue placebo prescriptions to unknowing patients and left the use of "deceptive" placebos to the clinical studies. While I had rarely prescribed "deceptive" placebos in the past, it became clear after this was not possible when I tried to prescribe one for a difficult patient with chronic fibromyalgia in order to not give narcotics that the patient was requesting.

The big question, of course, is what's really going on with the placebo effect? Is it not doing anything but having people "feel" better when nothing has changed in their bodies? Actually, there are powerful physiologic processes going on that are only recently coming to light and are cementing the mind-body concept as a real phenomenon. These include activation of brain regions responsible for pain control and anxiety, improving Parkinson's symptoms, reducing hyperactive and painful contractions in the bowel, improving blood flow to the heart, improving lung mechanics in asthmatics, reducing rashes and allergic responses and even modulating the immune system to mention a few. These are remarkable and measurable responses that are occurring in the *body*.

The placebo effect is also modulated by one's expectations which are influenced by past experiences, verbal instructions and by observing others in a similar situation. However, not all expectations are conscious. We now know that the pain-relieving effect of a placebo activates areas in the brain that control pain. However, the mechanism of lower blood pressure via a placebo is due to reducing the firing of the sympathetic nervous system to cause blood vessels to relax. Also, the placebo effect to improve immunosuppression in a kidney transplant patient to prevent rejection is entirely unconscious. The positive effects of a placebo can be enhanced by various methods. By the physician explaining in a very definitive way the benefit of a treatment while having a trusting relationship with the patient can exert a much more potent effect than simply giving the treatment. Most experienced doctors will know of this effect and use its advantage on a regular basis. This isn't lying but rather enhancing. I have purposely used this effect for decades to help lower blood pressure, improve diabetes control, enhance and prolong pain relief and alleviate anxiety, depression and stress while using the lowest doses of medicine possible simply by explaining the beneficial effects of treatment in a calm, positive tone that is trusted by the patient.

The placebo effect is not just limited to medications. Surgery and other invasive procedures also have been shown to have a profound placebo response. One of the most famous studies on this was done in 2002 and published in the *New England Journal of Medicine* by Bruce Moseley, M.D., who at the time was one of most respected orthopedists taking care of many professional athletes. His study, "A controlled trial of arthroscopic surgery for osteoarthritis of the knee," was a disturbing and astonishingly well done and conclusive study showing that all groups of patients had *the same* beneficial outcome if they either had: 1) the standard surgery of trimming damaged cartilage, 2) versus just flushing the knee joint with saline, 3) versus having nothing done except a small skin incision on the knee. The anger this study generated from his fellow orthopedists who were doing this routinely and making a good living on this procedure was enormous. However, based on this, patients and doctors had to rethink the need for this invasive surgery for arthritic knees and this practice has nearly ceased to be offered or performed these days.

What about the idea that placebos are just "tricks" and lying to patients and the effects are not "real" and would go away as soon the deception is revealed. To answer this, let's look at the work of one of the most important placebo researchers, Ted Kaptchuk, a professor of medicine at Harvard. As a young man, Ted studied acupuncture and practiced Chinese herbal medicine. He was impressed that many of his patients got better *before* he gave them treatments. He then went back to old Chinese herbalist texts and discovered the dictum that patients *should and would* feel better by just handing them the herbs, even before they took them. He then became fascinated with the placebo effect and has since been studying the effects in a rigorous scientific manner. The issue of non-deception or what is known as "open-label" placebo studies became important to him. He has published two studies on this. One in treatment of irritable bowel syndrome and another in cancer-related fatigue and both show a definitive improvement in the patients given a placebo while knowing it was in comparison to no treatment. I know of another open label study of migraine treatment where the group of patients who received the pill bottle labeled "placebo" did even better than the standard, proven medication for migraine. So, deception is not the primary or only factor working with the placebo effect. The effects are truly physiologic.

A point of clarification here is necessary. While placebos can have significant effects on various medical conditions, they are not useful for many. Cancer does not shrink or be cured by placebos. Infections are not cured by placebos. Broken bones, ruptured tendons, blocked intestines, blood clots, aneurysms, nerve damage, kidney failure, cirrhosis and many other serious medical conditions are not improved with placebos. But for many disabling, chronic and severely symptomatic conditions placebos can have an important and life improving effect without the need for invasive procedures or addictive medications.

So, what about the evil twin of placebos—*nocebos* or the *nocebo effect?* It also comes from the Latin meaning "I shall harm". These unwanted negative effects can wreak havoc on drug studies and established treatment by manifesting side effects and pain related to the expectations that the treatments are dangerous or *likely* to cause harm. The conscious and unconscious processes that enhance a response for placebos can then reduce or even produce a negative response for nocebos. For example, verbal suggestion that a medication causes side effects can produce that side effect much more commonly than would be predicted. Patients that have had an adverse reaction to one medication can have more frequent and more severe reactions to medications perceived as similar but in an entirely different chemical classification due to a nocebo effect. Also, patients that have heard of severe adverse reactions from others or read in the press or the medication inserts for certain medications more frequently have similar side effects.

Closely reading the medical insert given to patients when they get a prescription can be particularly problematic in inducing nocebo effects. This is the sheet of small print information that is given to patients when they pick their prescription from the pharmacy. It is given by law and unfortunately includes *every single* side effect that was reported by patients during the studies done for approval by the FDA, even for reported side effects occurring *less than 1%* of the time (generally deemed non-significant). The list is always long and alarming if one reads it thoroughly. In reality, medicines that have serious and frequent side effects are generally not approved or are given a black box warning at the top of the insert for definitively serious ones. In my career, I have spent a fair amount of time answering questions about side effects that occurred *before* patients even started a new prescription and then worsened after starting. Also, I've heard of fear and then stopping of an effective medication (such as blood pressure pill) due to a symptom occurring *years after* being on a medicine often after diligent reading of those inserts.

The occurrence of nocebo effects in the body is physiologically different from placebo effects. Different neurotransmitters and brain region activations have been identified. One area that has been shown to be active during a nocebo effect is the area of the brain associated with anxiety. For increased pain perception, neurologic imaging studies have shown increased pain signaling from the spinal cord to the brain. Nocebo effects are seen commonly in placebo-controlled studies of medications where one fifth of patients report side effects to taking the placebo pills.

In clinical situations, nocebo effects can be extremely annoying, time consuming and just bizarre. A patient that claims to be "allergic" to 14 of the most common antibiotics and has then a urinary tract infection or pneumonia poses a very difficult situation. When probed for what was the "allergy", I have heard patients recall various symptoms such as a headache, dizziness, nausea, itchiness, abdominal cramps, constipation, diarrhea, blurred vision, numbness, various isolated joint pains, hair falling out, pain while having sex and even nightmares as their *allergic* reaction. This is often followed by having been told (or believe being told) to "never take that medicine again". The patient with a long list of medication allergies and never having had a classic drug rash eruption to any of them is a typical *nocebo prone person* that doctors encounter. It is usually impossible to rationally discuss alternative explanations with someone that a certain symptom is not related to a medicine that they are convinced is the cause. Nocebo effects are seen more often in anxious patients, those with other unexplained symptoms and in those with greater psychological distress.

Recently, one well done study exploring the occurrence of nocebo effects on taking statin cholesterol medications was completed. Statins are a group of medications that powerfully reduce bad cholesterol by acting in the liver to suppress production. It has been known that in a very small minority of patients there is a risk of muscle inflammation and liver inflammation. This side effect and potential danger has been significantly publicized and known by patients and doctors. Doctors will often monitor laboratory tests to check for both issues particularly during the early phase of treatment and then at intervals afterward. The true incidence of a serious reaction has been estimated to be in the range of about 1 in a 1000 although this is likely an overestimate of the true occurrence. The most common symptom patients complain about with statins is muscle ache and in the vast majority of time the lab tests are normal or occasionally minimally elevated. Some placebo-controlled studies have shown the incidence of muscle aches is only slightly higher than with a statin and in many studies to be statistically the same. Yet, all physicians who prescribe statins see patients that are very aware of this potential side effect and report it as something to be very concerned about. The true side effect of *myositis* or muscle inflammation from a statin is one of ache and discomfort in *all* or most muscles in the body (as there inflammation throughout) and occurs at rest as well as with activity and it usually happens within a few months of starting, and also is continuous and not intermittent. However, most supposedly afflicted patients will report significant variations. Many will complain of one muscle hurting, lasting a few days or weeks, occurring years after taking the medicine and only with doing some specific activity, which is most definitely just plain muscle soreness. Often patients tell me they stopped the medicine and that they then felt better without discussing with me beforehand and are difficult to convince to give it another try. For patients who need this medication, it can be quite an important issue. Diabetics and patients who have had strokes or heart attacks can benefit enormously from a statin by preventing an early death. Strategies that have been adopted include switching a different statin, lowering the dose, or simply restarting the same medication to determine if that effect can be reproduced. All of which can be a difficult sell to the nocebo prone person. So, this newly completed study called SAMSON (*Self-assessment Method for Statin Side-Effects or Nocebo*, published 2022) expertly put all this to the test. The study showed that even though patients *do* get side effects, the rate was *equal* in the placebo group. The incidence of side effects for both groups was 10%. The design of the study was brilliant in that patients received numerically labeled bottles of the statin, placebo and empty bottles to be used for one month at a time randomly while at the same time using a smartphone app to record their symptoms daily. Patients were permitted to stop the pills if they were experiencing severe symptoms and then resume with the next bottle the next month. In the end, patients could see clearly the power of the nocebo effect as the placebo pills caused the same incidence of severe and mild side effects as the statin. With this unique nocebo study, doctors can now explain honestly that nocebo effects can occur and at the same time reinforce the high likelihood (90%) that no side effects will occur.

The story of Mary, a developmentally delayed 30-year-old woman who's psychologically remained as a 13-year-old, embodies an interesting combination of placebo and nocebo effects in regards to medical care. I first encountered Mary in the ER as an intern in Boston in 1983. She was brought in via ambulance in respiratory distress due a flare-up of asthma. Her wheezes could be heard across the room as she was breathing at a rate of two per second with short, shallow gasps. Her oxygen level was moderately low with an oxygen saturation around 85% (normal about 95%). From a clinical standpoint, she was on the borderline for needing prompt intubation and respiration ventilation but the second-year resident I was working with knew her from previous admissions and had seen her respond well to treatment with inhaled, nebulized bronchodilator medication so we held off. In fact, after 20 minutes of treatment which included oxygen, IV fluids and intravenous corticosteroids she was much better. For patients with a severe asthma attack, their sensation is like breathing through a straw while running up 10 flights of stairs as fast as one can. Which in severe asthma is what is happening as the small, medium and large airways are constricted to a fraction of their normal diameter and remain that way or worsen. There are many triggers for asthma attacks but some of the common ones are environmental allergies, cold air, exercise, emotional stress, a viral or bacterial respiratory infection. In Mary's case it was unclear what triggered this attack. She was in serious trouble but improved and needed to be hospitalized and monitored until this attack was resolved. For many severe asthma attacks, it can take several days or longer of intensive treatment to get the patient safely back to a normal state. Since I was on-call that night I was in charge with her admission and care during this hospitalization. In about an hour, Mary was much better but still wheezing when I saw her up on the medical floor. She was a bit shy but very smiley when I told her I would be taking care of her this time. She had been admitted many times in the past and several of the other interns and residents had taken care of her. "Oh Dr. Smith, thank you so much for saving my life!" she beamed. We talked about her asthma and her treatment and it was not clear what had sparked this attack. The next morning on rounds she still looked stable and improving and asked the names of all the other interns and residents in her room. She repeated each one while blushing. I told her how pleased we all were with her progress and that we would try to discharge her to home as soon as we could. While on rounds the next morning, I got an urgent call from Mary's nurse that she was much worse. We all rushed over to her room and sure enough Mary was wheezing up a storm and breathing quite rapidly. We all listened to her lungs for which she gladly sat up and took off her gown to allow us to. I ordered extra nebulizer treatments for her and an extra dose of cortisone and a monitored bed. Later that morning, she was doing better and was apologizing "for being so sick and a pain" again while blushing. I reassured her that it was not her fault and we'll get her better soon. This up and down pattern of improvement and worsening repeated over the next several days into the weekend but about a week after her admission she was able to go home and again was apologetic for "giving us a hard time".

A few weeks later, she was back in the ER with another attack. This time my intern colleague, John Hamil, admitted her and took care of her. We were on the same team and so we rounded each day on all the patients on the ward. John was an interesting, handsome and very sympathetic young doctor who planned on pursuing psychiatry after his internship. On rounds, Mary said "Hi, doctors…" to all of us in her bubbly, teenage crush, blushing way. She was quite ebullient with thanking John over his care. However, John, who was also the darling of many of the young nurses on the floor due to his good looks, became flustered with how Mary was not progressing. He was called to check on Mary several times a day because Mary's asthma had suddenly gotten worse. She remained in the hospital nearly 2 weeks when one of her nurses reported that Mary was always asking if Dr. Hamil was on the floor and then suddenly her next asthma attack would occur. Finally, after about 3 weeks, Mary was ready to be discharged. Our senior resident at the time was a woman who astutely noted this reaction and frankly acknowledged that Mary was "in love" with John. We laughed a bit and then went back to review her previous 10 or so admissions for asthma. It was quite clear that Mary's stay in hospital was always longer with a male intern than with a female intern in the range of 1-3 weeks for a male versus 1-3 days with a female. Teenage crushes causing asthma flare-ups! We then made a plan with all the interns and residents that if Mary needed admission in the future, one of the female doctors would be in charge of her care. This simple agreement kept Mary's future admission over the next 2 years to only a few days at a time as she no longer needed to invoke a "nocebo effect" needed to make her asthma worse to keep her involved with the young male interns she developed a teenage crush on. Yes, it's a bit convoluted but fits with the power of the unconscious mind to effect a change in health status in a real and dramatic way. In my interpretation, Mary's case represents initially the force of the placebo (along with treatment) to improve her clinical status dramatically after arriving in the ER many times nearly in respiratory failure and then improving rapidly in a half hour by pleasing her caretakers. Also an unconscious nocebo effect of wanting attention from her young male doctors in rapidly worsening her asthma when she knew she would be discharged home. Unfortunately, this story ends very sadly. In one of her severe asthma attacks, the paramedics attempted to intubate her in the field and placed the tube in the wrong position. Mary suffocated on the way to the ER and had a cardiac arrest that we could not revive her from. We were senior residents then and when we heard this terrible news, we all gathered around her bed and cried as if we lost a teenage daughter.

Thinking larger than clinical situations, aren't humans susceptible to "placebo" and "nocebo" effects in many life situations? Isn't falling in-love with its attendant glow that the other person is "perfect" as our brains are bathed in enhanced dopamine release, a form of placebo? Studies have shown people derive more pleasure from planning a vacation due its anticipated happiness than the actual trip, also a dopamine related placebo effect. The nocebo effects of real life include getting headaches, back or neck aches, dizziness, even nausea when anticipating something difficult such as an upcoming school exam ("what a headache") or a perceived difficult encounter with an adversary ("such a pain in the neck"). These responses are an intricate part of the human experience and we have much to learn from them.

CHAPTER 18

Taming the Amygdala

"I can't drive over the bridge to get to work," Sandra told me one day, somewhat matter of fact and concerned at the same time. "How long has this been going on?", I asked. "Well, a few months now and it's gotten worse and now I have to drive around which takes me an hour," she explained. When I asked her what exactly happens during these episodes, she recited a textbook example of panic attacks. "First, my heart starts racing and I begin to feel my head throbbing, then I start to feel tingling in my fingers, my chest is hurting and I can't breathe and I feel like I'm gonna die right there. So I have to stop the car and put my head down for a while before I feel somewhat normal and go back the other way." "Could I really die?" "I'm afraid I'm gonna pass out and have an accident," she added. This was a new development for Sandra. While she had a modicum of anxiety issues in the past and occasionally took a low dose of Xanax which settled her quickly, these full-blown terrifying panic attacks were new.

Sandra worked as an executive assistant at the same office for over 10 years. She was divorced for longer than that, had a grown son living not far away and had a steady if "annoying" boyfriend and at the age of 48 did not have much other stress in her life. She was always pleasant and talkative during our office visits and mostly saw me for various minor health issues.

"Did you try a Xanax for this?", I asked. "Well, a couple of times, afterward, but they just made me tired."

While nearly everyone has moments of anticipatory anxiety such as an upcoming exam/interview/athletic or musical performance, this is a natural neurophysiologic preparatory mechanism to be ready and focused on the upcoming task. The lens of life narrows down to thinking of the event at hand including the negative and the positive, often accompanied by sweaty palms, an increase in heart rate and an inability to think of anything else. Mental review of what is coming up occupies the conscious mind. For a smaller number, this anxiety becomes nearly or completely overwhelming. Stage fright is an extreme example. Sometimes the anxiety is so great that one's performance is actually much worse than what one could do under relaxed circumstances.

Panic attacks which contain many of the same sensations are a different animal and may be viewed as "anxiety on steroids". They come on as a bolt of lightning of intense fear seemingly out of nowhere. Often there is some external trigger like Sandra's bridge, although for her, previously going over bridges was no big deal nor was there a difficult specific memory or event in her life as a prior stress. Sometimes the trigger is an entirely new event, such as confronting the death of someone or some other intense experience. PTSD (post-traumatic stress disorder) is a common form particularly in combat veterans. Panic attacks can emerge during sleep and awake the person in a pool of sweat and the feeling of impending doom. They unravel quickly in a matter of minutes and are very difficult to stop once started. They can last many minutes but often up to an hour before the grip of emotional terror is released. The attack can be accelerated and worsened by hyperventilating which causes tingling and a feeling of near fainting due to lowered carbon dioxide levels in the blood. The median age of onset is 24 and it's twice as common in women than men. Young men, in particular, often go to the ER because they are convinced they are having a heart attack. It doesn't seem to affect children less than 10 much unless there is some childhood traumatic trigger and, fortunately, it does seem to fade with older age. I don't remember ever hearing about anyone over 70 having panic attacks. One seriously disabling offshoot of patients with panic disorder is the development of agoraphobia, the fear of going outside.

Modern neuroscience has advanced dramatically in the last few decades with the ability to study what is happening in the brain in real time with a technique called *functional* MRI imaging. This measures brain activity in various brain regions while one is having a real time panic attack. The amygdala is an area deep in the brain which has been associated with the monitoring and processing of the emotion of fear. Although recently it is found that emotional responses are *not* exclusive to any specific area of the brain. The amygdala is a relay station in the brain, sending and receiving various excitatory and inhibitory signals to various parts of the brain. One theory about panic attacks is that the amygdala *circuit* becomes sensitive to certain triggers and sends a cascade of stimulation to various other areas in the brain to start the process. One can look at it as a motion detector that turns on with the slightest of movement and then proceeds to turn every light in the house on. A hyperactive amygdala circuit is not so easily turned down.

From an evolutionary perspective, intense response to a perceived threat can have a life preserving effect, the proverbial "fight or flight response" is part of the amygdala circuit function. Of course, humans have a great deal of variability in how their nervous system reacts and so some take real danger nonchalantly and others go on high alert with the slightest hint of a threatening experience.

Treating panic attacks can also be tricky business. Just telling Sandra to "not worry about it, you'll be alright" is not a winning strategy for this condition. Like any ailment that is not continuous, the decision to treat and how to treat is based on the frequency and severity of the problem. Treatment for this condition has been well studied and there are two main approaches which both work nearly equally, namely, psychotherapy with a cognitive behavioral approach or medications. Medication treatment is divided into two types: acute treatment with quick acting anti-anxiety agents such as clonazepam or daily treatment with a medication in the class of antidepressant/antianxiety such as the popular SSRIs. Unfortunately, because of the paucity of properly trained mental health workers and minimal coverage by insurance companies, psychotherapy is rarely an initial option although many patients would prefer it to taking medications. However, because panic attacks

are such an intense negative experience with often very serious potential disability effects patients are usually more than willing to consider
medications. The biggest issue with using typical anti-anxiety medications is their dependence and abuse potential and of course this becomes
quite problematic in patients who have had prior or ongoing substance
abuse issues with any drug or alcohol. Therefore, those medications are
avoided. In general, most patients that go to the doctor for panic attacks
have been having them for some time and they are occurring regularly
and so medication treatment is best started with a long-term medication in the SSRI class such as sertraline. These medications which are
also commonly used for depression have some good advantages in that
they tend to have minimal side-effects and they work for this problem
generally at lower doses than those needed to treat depression. The other
benefit is that they often work much quicker for panic attacks than for
depression. Many patients start having a good response within the first
couple of weeks of taking them as compared to depressed patients taking
a month or two before benefit is noticed.

For Sandra, who wanted something in medication form right away,
we settled on a common SSRI at the low dose. Fortunately, she did fairly
well and had only a rare panic attack after a month or so. However, she
did find a different job that didn't require her to drive over any bridges
but she kept taking the medication as I recommended. Unfortunately,
panic attacks have a fairly high recurrence rate after they have been
controlled with medication, so patients usually need to take the medication for at least 6-12 months before trying to wean off them. Some
patients do fine off their medication but many will have panic attacks
again within a few months proving that they need their medication for
a longer period. There is no magic formula for deciding to try to get off
the medication but certainly a period of several months with no panic
attacks could be a starting point. Also, for those who need long-term
medication, sometimes many years, there is no way of knowing if they
need it unless they go through a trial period of weaning and seeing if
they recur.

Sandra took her medication and did well for the following 2 years
she was my patient. She changed jobs and changed insurances and

started seeing a different doctor on her new insurance after that but came back to see me about 8 years later. I asked about her panic attacks due to bridges and her use of medication and she informed me: "Oh, I don't need that anymore and stopped it a few years ago. I don't go over bridges much and usually have my partner drive over them when we go somewhere and it doesn't bother me!" This was a somewhat typical case for this problem and happily resolved after many years. However, in some patients the treatments are not as helpful and they need complex regimens with additional medications and cognitive behavior therapy to quell an over vigilant amygdala.

CHAPTER 19

Preventative Care Prevents What?

The phrase "Preventative Care" sounds so wholesome and nice and protective, doesn't it? It implies doing things to make one more healthy and to keep nasty diseases away. "An ounce of prevention is worth a pound of cure" is the old saying. One conjures up the notion that with the right amount we can hold off illness and death nearly forever. In articles that criticize the current health system in the US, particularly the costs, doing comprehensive preventative care is always associated with better overall health and less cost. However, the costs of our current "preventative care" strategy is extremely expensive and saves or prolongs life very little. Let's look at these conceptions or misconceptions to get a better perspective on the reality of this.

Clearly, there have been some remarkable preventions instituted in the last 2 centuries. In the early 1800s infant mortality was about 40% (yes, that's 4 in 10 children died during or soon after birth) and maternal mortality was about 1%, mostly from infections and bleeding. That certainly left a great deal of sorrow and kids without moms in those days. Thomas Jefferson and his wife had 6 children but only 2 survived to adulthood, she died of complications after their last child died in childbirth. The current infant mortality rate is about 1 in 1,000 for children and 1 in 10,000 for mothers. This very dramatic change has been largely due to improved hygiene and improved technical skill of obstetricians, advancing technology for monitoring complicated pregnancies and, for the past 80 years, the use of antibiotics to treat life-threatening infections.

The development and use of vaccines over the past 100 years is estimated to have saved nearly a billion lives in the world! It is truly remarkable that the world has ridden itself of one of its significant scourges, *smallpox*, so that no one now needs that vaccine. The current vaccine schedule for infants, children and adults is impressive and extensive, and also easily available to view on the CDC website and is backed by very strong scientific evidence of its efficacy. Unfortunately, the bizarre, unsubstantiated, anti-vaxxer movement that has grown worldwide and has begun to threaten populations with the re-emergence of preventable infections.

Besides improved safety measures (such as seat belts), strong public restriction and warnings to stop cigarette smoking, advice for healthy diets, regular exercise, sufficient sleep and stress management/reduction, what does modern medicine have to offer to prevent serious disease and death when one goes to the doctor for this service? Let's look at what we have to offer, how much benefit is proven, and also what patients perceive from seeing their doctor for a "preventative visit".

I came into the exam room where Arum was waiting for me, patiently checking his text messages. He was a handsome, 32-year-old software developer born in India, but his English was perfect and articulated his thoughts so well that he seemed more like a professional colleague than a patient. "I'm here for my 'annual', doctor. This is my first time here and this is a list of what is normally done and what I had done last year by my previous doctor" he stated as he handed me a printout of tests done exactly one year prior. I looked it over and asked, "Are you having any medical problems currently?" "None, I'm perfectly well, thank you." "OK, great," I replied. I went on to ask about any previous medical issues or family or genetic problems that he was aware of. Other than a couple of uncles with early heart disease, he and his family had been remarkably healthy. I went through the results of lab tests that were more inclusive than any I had seen before. Arum had switched jobs and medical insurance about 6 months ago and was formerly with a "concierge" doctor in San Francisco. He was very interested in not only keeping healthy but wanted to ward off any possible illness that may be lurking under the surface. On his own, he researched every possibility that could be identified and went through this analysis in agreement with his previously willing doctor. Besides the "standard" labs that most doctors order for "physical" such as a CBC (complete blood count), liver, kidney, glucose/sugar, and cholesterol panel, Arum had many more pages of tests including those for every possible endocrine disorder (thyroid, adrenal, pituitary, testosterone, growth hormone), every nuance of cholesterol subunits, along with every conceivable lab marker for cancer available as well as a full panel of nearly all vitamin levels. "Wow," I said, "this is an extraordinarily extensive laboratory analysis and extremely expensive," I said, thinking this likely represented thousands of dollars of blood tests. Then I added with some emphasis "fortunately, everything was in the normal range just last year!" In addition to lab tests, Arum had also had an EKG, echocardiogram and a treadmill test to evaluate his heart—all also normal. In the past few years, he had a brain MRI, endoscopy of stomach and colonoscopy, all in the name of "just in case" and for "completeness" according to his discussions with his primary care physician. "Wow," I said again and paused. "Well, I want to go over your physical examination but please tell me, what would you like me to do for you this year?" "Well, I think just repeating those tests last year should suffice, doctor, thank you." "Hmm," I said. Well, after a brief physical exam, I then spent the rest of our time going over the current scientific evidence and recommendations for testing someone in his health category (excellent) and age (<40) and it wasn't easy informing him that ALL the tests he had done were not part of a recommended medical evaluation as of 2020. However, I needed to first go into his understanding of what modern medicine can do and look for and predict in someone like him. While his personal Google research found all the possible tests available, it did not include an important aspect of prediction or need based on the level of incidence and potential harm from test results that are done for no reason. With scientific backup from the current and complete review collated by the US Preventive Services Task Force (USPSTF) we went over the current recommendations. On their website, there is a nice calculator to accurately inform anyone of the need or not of specific tests.

In Arum's case, the ONLY screening recommended was a blood pressure check and HIV test. He could be eligible for other STD testing if he had any risky behavior (which he denied). He asked why he didn't need to get even a cholesterol, diabetes or other "routine" lab tests like a check on his kidneys, liver, blood count, electrolytes or the ever-popular Vitamin D level? Why not check all his endocrine organs like his thyroid, adrenals, testosterone, etc.? Why not check for various blood markers of cancer such as PSA (prostate), CEA (colon), etc.? The "check just in case" argument is made both by patients and physicians often as a default to convince them that one is a "good doctor" or a "properly concerned patient". The reasons for not doing a mountain of tests has to do with answering a few important questions from a scientifically based data standpoint. These include: Is the screening test for a disease accurate enough to determine if the problem is present? Is there a sufficient chance (the incidence) that mass screening of various populations (age or sex) will identify those with a problem often enough to justify testing? And crucially, what should the time interval be for testing for potential problems that are asymptomatic (e.g. yearly or longer)? And, if a problem is identified, is there proven treatment that can eventually prevent death or serious complication of the problem without a significant risk of harm from the treatment (example—treating high cholesterol with medications in young people)?

Many folks are surprised, as Arum was, that in large data analysis of populations of folks under the age of 40 there is NO supportive data for doing any lab tests on someone who is well! There is an exception if one has a strong family history of diabetes, say one's parents and siblings have type 2 diabetes, then yearly lab testing is a helpful screening test to monitor and consider treatment for uncontrolled diabetes which is occurring more frequently in the younger sedentary, obese population. One of the biggest questions I have encountered is "what about my cholesterol, doctor?" Well, there are NO studies on medical treatment of younger individuals (<40) with statins for long periods of time analyzing the benefits or danger of treatment for 10, 20, 30 years or longer.

Statin treatment once it is determined to be necessary, is usually needed for lifetime. There is shown benefit from the "Mediterranean Diet" in lowering cholesterol and prevention of heart attacks, so it may be beneficial to know if one's cholesterol is elevated to consider this change. Also, regular exercise has been shown to protect against heart attacks and the more the better. So, these can also be recommended as the "best" form of treatment in a younger person.

Some genetic prone diseases are worth getting checked if present in the family. An unusual but treatable problem is hemochromatosis, a disease that causes buildup of iron in the liver and other organs. This can be tested easily and if identified and present is treated simply with intermittent blood removable to keep the level of iron in a low range. For women with a mother or sibling or several aunts with early breast cancer or ovarian cancer (under age 50), genetic testing for BRCA 1/2 is now recommended.

It is very common for patients to come in for a "physical" after hearing of a family member, friend or a horrible story about someone who was suddenly diagnosed with terminal, metastatic cancer or dropped dead from an aneurysm or heart attack or stroke at an age similar to the patient. Usually the visit starts off with "Doc, I want a *complete medical check* today" in an urgent and worried voice. My best way to get at the core of the concern is to then simply ask, "OK, what are you worried about and what do you want to check?" Then the full story of the recent tragedy unfolds quickly. Most patients are surprised and fortunately most are reassured that *their* individual risk of medical disaster at a young age is low and that current guidelines do not recommend any testing for most problems that are rare in a young person. Of course, some folks remained worried and "want everything done to check everything, *just in case*". These issues bring into play the very real limitations of modern medicine to predict the future of individuals with current testing and technology.

As a complex example, let's talk about one worrisome and devastating medical disaster, *cerebral aneurysms*. The prevalence in the general population of a brain aneurysm is about 2 in a hundred people who can have one or more. However, the rate of *an aneurysm rupturing* is about 1 in 10,000. The bad thing is that a ruptured aneurysm can either kill you or cause severe brain damage in at least half of those unlucky enough to have that event. Bigger aneurysms rupture easier. However, treatment of an aneurysm is risky business and difficult. The rate of post-surgical death or severe disability from a stroke or brain damage is about 1 in 5 (20%), quite high by any surgical standard. So, it is recommended to *not* screen anyone for an aneurysm (the screening test is a magnetic resonance angiogram using an MRI machine) unless there are 2 or more first-degree relatives who have been diagnosed with one. However, even with this limited recommendation the test found only about 9 percent incidence and a reduction of mortality after surgical treatment has not been definitively proven as of yet. The serious threat of the treatment possibly being worse than doing nothing has kept the aggressive approach of screening and surgery at bay.

Preventative care does not mean doing tests for all people at any time. There are several studies that have been shown to save lives and be cost effective if done at the right time and correct interval. Colonoscopy is one such test. While its alternative test, stool occult blood testing or the more advanced Cologuard looking for cancer DNA in stool, is an option, these are still not as accurate or complete or preventative. If one has a positive stool test, you then need to have a full colonoscopy. A colonoscopy has two great advantages. One, it directly examines the entire colon and if nothing is found then the patient is in the clear for quite a long time. Currently, that means 10 years before any other testing or colonoscopy needs to be done again. Second, if a polyp or abnormal finding is found, the gastroenterologist can then and there remove all the polyps and also biopsy anything that looks abnormal. Removing all polyps has a great preventative treatment advantage in that the vast majority of colon cancers arise from a polyp which can then slowly transform into a cancer, so no polyps, no cancer. Colonoscopy is currently recommended starting at age 45 (updated recommendation in 2021) for those without a family history or a genetic condition lending an increased risk. If so, then early testing is recommended, this means starting screening at age 40 or 10 years before the earliest age of onset in a family member. The risk for complications with colonoscopy is quite low while its benefit to detect early cancer, remove polyps and prevent death is well established. This is one preventative test proven to save lives and be cost effective.

Other screening cancer tests are not nearly as beneficial or as proven as colonoscopy. Certainly, screening for cancers of blood, kidney, pancreas, brain, bladder, liver, stomach, lung, or bone have *no* data to support testing in patients who do not have a family history or determined genetic risk. Even with close family members affected, it is very difficult to determine when and how often and how beneficial screening testing is to be used as most cancers occur (>95%) by random chance and not by genetic inheritance. In fact, it is estimated that most of us will develop a random cancer in our body several times during our lifetime and that our ever-vigilant immune system will detect it and get rid of it. This is the main reason why cancers mostly occur as we get older. Our aging immune system is not as robust as fighting off small cancers and they then can progress and develop into something more significant. While there are many biotech companies in 2021 trying to develop a "blood sample biopsy" for various cancers that might be detected early, nothing as of yet has been proven to be reliable as a detection lab test and even more important nothing is known about what can or should be done if one is detected as these would likely be very early and often non progressive cancer.

Let's look at two other cancer screenings and their controversial benefits, difficulties, limitations and current recommendations namely, breast cancer screening with mammography and prostate cancer screening with PSA blood testing.

Breast cancer screening has more data and more intense emotional reactions than any other preventative test. Since the adoption of modern X-ray mammography in the late 1970s there have been studies on trying to figure out whether it does any good for the past 40 years enrolling literally millions of women. The technical aspects of mammography have advanced over the years with *digital* mammography starting in 2000 and then *3D digital* mammography coming in 2011. Interestingly, the studies have not shown that the new technologies are actually superior to detecting suspicious lesions.

Before going into an analysis of all this data on mammography, it is important to point out that for many decades it has also been recommended for women to also undergo either "clinical breast examination"—that being done by a physician or "self-breast examination"—that being done by the patient. Unfortunately, none of the studies on regularly physically examining women's breasts has shown that it detects breast cancer any more frequently or earlier than not and as a result has not shown to save any lives. While it is a benign and relatively easy procedure, it can be falsely reassuring if normal or falsely alarming if a lump is found that appears to be new. All the breast examination studies did show a higher chance of finding a lump that required either another mammogram or biopsy or both but was not sensitive to detect new cancers overall. Currently in 2023, there is not a strong recommendation for this practice although some specialty medical organizations still promote it. Clinical breast examination done by a doctor would seem to be a good idea. However, physicians are not any better in finding abnormal lumps than women who self-check on a regular basis. The time and expense of doing "clinical breast exams" has been deemed a waste of medical resources for no benefit.

How well does mammography do in detecting breast cancer and more importantly preventing death from breast cancer? This is a complex topic and there are voluminous papers written on the collected data over the past 30 years. It is certain that since mammography became widespread in the early 1980s breast cancer was found much more frequently and at an earlier stage. Smaller suspicious tumors of less than an inch were found much more frequently. Overall, there has been a reduction in mortality from breast cancer over the past 40 years from about 7 per 1000 women to 5 per 1000 over the course of the time in women aged 50-60 years. However, there have also been significant improvements in treatments during this period so it has not been easy to separate which has been more important. The other issue is that many small cancers do not progress although the treatment for these, which is often quite aggressive with surgery and chemotherapy, can contribute to overtreatment or overdiagnosis as all of these are classified equally as a "breast cancer". The best overall estimate of the benefit of mammograms was nicely summarized in the *New England of Medicine* a few years ago. They summarized the available data in an easily understandable format in the age group of women in the 50-60-year age range (where some studies have found some benefit). In analyzing women younger than this, the studies are inconclusive in conferring *any* benefit to mammograms in regards to the rate of death. That is because women under age 50 are generally pre-menopausal and breast cancer is much more uncommon and tends to behave differently and more aggressively than in an older woman. In the 50-60 age group in women who do *not* undergo mammograms their rate of death from breast cancer is 5 in 1000. In the same cohort of women who undergo mammograms every other year (the current recommendation) the mortality rate is 4 in 1000. So, one woman's life out of a thousand tested is saved after 10 years of biannual mammography. The question is, is this benefit worthwhile? Considering that about 1 in 10 mammograms are read as "abnormal" and in need of further testing, biopsy or surgery and that about 1 in 10 of the abnormal mammograms shows some form of early cancer we are talking about a significant amount of anxiety and medical cost. The real question is: does mammography catch an early breast cancer at the right time that its removal would *truly* cure the patient? Given that many early breast cancers do not progress at all or very slowly and that there is an indolent form known as Ductal Carcinoma in situ (DCIS) which progress only in half the cases, many of these treated cancers have no impact on future life expectancy or if treated at a later stage (discovered by a lump) would be equally curative. Also, as mammography only prevents a small percentage of deaths, it does not detect cancers that have already spread and will be deadly regardless. The current recommendation from the CDC is for women to have mammograms every 2 years beginning at age 40 until age 74. A discussion of the risks versus the benefits is recommended due to possible false positive or false negative results and radiation exposure. For women over age 74, where breast cancer becomes significantly less common and less deadly, there is no benefit to continued mammography shown in scientific studies. These recommendations are for "average" risk women. Those with family history of breast cancer or a possible genetic risk such as BRCA mutations are recommended to be screened earlier than 40. In my view, while I support the recommendations for women getting mammograms, it is far from a great screening tool. However, it is the only one we currently have. With the limitations of catching a dangerous early cancer, the significant amount of false positives, the expense and difficulty of evaluating every "abnormal" result it doesn't serve to be reassuring or that helpful overall. Many experts and even some countries have claimed that mammograms are not useful enough to recommend them. This limited benefit hasn't stopped the very aggressive marketing and sometimes shaming of women demanding that all get and have access to mammograms by various organizations.

Let's move to a parallel situation involving men. Namely, prostate cancer screening with the use of the blood test PSA which stands for prostate specific antigen. While prostate cancer is the leading cancer diagnosis for men in the US, it is the second leading cause of cancer *death* in men (behind lung cancer). Like breast cancer in women, prostate cancer death rates have decreased nearly 50% in the past 30 years since PSA testing became widespread. This decrease is due to increased detection of early and sometimes benign (minimally progressive cancers) and also due to advances in treatment (like breast cancer). Unlike breast cancer, prostate cancer increases in men as they age but most are unlikely to have symptoms or to die from having it. In autopsy studies of men who died of other causes, prostate cancer is present in 30% of men aged 50 and rises to 70% for men in their seventies proving that prostate cancer is a common and slow growing indolent disease for most elderly men. These percentages are much higher than those actually diagnosed with the disease. In the US, the lifetime risk of dying from prostate cancer for men is 2.4%. So, the vast majority of men die of something other than prostate cancer.

The PSA test was discovered by Richard Ablin, PhD in 1970 while working on the immunologic aspects of prostate cancer. While this protein was initially found to be produced by prostate cancer, it was later found to be produced naturally by the prostate gland. It does not have any immunologic or cancer promoting properties. Its main correlation is that the level of PSA went down after the removal of a cancerous prostate. The FDA approval in 1986 was for monitoring patients *after* treatment of prostate cancer to determine if there was a recurrence. This is still its main function today. If there is a significant rise in the PSA after surgery or radiation treatment, then it is nearly certain due to cancer recurrence and the possible spread to other tissues. In 1994 the FDA then approved the test as a screening tool for men over the age of 50, although physicians and mostly urologists had been using the test off-label before this to screen patients. The contested issue at the time of approval for screening was that it was well known that the *false-positive rate* of the test was 78%! This means that the test *wrongly* classifies someone as having cancer 4 out of 5 times. It was an apparently very hotly contested debate at the time for the advisory board of the FDA but ended up passing and became a standard "preventative" test until an extensive review in 2014 changed the recommendation to be a "discussion of the risks versus the benefits with the patient and the physician and to not routinely do this test". So, it is no longer on the checklist of things to be done reflexively. However, it is actually still done very commonly and matter-of-factly by most primary care physicians and urologists today. What's the problem with this and why is it done so frequently? Well, the problem is that this test is reported as a level of PSA in the blood (<4 is generally thought to be OK) which, unfortunately, has no definitive level telling if cancer is present or not. This means that even at a very low level, e.g. 0.05, a man could still be harboring an early cancer and that at a very high level such as 30 there may be no cancer as a normal or inflamed prostate could just be overproducing this protein. An abnormal level typically triggers a trip to the urologist for a biopsy for which it is standard to get 12 core samples from different parts of the gland. If a cancer is found, the sample then undergoes an additional complex laboratory evaluation and then other tests are done to determine if cancer has spread to outside the prostate. The problem then becomes the treatment. There has been a growing consideration to consider no treatment in early, low grade cases over the past 10 years, as it has been found the majority of these will not progress to invasive or metastatic cancer and the "watch and wait" approach is as scientifically beneficial as the definitive treatment approach. The issue with attempted curative treatment is that the choice is either surgery to remove the entire prostate or radiation treatment to destroy the entire prostate and both result in a significant amount of morbidity or bodily harm. The two most common side effects of either treatment are impotence and urinary incontinence, both of which can become life-long problems for the treated patient. The usual counteracting force in a man's mind when he hears the word cancer is to "get that thing out of there ASAP!", so the discussion of "we can wait and see what happens" is mostly untenable even though it has no downside or side effects. So how good is PSA screening for men? After an extensive re-evaluation in 2018 the US Preventative Task Force changed its recommendations to strongly advise: 1) no screening in men over the age of 70, and 2) not recommend screening in men between 55 and 69 until a discussion of the risks and benefits had taken place. They recommended no screening in men under the age of 55. However, they were careful to point out the men who had a family history of prostate cancer and Black men (who have a higher incidence) should be considered for early screening. The reasoning behind this change is that the data did not support a reduction in the death rate from prostate cancer in screening in older and younger men as noted above. Interestingly, the data showed a very mild reduction in mortality for men aged 55-69. About 1 in a 1000 men screened over a 13-year period which is similar to the effect for mammogram screening for breast cancer in women of similar age. However, in real life the answer from patients to the question of "Do you want to have a blood test for possible prostate cancer?" is always "Why not?" and "If it doesn't cost anything, sure" is commonly heard. So, even though the accuracy is low, the finding of a low-grade cancer can be benign and harms from treatment are significant, this test will likely continue for the foreseeable future until a more accurate screening test is discovered (if one actually exists). Tellingly, the discoverer of the PSA test, Dr. Ablin, has condemned using it for screening as in his analysis he found it not specific or accurate enough. In 2014 he wrote a book supporting his position and its history called *The Great Prostate Hoax* criticizing the billions spent on the testing and medical service involved in its use.

Let's shift back to women with the screening for cervical cancer. The famous PAP test was universally adopted in the 1950s after being developed by the Greek pathologist George Papanicolaou in the 1940s.

He was able to definitively identify uterine and cervical cancers under the microscope in comparison to normal cells. The use of this brilliant, simple and inexpensive screening test led to the remarkable reduction of cervical cancers and deaths from this disease by 70% since its routine adoption by western countries! The standard of care had been yearly PAP testing for all women. The next major advancement in the knowledge of this cancer is when the German physician, Dr. Harald Zur Hausen, proved that cervical cancer was due to an infection of the HPV (human papillomavirus), a sexually transmitted virus after working on this for over 2 decades. Dr. Zur Hausen co-shared the 2008 Nobel Prize for his discovery. This led to the development of a test for the virus in cervical tissue and an effective vaccine that was introduced in 2006 and improved and expanded to its present form in 2014 that includes 9 subtypes covering the vast majority of cancer-causing strains (Gardasil 9). HPV infection has been known to be the cause of sexually transmitted anogenital warts for quite some time before being proved the cause of cervical cancer. It is a treatable problem by locally removing the warts but is not a curable condition. HPV is now also known to be the cause of most oropharyngeal cancers, anal cancers, and most vaginal and penile cancers. Since the introduction and extensive use of the HPV vaccines over the past decade it has been shown to be very effective in preventing HPV infections and its widespread use will most likely also greatly reduce the incidence of those cancers caused by it over the coming decades. The vaccine is recommended to be given to girls and boys starting about age 12 in order to prevent infection before becoming sexually active. As there is an accurate test for HPV, women who test negative for the virus are eligible to get vaccinated up to age 45. Even though the PAP test has been well ingrained into women's health for over half a century, the landscape and recommendations are changing in light of the power of HPV testing directly and the vaccine. HPV testing is somewhat similar to a PAP test in that a sample of cells is taken from the cervix but it is tested directly for the presence of the virus. One can also get cells at the same time to perform a standard PAP test and many times both are done. Because of the complexity of newer testing accuracy, women are no longer recommended to get yearly PAP tests. Currently, the schedule includes NO testing (PAP or HPV) for women less than 21 years old due to the very low incidence of cervical cancer and because HPV infection takes many years to induce cancer. After age 21 until age 29, there are two options—1) PAP testing every three years or 2) HPV testing at age 25. Women aged 30-65 have three options: 1) HPV testing every five years, 2) Co-testing PAP and HPV testing every five years or 3) PAP testing every 3 years. For women over 65 years, it is safe to discontinue any testing if all testing over the previous 25 years has been negative. However, some experts advocate continued screening until age 74 or even age 80 if there has been no prior screening. These recommendations are for women with average risk (no family history, not immunosuppressed). Certainly, this is much easier for women than the previous practice of yearly PAP tests for life which in my experience many older women found painful and unnecessary. Cervical cancer is actually somewhat unusual for general physicians practicing in the US. In my 35 years of practice, there had been only a handful of women I directly cared for who had the disease. And in nearly all, they were elderly, immigrant, women who never had any prior screening and unfortunately, had their cancers discovered at a late and deadly stage. One side note is that women who have had a hysterectomy (which most commonly includes removing the cervix) *never* need another PAP test afterwards, which, unfortunately, has been done for the "just in case" rationale.

The most common cancer in the world for both men and women is lung cancer and the greatest risk factor is smoking. The risk increases with the number of cigarettes per day and the number of years one smokes. Quitting smoking cuts the risk of future smoking depending on the length of time one is smoke free. So, for someone who quit 15 years ago their chance of lung cancer is reduced by at least 80 percent! Since lung cancer is the leading cause of cancer related death, there has been a steady push to try to screen for early, treatable lung cancer as later stage lung cancer has nearly a 100% mortality rate even with new treatments. About 75% of new lung cancers are diagnosed at a late stage.

In the 1970s, researchers looked at screening with plain chest X-rays in smokers but could not find any reduction of death rate as compared to no screening, so this was abandoned. As CT scanning became more available, the current technique of Low Dose Chest CT scanning (LDCT) has been used as a screening tool. The USPTF (US Preventative Task Force) first recommended routine screening for current or former smokers in 2013 and has recently revised its recommendations in 2021. The current recommendations include: all persons aged fifty to eighty who have a twenty pack-year smoking history (smoking one pack of cigarettes per day for twenty years or the equivalent) and either are currently smoking or have quit less than fifteen years prior should undergo yearly LDCT scanning. The recommendations include a discussion of the potential benefits, limitations and harms of regular screening. These recommendations were devised based on a significant accumulation of international data and discussion in detail of the limitations and hazards of screening. The overall benefit of screening has been determined to be about a 20% reduction in lung cancer mortality which is due to finding earlier stage cancers. Although this benefit is limited, it is in contrast to the five-year survival rate of all lung cancer patients which is only one in five or 80% mortality rate. Of course, as we have seen with other screening tests, there are the problems of false positives where the scan shows a problem that is *not* a cancer, the potential of complications from a lung biopsy or surgery and the psychologic distress of getting the news of a possible cancer. Unfortunately, finding a small cancer also does not necessarily mean that it has not already spread as the biology of lung cancer is not easily predicted based on a CT scan. Like many areas in medicine, this is a complex topic, and the answer is not a simple one to screen or not to screen when the test is not as accurate as one would like. It's important to understand the limitations of the technology for screening as we currently have in modern medicine.

What about screening for the most common killer in the world, cardiovascular disease? Cardiovascular disease includes heart attacks (coronary artery disease/blockages), strokes and "other" vascular (blood vessel) problems such as blockage of an artery in the aorta or legs. In this category we are talking about folks who have NOT had a cardiovascular event or defined problem and also do NOT have any definitive symptoms suggestive of a current problem. Those patients with disease require definitive testing and ongoing treatment and monitoring for their medical condition. The risk of having significant cardiovascular disease increases with each additional known risk factor such as: cigarette smoking, hypertension, diabetes, high cholesterol and a family member who had a cardiovascular event at a young age (<60).

There are several different tests that are available to screen for coronary heart disease that vary from the simple EKG (electrocardiogram), to exercise stress testing, pharmacologic stress testing and the newest test, CT scan coronary calcium scoring.

In regards to screening special circumstances, let's separate out those people in whom there is public safety or high-risk activity that a regulatory agency has determined the need for routine evaluation to prevent a disaster, for example: airline pilots, bus drivers, scuba divers.

There is general agreement from the main medical organizations who have looked at the predictive ability of the simple resting EKG in that it provides *no* value in screening patients for coronary heart disease and do not recommend its use as a screening tool. This does not include the possibility of rhythm disturbances or intrinsic electric heart abnormalities. The problem with the standard resting EKG is that up to *half* of individuals with normal coronary arteries can have EKG abnormalities. Conversely, about a third of those with severe blockages will have a normal EKG.

The most common test to screen for coronary disease in order to prevent a heart attack is the exercise stress test. This can be done with or without echocardiography which enhances the positive predictive capability of detecting unknown coronary blockages. This test indirectly identifies coronary blockages by seeing changes in the exercising cardiogram at a progressively higher level of physical effort. Most stress tests are done either with someone walking on a treadmill or pedaling a stationary bicycle. If a patient cannot do either exercise due to arthritis or severe physical deconditioning then the test can be performed by injecting a radioactive substance that causes the heart rate to be increased and the result can show areas of likely blocked coronary arteries.

In evaluating the data on doing exercise or pharmacologic stress testing on asymptomatic individuals without known heart disease, there is an increased predictive value of a fatal heart attack in men but not necessarily in women. However, the predictive value of current cardiovascular risk calculators which take into account the age and various risk factors mentioned, physicians routinely prescribe preventative treatment with statins, blood pressure medicines, diet and lifestyle changes which substantially reduce the individual's chance of a heart attack. Therefore, all the major organizations (US Preventative Task Force, American College of Cardiology, American College of Physicians) do NOT recommend stress test screening for *asymptomatic* persons.

It is important to note that finding any significant abnormality on stress testing, the next decision to be made is to proceed with coronary angiography or not. This is an invasive procedure that is *not* used as a screening test but is a diagnostic and treatment modality for coronary artery blockages using current stenting technologies.

Over the past 10 years there has been a rise in use of a CT scan of the heart to obtain both a score of the calcium buildup in the coronary arteries and to determine if there are blockages by this noninvasive technique. Currently, there is consensus on its recommended use in screening certain individuals, namely, in those with moderate risk asymptomatic individuals over the age of forty and less than seventy. It is not recommended in low risk or high-risk patients (as they need more definitive testing) or in patients outside the above age limits. The results are used as a way to determine if an asymptomatic individual will benefit from therapeutic measures such as statins and are not used to determine if someone needs an angiogram.

In summary, currently it is not recommended for asymptomatic patients to undergo regular stress testing as a screening test for possible coronary artery disease. Screening for cardiovascular risk and active treatment of high blood pressure, elevated cholesterol, diabetes, smoking cessation, improved diet and increased exercise are proven to reduce cardiovascular events and death.

An important tool that I have mentioned is the use of the *cardiovascular risk calculator*. It is easy for one to do this with a simple internet search. The data used are: age, gender, race, blood pressure, total cholesterol, HDL cholesterol (good cholesterol level), and presence or absence for hypertension, diabetes, or cigarette smoker. The likelihood of having a heart attack or stroke over the next 10 years is calculated as a *percent such as 5% (low), 15% (moderate), 30% (high)*. What this means is that if one has a 10% chance of a cardiovascular event over the next 10 years, the odds are 1 in 10 of an occurrence. To frame this another way, one would have a 90% likelihood of *not* having a heart attack or stroke. This calculator is used *only* to recommend a statin to lower cholesterol. There is some controversy on the cut-off of when to prescribe a statin. The conservative recommendation is 7.5% or higher but other experts such as Rita Reddit at UCSF recommend a cut-off of 10% or higher. Still, the majority of either group would not have a heart attack or stroke over the next ten years. The use of statins has been well proven to *half* the risk of heart attack if taken regularly. A powerful reduction but in the real-world calculation with a risk of heart attack of 10%, one hundred patients would have to take the medication regularly for 10 years in order to prevent 5 heart attacks or strokes by the end of that period. Therefore, 90 patients would have not been any different from taking the medication and 5 patients that took the medication would have a heart attack or stroke anyway. This does not mean statins are not important in preventing cardiovascular events as they are a definite method of prevention. However, it's important to point out that all the risk calculators do not include the interventions of diet or exercise to mitigate one's chances of avoiding a heart attack or stroke. There is actually good scientific data that following the Mediterranean diet which is mostly plant-based and low in saturated fats can reduce one's risk by about 25%. For exercise, the reduction in risk is up to about a third (25-40%) for those who do moderate exercise 5 hours per week. So, the combined effects of proper diet and regular exercise can have a similar risk reduction as taking a statin daily. There is not much current data on the overall reduction of cardiovascular events on doing all these in combination but it is likely there is an additive effect although to what degree is not well studied.

Since most cardiovascular events occur by sudden blood clot in a coronary artery or brain artery, many experts have advocated the use of aspirin as a prevention. There is sound evidence for those who have established coronary disease or prior strokes or significant peripheral arterial disease to take aspirin daily but for everybody else taking aspirin does as much harm (bleeding risk) as good and is no longer recommended for general use.

So where are left with the good 'ol *annual exam* or *yearly physical* or *routine checkup* or *wellness visit* or *preventative care* or anything else that a visit to the doctor when not sick is called? Well, in an excellent review of the topic in the journal *JAMA* (*Journal of the American Medical Association*) in 2021 concluded that general health checks, while not proven to reduce mortality (death) or heart attacks or strokes, were able to identify chronic diseases such as high blood pressure and diabetes. Also, they did assist in patients having preventative measures updated and helped reduce risk factors for disease and were associated with happier patients. The overall recommendation was to offer physicals to patients at high risk of disease occurrence and generally lower health. However, a precise schedule for these visits is not known and the cost and utilization of the healthcare system for these has not been determined to be beneficial to society in general. One benefit that is difficult to measure but likely important is the enhanced interpersonal relationship between doctors and patients from regular checkups.

CHAPTER 20

The Brown Journal

As I sit here at the end of 2021, the end of my first year of retirement trying to write this book, I quietly notice that there are on my desk the last 2 issues of the *New England Journal of Medicine* waiting for me. The *Journal* started in Boston as a quarterly medical and philosophical publication in 1812 then to a weekly edition in 1828. It was purchased in 1921 by the Massachusetts Medical Society for $1 and then changed its name several years later to its current title. It is and has been predominantly a journal that publishes peer reviewed medical scientific studies, up to date reviews of medical topics, unusual case studies reviewed by an expert, editorial opinions on its articles and views of opinions on a variety of medically related topics. Its cover page is white with the name, date and logo and the list of articles. It does get financial support from advertisements (largely drug companies) and subscriptions and contains at the back a classified ad section for physician job openings around the country. Like all print journals, magazines and newspapers the *Journal* joined the internet age in 1996 and has opened its archive to the public for all its non-current articles.

My first real interaction with the *Journal* occurred during my internship when I was in my first year of Internal Medicine residency at the Faulkner Hospital in Boston. On rounds with the senior residents and chief of staff, there were mentions of certain recent or past studies that could apply to a specific case we were treating. It was astounding, fascinating and somewhat unbelievable how others had the time and memory to absorb all this medical data and then speak of it with confidence, articulation and analysis that seemed way beyond my chronically sleep deprived brain. Being able to recall and cite a *Journal* article was the height of medical intellectual ability and also somewhat showmanship as it was and still is the most prestigious medical journal in the world well ahead of the British journal *The Lancet* and *JAMA* (*Journal of the American Medical Association*). To be published in the *Journal* is such an honor, it can make one's career complete. Being in Boston and having a certain number of prominent medical institutions closeby and being in a teaching hospital associated with Tuft's and Havard's medical schools, some of the senior staff physicians knew of and knew personally some of the authors of these prestigious studies. In some way, the *Journal* felt like *our* own and we understood its importance quite well. We became more directly aware when copies of important articles relative to specific cases appeared during morning rounds for us to review and to briefly discuss. While there was always a copy of the most recent and the past years *Journals* in the hospital library where we could make a copy of certain articles, nearly all the medical residents eventually subscribed to the *Journal* themselves. Fortunately, the cost for a subscription was and is quite affordable for physicians in training. Its arrival each week in the mail seemed to occur so quickly that we usually found them stacked on our desks awaiting to be read. As the mailed version was always wrapped in brown paper that needed to be torn off to get to its white cover, that stack of unopened *Journals* became known as the stack of "brown journals". For many years now the *Journal* arrives in the mail wrapped in clear plastic, but all older internists are knowledgeable of its slang name when we chat about the not-so-old days.

The editors of the *NEJM* were held in the highest esteem and often spoke and wrote about political issues related to medical care and the ethics of medicine and publishing scientific studies. Arnold Relman was the editor-in-chief during my residency and beyond. He held the post for 23 years from 1977 to 1991. He was an early advocate for single payer health care as the costs for care began to skyrocket and he coined the phrase "Medical-Industrial Complex" as the corporate takeover of many aspects of the profession crept in. He also brought to the *Journal* and medical publishing community the concept of "conflict of interest" which meant that authors had to disclose any financial incentives in their research to make publishing more transparent such as support or payment by a drug company. He was a beacon and a clear voice for medical care and physicians.

Each week the *Journal* included a problem-solving case from the famous Massachusetts General Hospital. The case would proceed in the exact way it unfolded when a patient came to the hospital. For example, "a 60-year-old woman with chest pain and a fever presented to the ER." What was fascinating was that as a physician in training, one could follow along with the chronological details of the case as the guest expert would analyze each step and discuss in detail the history, the diagnostic findings and the possibilities. This would include at each stage all the possible diseases that the patient *could* have, known as the *differential diagnosis*. Just by following the rationale as the expert considered the possible causes and eliminating others was itself a big learning experience in deductive reasoning. The hook of this is the expert did *not* know the final true diagnosis and he or she had to work through the case to get to the crucial point of deciding what specific lab test, radiologic exam or even a biopsy would give the answer. The end of the discussion of all the relevant information often ended with "and a diagnostic procedure was performed". One could feel the heat rising as the expert gave his answer and then gave his opinion on the final diagnosis and a discussion of the rationale. Obviously, if he was wrong this would be a big professional embarrassment. However, and amazingly, it was quite rare that they got it wrong! Most of these cases are either so unusual or have such disparate symptoms they can be quite difficult to solve.

During my second year of residency, we heard that our Chief of Medicine, Andrew Huvos, M.D., was selected for a case study that would be presented and then printed in the *Journal*. The case presentation takes place usually a few months before it is printed and occurs in real time with all the physicians involved with the case, the experts and case moderator meeting together at the Mass General Hospital conference room. The actual case presentation is the same that occurs at "Grands Rounds" at all teaching hospitals around the country where an interesting or unusual case is presented with the history, physical findings and laboratory and radiologic data in order to tell the story. Dr Huvos was going to be given a case in his specialty, cardiology, to solve. "The Eggman" (as he was called because his name was close to the Spanish word for egg, *huevos*) presided over daily morning rounds in his office. He was a quiet, soft spoken, introspective man originally from Hungary who usually sat listening attentively with his hands in an open prayer formation as he tapped the tips of fingers slowly together while listening to anxious residents present the patients who were admitted the previous night. This daily exercise created such a sense of need to perform and to be precise that it drove motivation to do all the correct things the night before and to prepare the presentation in such a way that there would be nothing left out to ask about. Unfortunately, disheveled, sleepless interns and residents were prone to forget at least one important aspect of the case. However, the rested, relaxed "Eggman" who seemed to know everything in general Internal Medicine could go right to missing data elements directly after the intern had finished. I recall many of these that had a short pause of silence and then he would ask the pertinent question such as "and what was the BUN (blood urea nitrogen level)?" After which one would fumble through the sheets of loose paper to find it while a facial flush grew to bright red as the rest of us cringed in our seats understanding the importance to the case. With these background experiences, we all awaited with great anticipation Dr. Huvos' case in the *Journal*. When it finally arrived on its usual Thursday delivery in the mail and we saw his name under the case title, all of us went right to it to read every word but first we had to check if he got it right and when we saw the final diagnosis matched his, a little cheer and pump fist went out. His case was a ridiculously complex cardiology case of a woman with a disease most had not encountered or even knew about, namely *Pulmonary Veno-occlusive disease*. This is where small blood clots slowly occur in the veins of the lungs causing blood flow problems, heart failure, shortness of breath and oxygenation problems. To get to the correct diagnosis one needed to understand the intricacies of the internal heart pressures and blood gas measurements as well the details of the echographic details and all the other radiographic and lab tests to get to why this woman was experiencing the common symptom of progressive shortness of breath in this very unusual way. His explanation in the *Journal* was a brilliant masterclass in understanding the interplay of heart and lung physiology. The next morning in daily rounds we all congratulated him and gave him a standing ovation which he demurely thanked us and went on with the cases at hand. Afterward the chief resident asked him to please go over how he was able to figure out such a tough case so well. "Well......" he started off slowly and methodically and then went through the important points again in a step wise, logical way that we all seemed to understand clearly. Truly one of the most memorable teaching points that would have almost no impact on our careers as internists. However, because of being exposed to this rare disease we could then include it in our differential diagnosis of complex cases in the ICU while trying to impress him or the other cardiologists in our hospital on rounds. The Eggman was our hero for that entire week and also for our entire residency because of that one case study in the *Journal!*

Every week the *Journal* published a group of letters sent in as a discussion dissenting opinions of previous recent articles but also some on various interesting topics and short unusual cases. Although not as prestigious as having a formal scientific study published, having a letter published amongst the hundreds the *Journal* received each week was quite an honor in itself. Many of these short letters were concisely written and provided other insights and thoughtful criticisms of important published studies but also had a flavor of literary panache when writing about random topics and experience in medicine. One of our admitting physicians who held board certification in dermatology and internal medicine had a letter published and it became the talk of the lunch table. Our discussion, however, quickly shifted to get a letter published on the various sexual escapades of one of our beloved residents, Ramon. The hilarious depictions of his physical exploits with a certain, sweet, attractive, shy radiology technician were infamous and we anxiously awaited for the next installment in order to live vicariously at our Monday lunch. Per Ramon, most of their physical encounters occurred on the carpets of their apartments. Ramon was complaining how his knees were getting raw and it was becoming difficult for him to perform. We chided him, "Yeah, did you have any other symptoms, Ramon, such as a fever or flushing or sweating?" we asked while doubling over with laughter. "Well," he answered while slowly rubbing his chin, "I think I do definitely have some elevated temperature after we are done." "Well, this seems like a reportable case to me," Mark Hammel, one of colleagues, noted. Thus we engaged in writing a well constructed, scientific appearing letter documenting the systemic inflammation of certain physical activities performed on a rug and submitted it properly to the *Journal* for review and publication. Of course, Ramon was delighted with the prospect and even more so when we began calling him Rugmoan with an emphasis on the second syllable. Needless to say, it was never published but we did get a nice letter from the *Journal* thanking us for our efforts.

My relationship with the *NEJM* became somewhat personal after I started dating a woman I met at a Halloween party in Boston. She was the administrative assistant to Maria Angell, M.D., who was one of main editors at the *Journal* and who worked closely with Dr. Relman. Unfortunately, I couldn't get any inside scoops or advantage to get published from my loyal girlfriend. While my relationship ended after about a year, Drs. Relman and Angell eventually married after 40 years of work together and continued their alarming and informed opinions on the negative aspects of the structure of American medical care well into the 1990s and 2000s.

Years later, when I was looking to move from sunny Southern California to the Bay Area, I consulted the classified ads of the *Journal* and actually was offered a position listed there for a job in San Francisco. Thus facilitating my move to the Bay Area which began over 30 years ago.

The purpose and mission of the *Journal* has always been to provide the latest, most important, medical research and analysis to the practicing medical community worldwide. It has reported on such important events as the AIDS epidemic in the 1980s when the identification, testing and treatment were in its infancy. It is well known for publishing important scrutinized questions of treatment often with several lead articles defining a new paradigm of care. A simple example is the publishing of 4 large, well conducted studies in the same edition on the question of whether all adult patients should take aspirin on a daily basis to prevent heart attacks. The answer went against popular opinion in that those without heart disease or diabetes had no measurable benefit over the possibility of a serious complication such as bleeding. The tactic of publishing two or more research studies on the same topic to push forward the science of medical care has had a more significant impact on treatments being updated more rapidly than a single study can do. Quite plainly, doctors listen more attentively when there is growing preponderance of evidence for a specific treatment.

In general, the *Journal* has steered clear of political debate but for one of only 4 times in its history. All 35 editors condemned the handling of the Coronavirus pandemic by the Trump administration in the fall of 2020. They correctly pointed out that this "crisis was turned into a tragedy" by poorly handling testing, protective equipment supplies and preventative measures and by undermining our institutions the FDA and CDC. They bluntly stated the fact: "By relying on uninformed, opinionated non experts they were directly responsible for tens of thousands of excess deaths", by noting the administration's "dangerously incompetent" behavior.

For over 40 years my medical training and career has included the *Journal* in a real and professional moving way. The longest relationship of any type of publication in my life. Of course, like everyone, I don't have time or interest to read every article as many of the studies are in very specialized areas that don't have an impact on my need for a certain knowledge base. But, I do review the table of contents to see what is relevant or interesting and do read the conclusions of studies that have importance. I still like going through a case that seems interesting and also an occasional letter to continue my appreciation of the process of thinking in a medical analytic way.

While I initially paid for a subscription, when it ran out it began to arrive for free. This is not uncommon for medical journals to keep or increase their circulation numbers up. I don't plan on informing them that I am retired and may not need their generous support of my ongoing medical education. So, I guess I will continue my relationship with the *Journal* for as long as I am around to enjoy it.

CHAPTER 21

Shrinking and Shrinks

My four years of medical school followed by three years of internship and residency in Internal Medicine included only a six-week rotation in psychiatry to prepare for a lifetime of interaction and need for treatment of those suffering from mental health problems accompanying my patients over the next 35 years. That six-week rotation gave little clue to helping the real world of disabling anxiety and depression that was commonly present in my waiting room. For our rotation, my medical school mates and myself determined that it would be a "fun" escape from inner city hospitals to spend the rotation at a 1,000-bed inpatient psychiatric hospital for Veterans in rural Pennsylvania where we were housed and fed for free.

Coatesville, VA hospital opened in 1931 on a sprawling campus of buildings and facilities on 125 acres of land that included local farmland about an hour's drive west of Philadelphia. Its mission was to provide neuropsychiatric care to veterans. It was both a residential facility for veterans suffering from common disabling psychiatric diseases such as schizophrenia and manic depression of which there was no medical therapy until the 1950s but also included *shell shock* from war experience, namely PTSD (post-traumatic stress disorder). It expanded over the years after two world wars to become a significant residential facility where the severely incapacitated were housed and treated mostly as long-term institutionalized patients. The large amount of land for farming and animal husbandry allowed patients to use the land as therapy in a physical and mental manner while making the hospital partially self-sustaining. Unfortunately, due to a combination of changes to food procurement, growing civil rights for patients and newer medications for psychotic disorders shifted patient activities entirely away from the outdoor farming aspects during the 1960s and '70s. The scene that my medical school mates and I encountered in the early 1980s was one of long-term institutionalized, psychiatrically disabled patients who unfortunately had very little to do all day except to sit around smoking cigarettes between visits to the canteen for meals or visits with the physicians and the medical students in individual and group therapy. Patients were typically on a weekly schedule of individual and group therapy sessions that we attended and learned of their chronic conditions. At that time, most of the residents were from the more recent wars: WWII, the Korean conflict and Vietnam. Many of these patients had had difficulty with substance or alcohol abuse that made their psychiatric problems more complicated. Most had been residents for many years, some for decades, so there was a significant age range of young men in their 20s to those in their 70s.

Our schedule for the rotation was Monday to Friday 9-4 with weekends off. Since it was over an hour's drive, we usually drove out on Monday morning and stayed on campus during the week returning to Philadelphia on Friday afternoon. We were housed in one of the dormitories near the patients' housing. Our meals were taken in the same cafeterias of the veterans and at 8 in morning we found ourselves in line with the varied male patients displaying their mental health issues in plain sight while we were encased in a cloud of stale cigarette smoke. The food was downright awful and included the typical American diner style cuisine such as fried eggs, bacon, hashbrowns all dripping in oil with canned fruit and bitter, burnt coffee. However, for medical students free is free. Occasionally in line, we would encounter a patient we had seen in the clinic the day before and the reaction would be varied. The man might recognize us and nod or say hello, or it could be an awkward shyness and cowering away, or a boastful "hey, you're my new doctor, right?", or even a whisper asking for a cigarette or help "getting out of here". Seeing patients in the clinic with the staff psychiatrist was mostly an exercise in repetition of previous interactions. The patient's chart was usually many inches thick and of many volumes of various notes from the different staff that documented their clinical experience. Our teaching included mostly trying to understand the psychiatric disease classifications and the various medications the patients were on and the reasoning for the specific prescriptions. Many sessions with the patients were verbal battles during which the patient wanted to have more of a specific medication (usually tranquilizers or sleeping pills) or to change their medication to something else or to a previous one that they believed would help them more. Many of the severe, chronic schizophrenics still suffered dearly from auditory hallucinations and an inability to be present in the real world that the various medications available could only slightly tame. There was often an issue of whether the patients were actually swallowing their pills when their symptoms and behavior became more difficult. None of us there were interested in pursuing a career in psychiatry and this situation of institutionalized, chronic psychotic patients certainly confirmed our direction away from this discipline. After the clinic we were free in the evenings. I often would go for a jog around the campus and out into the local area for exercise. As it was springtime, it felt wonderful to get out into the fresh clear air in the rural countryside to clear my mind and refresh my body after a long day of difficult patients. I could see the extensive grounds where in the past patients worked the farm and took care of animals, all now managed privately. While our experience was not as dire as that portrayed in the 1975 movie *One Flew over the Cuckoo's Nest* which was set in the 1950s when frontal lobotomy was a more accepted treatment for severe mental illness, there was a pall of oppressive energy and little expectation of significant improvement in the vast majority of these patients. Our planned escape to the countryside turned into seeing the entrapment of severe mental illness on its unlucky victims. The patients were essentially there because they could not survive anywhere else. They did not have the mental capacity to take care of themselves, to work or to find housing and the vast majority did not have family that could undertake such a commitment. However, over the following ten years starting in the Reagan administration, many of these same patients were "released" into the public after the passing of the Mental Health Systems Act of 1980. Most of these patients could not navigate the "real" world and could not get to the treatment that helped, forcing many of them into a world of homelessness and substance abuse and early death. A problem that persists today, 40 years later.

Some evenings we went out to the local restaurants and bars. There we found the locals, many of whom worked at the hospital. In general, the hospital offered a better job than most in that area. On occasion, a patient would "leave" the hospital and be found drinking in one of the bars. One evening while we were relaxing at a local bar, the Bongo Club, we spotted a patient we had seen in clinic. This young, inebriated, manic-depressive man was quite animated and gregarious and came over to clink glasses in between playing darts and drinking shots of Jack Daniels with his beer. The bartenders were relaxed about the issue and called the hospital security to escort him back to campus. Yes, there was a locked gate, so it required some finesse to get out into the real world. Occasionally, someone would get far away after hitchhiking out of town on the King's Highway but we never heard of anyone permanently getting away. Personally, I was quite impressed with the earnest dedication of the staff who worked there. The nurses, physiotherapists and aides all looked after these men with great compassion and care. Our favorite day there was "Olympic Day" in which all sorts of outdoor activities and games were set up for the patients who were mostly quite excited to participate. Simple sports such as badminton, horseshoes, volleyball and crafts were set up around the campus and we helped out at various stations. There was an obvious fun "playground" atmosphere where many older patients wore smiles and sweat. The day was capped off with a BBQ including watermelon and ice cream and to me it seemed that more of this type of active interaction would have the best benefit for many of these unfortunate patients. The unavoidable impression of encountering these patients with severe mental illness is that their life is filled with discomfort and pain. Somewhat similar to those with chronic pain which has no obvious source but which is nonetheless relentless. Psychotic patients struggle with their minds flooding their consciousness with outside thoughts, fears and threats not present in reality. It is a continual barrage that is inescapable but can be mitigated and significantly lessened by many of newly available pharmacologic treatments. When the medications are effective it is visually apparent on the face of the patient that they are more relaxed and in a happier state of being and able to engage in normal conversation without the torture of intrusive thoughts jamming their consciousness.

Alas, in researching this essay I discovered Coatesville, VA is scheduled to close soon after 90 years due to downsizing into a smaller outpatient facility just outside Philadelphia while it had transitioned itself to a predominately outpatient clinic.

While over the next 38 years after this rotation, I would occasionally encounter a patient who was suffering from severe psychotic disorders which required specialty treatment, the common psychiatric issues such as anxiety, depression, phobias and mood disorders predominated my experience. However, the "elephant in the room" was that most of these problems were hiding under the surface and manifesting and amplifying their medical problems and complaints. This along with the stresses of life including: relationship difficulties such as divorce or abandonment; job difficulties such as harassment and cruel treatment; family conflicts; chronic low self-esteem due to childhood development problems; and hidden effects of childhood traumas such physical, sexual, and emotional abuse played a significant part of their perception, reaction and response to treatment of their medical issues. Not many of us do not have life or personal issues that can influence our emotional state which can affect our sense of physical health. The simple association that mental health has an effect on physical health and vice versa is a fact of human experience.

These connections of the mental and the physical state can be obvious in some instances. For example, when in the grief of loss one can experience various physical symptoms such as headaches or stomach pain as well as the disorientation of sleep loss. In many or most other situations the delicate interplay of the mind and body is much more subtle and hidden at first. These effects, of course, are mostly not on the radar in young physicians as the most important focus is to get the "right diagnosis and the right treatment". It takes time to see the human condition as an interplay of all factors of one's life, even if the medical conditions are acute and severe. Naturally, the urgence of quickly and accurately evaluating someone with life threatening illness in the ER or the ICU puts one's entire focus on treating directly the heart attacks, strokes, low blood pressure from sepsis, gastrointestinal bleeding, acute poisoning, etc. is what matters most. However, in the typical world of primary care office settings, there are few sudden life and death situations. Moreover, patients don't come to the office with a "disease" per se but only with a "complaint" of something not feeling right. My job is to interpret accurately whether these symptoms are life threatening such as chest pain possibly indicating a heart attack; or other pains possibly indicating a cancer; or a common treatable problem such as an asthmatic wheezing; or a simple problem that will resolve itself such as a cold. Of course, there can be symptoms without a medical disease caused by psychological distress which can mimic any disease.

This sorting out of complaints is the most complicated part of the job and may require medical tests and evaluations but what also is needed is a sense of the person, especially important if one has interactions over time clarifying an individual's personality and responses. One memorable example is my long-term patient Lolo. I had treated Lolo's husband for his diabetes for some time before she came to see me after complaining her previous doctor was not taking her seriously enough. Her response to the question, "How are you feeling?" became the same for each subsequent visit—"I don't feel good, doctor!" While this reflected how she was feeling emotionally to what she was feeling physically, I had to explore what wasn't feeling well in her body. There were a myriad of physical symptoms that were offered for my review. Sometimes only one—"I have a headache" but often several "and my stomach and back hurt." After exploring the details of each complaint to determine the possible and then probable causes of her symptoms, such as migraine headache versus tension headaches versus other rare possibilities, Lolo would invariably ask after my questioning but not before my examination was done: "Do I have cancer, doctor?" More specifically she would ask "Do I have brain cancer" after having a headache last week or "Do I have stomach cancer, doctor?" for a complaint of abdominal bloating and gas. I was asked "Do I have leg cancer, doctor?" for a pain in the knee from kneeling down while doing housework. I would then need to perform my physical examination and proceed to categorically and without a doubt assure her that she was not suffering from any of her feared cancer phobias. Fortunately, she was able to be reassured with my detailed explanation of why she didn't have cancer but would end with "but doctor, I don't feel well". This was an obvious opening to the psychodynamic of asking what was behind her fear. Her responses were sometimes vague but often tied with an ongoing life event or stress. If she heard of a relative who was diagnosed with cancer, she would be concerned she also had the same one. Many times her symptoms corresponded to stress issues related to family conflicts and she had many in her life. Over time, I found out that Lolo was a daughter of Holocaust survivors who were emotionally absent and abusive who disapproved of her choice of husband which required that they elope and were then outcast from the family. She was terribly conflicted with her own sons' choice of wives. She was a victim of mistreatment of her boss at her work at a school cafeteria. There was difficulty with all her relatives and many others in the world but her saving grace was her entirely devoted husband who knew of her mental torture and tried to help and calm them as best he could. Lolo suffered from chronic anxiety and low-grade depression and with each visit it became obvious that she was in need of medication and counseling to help her cope.

Lolo is not such an unusual patient in a primary care practice. All of us have our "crazy" patients that can have nearly every symptom at various times and which can take up enormous time in the office and with phone calls and with testing and referrals. One might label these patients "hypochondriac", a term that semantically means "under the cartilage of the ribs". For myself, it was very important to get the details of their experience in order to sort out importantly if it corresponds to a specific, significant medical problem or is a physical symptom that is enhanced by the anxiety and individual meaning that patients have along with their physical sensations. Certainly, patients are not making up their symptoms, their experience is real. It may be that their symptoms are a heightened awareness and focus of common everyday bodily sensations. As all of us at times may experience a throb in the head, a tingling sensation in the hand, a discomforting bloating feeling in the stomach, a pain in neck, head or back, even a sensation of dizziness when standing for a few seconds accompanied by a mild visual difficulty or a feeling of being off balance. These are all part of the experiences of the human body. For those that then interpret these intermittent feelings as something dangerous, life threatening and fearful, the appearance of any concerning bodily sensation cannot be ignored and discounted but rather is amplified to a level of near panic which can prolong or exacerbate the symptoms. An interesting example is the infamous "second year medical student syndrome". As medical students beginning to learn about human pathology, diseases and associated symptoms in their second year of classroom work (the first year is taken up with understanding the body anatomically and physiologically in its normal state), many believe that they have some of the most rarest of diseases because they have noticed one or a few of the symptoms occurring randomly and intermittently in their bodies. Especially, since most rare and serious diseases can have common symptoms. For example, kidney cancer may manifest as back pain, but because back pain is so common it is rare for that to be the case.

Lolo was a tough case and in getting to the root of her real problem, her psychologic distress and anxiety, I had to patiently go through her physical symptoms and give her a definitive and confident answer that she was not suffering from cancer. Occasionally, I had to do a lab test or X-ray to confirm the negative. After this detailed explanation, it was important to explore the underlying concerns which actually were easy to access by just asking. Lolo was pleased to hear that she didn't have cancer, it was in talking about her anxieties and stress where the true therapeutic effects of the visit occurred. While I was not a trained psychologist, my "on the job" experience and life experience allowed me to calmly discuss and offer a sympathetic perspective and even practical suggestions for dealing with the emotional impact of her experience. For Lolo and many, however, these intrusive, persistent feelings were part of daily life and took their toll so prescribing medications to help alleviate the pain of persistent anxiety and its resultant depression was important treatment. I prescribed various modern non-addictive medications to Lolo over the years with some positive impact. That is, when she took the medication.

Many people are fearful of medication for the mind, thinking that they are for the "seriously" ill or for "crazy people", or that medications will make them either crazy or zombies. It can take a fair amount of discussion to get patients to take these daily for several weeks before they have a positive effect. Of course, the other side can be that patients will stop their medications after they feel a bit better thinking they don't need it, only to relapse within a month. Most patients on antidepressants need them for 6-12 months before thinking about weaning off and many will need medications for much longer or even lifelong if their disabling anxiety and depression recurs. The good news is that there is no long-term danger from taking them. I'm not talking about tranquilizers or sedatives here that are addicting but the class of medications used for anxiety/depression on a daily basis. Fortunately, there are many of these from the older sedating types taken at night to the newer SSRI types typically taken in the morning. However, all medications can have side-effects and each person doesn't respond to the therapeutic effects so it can take some time to find the right fit for efficacy with minimal side effects.

Lolo improved when she took her medication regularly and I could mostly tell when she had stopped it based on the depth of her mood and anxiety on her symptoms. I used humor as one of my techniques to get to the source of her symptoms and to alleviate her torpor in a short time. After going through the exam and explaining why she didn't have cancer this time, I would try to playfully joke with her to let her see herself for a moment—"You know, finger cancer is nearly impossible, unless you have a lump!" Eventually, after many non-cancer explanations around her body, I settled on a pre-emptive question when I greeted her with her tell-tale distressed face: "So, Lolo, what cancer do you have today?" While this was wise-cracking close to the limit, I knew her well and seeing her smile and laugh helped to lower the intensity of her distress. Of course I listened to why "I don't feel well," but laughing did open the conversation to go over the underlying psychological processes and reactions she was experiencing. The danger with these patients is to preconceive that every symptom is not related to a serious physical problem. It was crucial to keep this bias in mind. When Lolo complained about classic gall bladder symptoms of pain and nausea in her right upper abdomen after eating a heavy meal, her ultrasound revealed gallstones and required a laparoscopic surgery. When she started having chest symptoms that could be cardiac in origin, I referred her promptly to the cardiologist where a blocked coronary artery required stenting. So even "crazy" patients can have medical diseases. I attempted to refer her to a psychiatrist or psychologist but she wouldn't pursue it. "I like talking to you, doctor. You make me feel better" she said. So, in her case I became a combination of counselor and physician.

Over time and with detailed observation, one can know patients' psychology and physiology which influences the approach to help them in both areas. For some patients, being a bit authoritarian and vocally forceful or instilling a sense of urgency or fear is best to get their focus on an important medical situation. "I don't mean to scare you, but this diabetes you have can affect nearly every part of your body and will kill you early if you don't pay it the attention and care that is necessary to get this under control!" Some patients who take health and medicine nonchalantly need to be brought into the reality of their situation. Others who are suspicious and critical of medical treatment need a more gentle approach and slow convincing of what is best for them along with complete understanding of what to expect. Others who are shy and fearful of being ill and then are unable to follow what is needed for their treatment need a more reassuring and comforting tone to be able to understand and participate in their care.

Many patients needed more intense and professional counseling than I could provide. Some of these sought this on their own, most were attempted to be referred to a mental health specialist. Unfortunately, the medical system kept this aspect of care out of reach for most due to the complexities and inadequacies of the insurance system. I found out the hard way in billing Medicare for services that were listed as mental health problems such as depression and anxiety. I was paid at a rate of 50% in comparison to treating medical problems such as back pain or hypertension! This was due to the rule established in 2002 by the *Medi-*

care Mental Health Outpatient Payment Reduction Overview. Since all other insurances in general follow the Medicare guidelines for reimbursement this led to less payment across the board. After I discovered this, I asked my psychiatric colleagues about this and there was a resigned universal "yes, that's the way it is". In addition, the patient is liable for a higher amount of the copay for any mental health service. Because psychiatrists have special training in counseling they can bill under a different set of codes but these are all at a relatively low level of reimbursement for the time spent. So, simply many psychiatrists and psychologists limit or exclude patients with insurance from their panels in order to make ends meet from a financial standpoint especially in urban areas. There was always this game of patients having insurance coverage when they inquired about it but were nearly unable to find a counselor that would see them under their insurance. So, of course, most patients did without any mental health services unless they were willing to pay out of pocket. Therefore, my limited but compassionate counseling was what many patients relied on.

I have worked with many psychiatrists over my career in different situations. For a time working in a back care clinic where many patients had complex psychological and chronic pain issues to then private practice where patients needed expert treatment for deeply disturbing psychological problems that coincided or clashed with their medical issues. While one may have the preconception that psychiatry is a mysterious, strange and fearful discipline, my impression is that their work is based on being as practical and direct as possible. While psychiatry has definitive classifications of problems there is a fair amount of variability as each patient brings his or her own flavor of psychological distress. These can range from acute situations to long-term or lifelong which all may be influenced from developmental childhood traumas such physical/sexual abuse or abandonment. Of course, psychiatric problems can be significantly inherited as well. Chronic depression and anxiety often have a genetic basis if one's parents also suffered a similar fate. Psychotic diagnosis such as schizophrenia and manic depressive disorders have genetic factors predisposing one to this unfortunate malady. Addictions to alcohol and other drugs have an innate neurophysiologic predisposition that can become full blown depending on the timing of the exposure and the strength of the genetic trait. For example, children of alcoholics exposed to alcohol in significant quantities in their teen years have a much higher chance of becoming lifelong alcoholics compared to their peers without alcoholism in their parents.

Psychiatry, obviously, is not like treating a strep throat. A simple prescription does not cure the condition forever. All psychiatrists employ a combination of counseling techniques (of which there are many) and medications to help their patients attain a more balanced, adaptive and happier life. Certainly, the push has been more in the use of pharmacology over the last few decades with an increase of various medications and combinations of medications that are not addicting along with the low rate of reimbursement for counseling.

Psychiatrists have to work with the individual and life situation in order to create a trusting bond and figure out a way to improve their psychological state. The research on improving non-psychotic illness has not sided with either talk therapy versus medications as a better method. For many or most a combination of the two treatments has the best chance of significant long-term improvement.

The problem all primary care providers have had is in getting patients access to the limited number of psychiatrists that provide care under the patients' insurance. It seems ridiculous and odd that in a cosmopolitan and advanced area such as the San Francisco Bay Area there is such a huge shortage of available mental health counselors. This shortage is compounded by the fact that many patients choose to see a counselor and pay out of pocket which further limits availability time and disincentivizes mental health workers to take insurance-based patients. The large organization I worked for at the end of my career, Palo Alto Medical Foundation, which had hundreds of thousands of patients in the northern peninsula area had no psychiatrists on staff, requiring us to try to find and refer someone for treatment outside their system. Needless to say this was a continual exercise in futility. Fortunately, there were a few of my psychiatry colleagues that were willing to squeeze a patient in their busy schedule for an urgent consult and treatment.

I will be eternally grateful to Frank, Tim and John for helping me help my patients over my 25 years of private practice. These three were especially available and insightful for those patients that needed expert psychiatric care.

The problems of limited access to mental health are complex as noted above but also reflect a societal decision to undervalue and ignore the needs of people with psychological illness. Like medical illness, psychiatric illness is not a choice but a fact of human experience. Not recognizing the issue as a crucial part of health care serves no-one and in the end costs more to society in visits to the ER, police calls, and lost productive lives.

CHAPTER 22

The Rise and Fall of Cardiac Surgery

At a quiet lunch in the doctor's cafeteria in the fall of 2008 I was having a pleasant conversion with Bud Bronstein, M.D. He was telling me of his impending move to the Santa Cruz area to take over the directorship of the cardiovascular surgical division of a local hospital there. Bud and his wife had a second home near the beach, and I pleasantly recall visiting him there once. His home had an obvious peaceful, unhurried vibe which included a dense garden and light-filled rooms. Bud was close to retirement then in his mid-60s and had a long-interesting career as a cardiac surgeon mostly at the hospital I worked at. He was an excellent surgeon and had a warm, natural caring demeanor which helped his patients get through the rigors of coronary bypass surgery and other heart surgeries. He came of age as the technology and treatment of cardiac diseases was advancing and becoming routine by the late 1970s when I was in medical school. Bud's new job would include supervising and coordinating the protocols for all the cardiac surgery at his new hospital which still had an active program and was recruiting cases from the Kaiser health system closeby. He would be doing some of the surgery and assisting the other cardiovascular surgeons there. The move was also prompted by the fact that he and all the cardiovascular surgeons at Seton Hospital were at the nadir of their careers of having operations to do. As a response to the declining volume, they all had extended their staff privileges to several hospitals in the area and were learning the newer techniques of cardiac surgery but still, their practices were severely declining from a caseload and business standpoint as the advancement of treating coronary artery disease by cardiologists with angioplasty and stents had nearly taken over. With safer, faster and equally effective treatment, patients no longer needed to undergo getting their chest "cracked" and being put on a circulatory bypass machine while having their heart stopped and suffer all the difficulties and complications of coronary bypass surgery.

The leading cause of death in the developed world has been from cardiovascular disease for most of the 20th century and still continues into the 21st. Myocardial infarction, e.g. heart attacks, remains the leader followed by strokes. The treatment techniques of bypass surgery and angioplasty developed in near parallel in the 1950s. Starting with the development of the cardiopulmonary bypass machine by John Gibbon, M.D., a graduate of my alma mater, Jefferson Medical College. This was followed by the first coronary angiogram in 1958 by F. Mason Stones, M.D., who accidentally put a catheter into a coronary artery and injected dye when he was trying to check the aortic valve and discovered the anatomy and imaging of the right coronary artery.

The cardiopulmonary bypass machine is an extracorporeal (outside the body) blood pump that filters blood over an oxygenating membrane mimicking exactly what the heart and lungs do while allowing blood to be diverted from the heart so it could be operated on by surgeons was a brilliant first step. The surgical advancement of using the bodies' own veins and arteries to bypass a severe blockage in a coronary artery by attaching one end to the beginning of the aorta and the other beyond the blockage was first successfully done in a patient by the Argentinian surgeon Rene Favoloro at the Cleveland Clinic in 1967. These technical factors when combined with the diagnostic coronary arteriogram where radiopaque dye was injected into the coronary arteries revealing the exact location of the blockages and how severe they were gave all the tools to start a new age in medicine for treatment of its deadliest disease.

By the time I started my clinical rotations in medical school in 1980, coronary artery bypass surgery was very established with teams of surgeons, residents and fellows (doctors in training to be surgeons). By then it seemed that bypass surgery was an advanced, factory-like program in many hospitals around the US. During my time on the cardiac surgery service at Lankenau Hospital in suburban Philadelphia, there were 6 surgeries scheduled every Monday, Tuesday and Wednesday. This was quite lucrative for the hospital and the surgeons, as this was a highly regarded procedure for which surgeons could charge and receive up to nearly $20,000 per surgery in the era before managed care.

The cardiologists were also making dramatic gains from the use of the new technique of coronary angioplasty whereby using a similar catheter used for a diagnostic angiogram, they fitted a small inflatable balloon on the tip to open up a blocked coronary artery without surgery. Andreas Gruntzig in Switzerland pioneered the procedure in 1977. The following year two cardiologists performed the first angioplasties in the US. Simon Stetzer, M.D. in New York, and Richard Myler, M.D. in San Francisco, did them on the same day! These two titans of early angioplasty would end up working together at Seton Hospital in the San Francisco Heart Institute in the '80s and '90s where Bud and I would practice as well. Bud came on staff during this time, filling the need for the large number of patients that would need bypass surgery. Initially angioplasty was limited to treating only one blockage in the heart and all other patients would be recommended to have surgery. Also, early angioplasty had a high recurrence rate as only using a balloon to dilate a narrowed coronary artery blockage would only be temporarily opened in a significant percentage of patients. Thus requiring the procedure to be repeated sometimes many times and if still blocked would then be referred to undergo surgery. These failures along with multivessel blocked coronary vessels in the same patient kept Bud quite busy. Bud and his cardiovascular colleagues were also in demand by the large backload of patients that needed valve replacements from diseased heart valves such as from rheumatic fever, congenital deformity or aging calcified valves as none of these patients were able to be treated before the era of cardiac bypass.

However, with the field of cardiology and angioplasty advanced as they developed several additional technologies including lasers, rotational blades to bore through the blockage and finally stents (wire mesh tubes) to keep their procedures from failing. Stenting after angioplasty is now the standard and has a high rate of success especially with using drug coated stents that prevent blood clots from forming after insertion. Since the mid-1990s stent technology has allowed cardiologists to treat longer and more complex coronary blockages and to also treat several blockages in the same or different arteries at the same time. These advances led to a dramatic decrease in the need for bypass surgery with its long operation time, long recovery time and multiple possible complications.

Coronary artery bypass surgery while being a major advance is also fraught with potential very serious complications. Among them is an infection of the sternum, the bone in the front of the chest that must be sawed through to access the heart. This is a particularly difficult infection especially when the bone is infected. Other serious problems include bleeding in the chest after the surgery, blood clots in the legs and strokes to the brain as well as a particular neurological condition known as "pump brain". This last issue seems to be due to the effects of using the bypass pump and is likely related to small bits of material including microscopic air bubbles reaching the brain and causing the patient to have a cloudy state of mind, confusion and memory issues for some time after awakening from the anesthesia. Sometimes this side effect can be permanent.

One can see the collision course of care that developed here. On the one hand the cardiac surgeons had established themselves as the definitive caretakers of coronary disease and any other structural problems of the heart that needed surgery. On the other hand, the cardiologists caught up with their technical advances and were able to match bypass surgery with less costs, minimal hospitalization, less trauma to the patient and less complications. Quickly in the late 1990s angioplasty equaled and then overtook bypass surgery as the definitive procedure for treatment of coronary artery blockages. And in 1997 there were over 1 million performed worldwide as it became the most common medical procedure.

Of course, the bottom line is what works better. Coronary artery bypass surgery declined significantly from its heyday in the 1980s as it should have because there were too many surgeries done on minor arteries with one blockage which did not pose a threat of death. However, it remains proven that patients live longer and have less heart attacks after a multivessel bypass operation as compared to angioplasty. So it still has an important place for patients with severe, extensive coronary disease, especially patients with diabetes or left anterior descending coronary artery disease ("the widowmaker").

Interestingly, while angioplasty may have some protection against a patient having a heart attack in the future, its major use is with the treatment of angina due to 1,2 or 3 accessible blockages. The other significant use is emergently treating someone who is having a heart attack. Angioplasty along with directly placed clot busting drugs (blood clots in a coronary artery are the cause of a heart attack) can prevent a heart attack from developing, save heart muscle and prevent death. Most hospitals now have advanced protocols to have patients undergo an emergency angioplasty within 90 minutes of arrival in order to maximize this benefit.

In parallel to the procedures to treat coronary artery disease, the other great advance of modern medicine is the use of medications. Particularly with the introduction of statins in the late 1980s. This class of medication along with newly developed medicines for blood pressure and antiplatelet treatments can dramatically reduce the risk for heart attack and stroke in patients. The benefits of long-term drug treatment reduce the need for angioplasty and bypass surgery.

Bud saw his very busy practice begin to disintegrate and go from about 10 cases per week to 1 or 2 over the course of the next 10 years from the turn of the 21st century. Not only that but the surgical cases were much more difficult in that patients referred for bypass surgery were much sicker and had more complicated coronary disease with most requiring many blocked coronary arteries that needed bypassing. This along with the severe drop of other heart surgeries such as valve replacement as the cardiac surgeons had done a great job over the past 20 years operating on everyone that was in need and so the only valve replacement cases were those that occurred in the population after all that backlog was dealt with.

Not only was there a very significant drop in caseload but reimbursement began to fall precipitously in the 1990s for all procedures and surgeries as managed care and Medicare began to reduce costs. While in the early 1980s, cardiac surgeons were getting over 10 thousand dollars per case, their reimbursement by the late 1990s fell to less than $2000 per case and continued to fall afterwards.

Cardiac surgeons practices were "withering on the vine" and some suspected the demise entirely of the specialty in the early 2000s. The surgeons were stuck with very little to do except to accept any case they were offered no matter how difficult it was going to be. It was an odd scenario as just 20 years earlier this group of physicians were considered the major heroes of modern medicine. From a primary care standpoint, I felt a bit sad for them but could do nothing to offer them more surgical cases. The indications for surgery and their need had changed dramatically. Some of the cardiac surgeons left for different parts of the country where there was less competition and a bigger need and many expanded their practices to be available at all the hospitals in the region.

All this caused a severe drop in Cardiovascular Surgery training programs around the country and the world. Today, there are now only about 20 positions per year offered in the US mostly as a combined Cardiothoracic (heart, lung and chest) training program so that these surgeons can also treat lung diseases such as lung cancer.

Bud had done well and immensely enjoyed his career which mostly coincided with the boom of cardiac surgery of the mid-'70s and '80s. He was OK with doing less but still loved being involved with one of the most dramatic advances of modern medicine. His move to his new location fit well with the changes in his life and the field itself. I missed him dearly when he left.

The cardiac surgeons have also not stopped innovating their skills. Many open-heart operations are now done "off-pump". That is, the heart is beating during the surgery but they are able to use a simple device to keep the section of the heart where the bypass is being done still. This cuts down on the expense, complications and time of the surgery and as well as less equipment. Also, certain aortic valve replacements can now be done using catheters through the femoral artery. An amazing technical advance in which there is no need to open the chest wall or put the patient on bypass.

I suspect this is the future of the field of cardiovascular surgery as it has been for all of surgery over the past 30 years which has seen less cutting, quicker recovery, less complications and better long-term outcomes. Stay tuned, we are all bound to benefit!

PART 4

A Career of Epidemics Ending with a Pandemic

CHAPTER 23

HIV/AIDS

January 1984 and I am a second-year resident doing a 6-week rotation in the ICU in Boston. Along with another resident, intern and senior resident, we have about 20 patients in the three ICUs on the fourth floor of the Faulkner Hospital to take care of. We were perplexed by this very unusual case of a young man in his early 30s with multiple brain abscesses. He had come in with confusion and a fever and a CT showed these infected areas on the outer surface of his brain. He had never been ill in his life up to this point. He was septic with a bacterial blood infection from his brain abscesses and required intravenous medication to raise his blood pressure to a safe range. Slowly, he began to respond to an extensive regimen of antibiotics but needed to have these abscesses drained by the neurosurgeon several times. Then when we thought he was getting better, he developed an odd pneumonia and then died before we could figure out it was caused by pneumocystis, a very unusual bug for a young person.

We had all read the articles that had been in the news about this new syndrome labeled the "gay plague" in which young homosexual men were dying of unusual infections who also developed an acquired immunodeficiency but the cause was still unknown. We suspected this young man was part of this new medical phenomenon. Research was moving swiftly to identify the agent and nearly simultaneously in Paris at the Pasteur Institute and at the National Cancer Institute in Washington, two groups identified a likely virus which turned out to be the same retrovirus and cause of HIV/AIDS in April, 1984. Remarkably, soon after this discovery, there emerged a blood test that could identify who was infected with this unique virus that was spreading quickly through the gay men communities of North America and Europe which was later discovered had jumped from chimpanzees to humans after several mutations of the virus in Africa.

Even more remarkable in the early stages of this story is that a medication, azidothymidine (AZT), was found to be effective treatment after the biology of this new virus was found to contain a unique and important enzyme for its replication named *reverse transcriptase*. AZT had been abandoned 20 years earlier after failing to be an effective cancer drug. This drug directly inhibited the enzyme for reproduction and therefore could contain the spread of the virus in the body and transmission to others. So, within a few years this rapidly expanding viral disease had been identified, its biology of transmission was worked out, its effects on the immune system to drastically weaken it was discovered and an effective medicine was approved by a rapid process in March 1987. Initially, AZT seemed to be an incredible treatment. Although with significant GI side effects, the early clinical studies found it reduced deaths and opportunistic infections, prevented progression of infected individuals to full blown AIDS and prevented transmission to others including pregnant women to their babies. However, these fantastic results were soon tempered when it was discovered that the HIV virus could mutate and render the medication ineffective in most infected patients. Research into other medications was intense and by the early 1990s several other antiviral drugs were developed based on the growing knowledge of the biology of the virus and how it infected specific cells of the immune system. Along with this, reliable and accurate blood tests were developed that could quantify how much virus a patient had in their blood and measure the effect on the circulating immune cells. The story of the scientific advancements in just a handful of years is one of particular marvel and was entirely unique in the history of medicine. This all occurred in the early technological development of being able to genetically analyze viruses and their proteins and to match these findings with drugs that could treat the infection. 1995 was a pivotal turning point in this worldwide epidemic when it was shown that a combination of drugs were vastly superior in treating AIDS and in preventing infected asymptomatic patients from progressing to the full-blown disease. New medications were developed in different classes that attacked specific processes of virus replication and infection of the immune system. Since that time, treated HIV patients have been able to live a near normal life and lifespan with a chronically controlled infection by medications and monitoring. However, even with these advancements the worldwide death toll of HIV since its start 40 years ago is *over 38 million*. A larger devastation has occurred in resource poor areas of Sub-Saharan Africa, Asia, the Pacific Rim, Latin America and the Caribbean compared to North America and Europe and the demographics have shifted to predominantly Black and Latino populations since the mid-1990s.

When I moved to San Francisco in 1988 in the Upper Market district near the Castro area, I found myself living close to one of the epicenters of this epidemic which was visibly evident from the street. In the Victorian building where I rented a flat, there were 4 apartments of which two were occupied by gay men who were in the later stages of AIDS. These middle-aged men looked like many similarly afflicted in the neighborhood—gaunt, shuffling with a walker and a helper, obvious visible skin tumors, sunken eyes and looking extremely fatigued. These unfortunate men looked to be right out of a concentration camp and there were a lot of them around. At that time, the life expectancy of someone with AIDS was only about 6 months even with treatment with AZT.

My interaction with this epidemic was largely not from the medical side but from the social/community side. My work at the time did not involve any direct care of HIV patients as I was working at a spine center across town. However, two physician colleagues died of AIDS within the first two years I was there. At their memorials, their close friends related to me the hundreds of similar events they had attended over the past several years. The devastation of the gay community was almost inconceivable as thousands of young, bright, working men were laid dead in a short period of time. The response to the epidemic by the gay community was nothing short of miraculous and extraordinary.

The support for each other in every way was truly inspirational from a humanistic standpoint. From coming to the aid of companions and family, to financial help and psychological support of each other in this relentless time of grieving and loss showed a level of compassion that I have not come close to seeing before or since. This extraordinary sense of community and assistance increased with the need. Importantly, the gay community became intensely committed to preventing the spread of this deadly virus with appropriate and effective methods of safe sex practices and use of condoms that significantly slowed the spread by the early 1990s.

In the spring of 1995, in anticipation of starting my own private practice, I took a course offered by UCSF (University of California San Francisco) which was one of the leading centers of research and treatment of HIV/AIDS in the world. This was an exciting new time, as new treatments were becoming very effective for the control of the disease and I thought I would need to become familiar with the current knowledge of this disease if I was going back to general internal medicine. It was an enlightening course about all that was known at the time from many of the world's experts. The care of HIV/AIDS patients in San Francisco and elsewhere was largely done by infectious disease (ID) specialists. However, there was a cadre of primary care physicians who, prior to the epidemic and continuing through it, were taking care of the gay population of San Francisco. These were mostly gay men and women who were Family Practitioners and General Internists and involved with the gay community and interested in medical issues specific to them. As AIDS progressed, they found themselves with a growing number of these infected patients of which there so many that they could not all be cared for by ID specialists. Their expertise and experience evolved with the disease and they became familiar and competent in the evaluation and treatment at the front lines. These were some of the most competent physicians in the world on the course, complications and treatment of AIDS from the mid-1980s onward. In other parts of the US and the world, generalists rarely directly treated gay and AIDS patients and when they did they quickly referred them to an ID specialist.

Seeking to get some insight into the real issues and potentially treating AIDS patients, I was introduced to a respected family doc working in the Castro district who very kindly allowed me to shadow him in his office practice for several weeks to directly observe the current state of affairs in regard to AIDS. What I discovered was that treating HIV/AIDS was the most complicated medical problem that one could encounter. From the medical side, there was a need for a regular battery of blood tests to evaluate the infectious and immune status of the patient which would guide which combinations of medications to use. Then, there was the constant evaluation of response to treatment and the side effects these medicines caused. In addition, many patients developed other medical conditions such as hypertension, diabetes, a physical wasting syndrome, chronic fatigue, strange tumors and other metabolic and endocrine disorders in relation to HIV. Then there were the various opportunistic infections to be on a constant vigil about and could be difficult to treat in the face of a faltering immune system. The psychological impact of this disease was enormous while the patient also experienced loss of friends and loved ones. It was clear that the patience and compassion these primary care AIDS doctors gave to their patients was truly heroic.

As my primary care practice grew, I began to see HIV patients but fortunately their complex regimens were handled by our local infectious disease specialists so my function was largely to care for any other medical conditions that the patients had. From a general practice standpoint, those patients fit into the category of chronic medical conditions that had their own set of protocols somewhat like diabetes, hypertension and heart failure patients. Unlike other patients, however, the vast majority of HIV patients kept themselves extremely informed on their disease, treatments, side effects, and natural progression of their life-long infection which made interactions and visits much more of an involved shared decision-making process which for me was always a better experience.

There are significantly fewer HIV infected patients these days than during the period from the mid-1980s to 2000. Currently, the medication regimens are quite refined and effective so that HIV/AIDS is a very stable and predictable problem but is still handled by ID specialists.

However, there are still one million new HIV infections worldwide and 30,000 in the US every year. The most recent development has been in using medications as a pre-exposure prevention of infection (PreP) first approved in the US in 2012. In individuals who are at risk for contracting HIV, combination medications taken daily can nearly eliminate the risk (~99%) of getting infected and this has become quite popular in younger gay men. While this works very well if one is compliant with the prescription, there is concern that many only use it as a "morning after pill" which is likely not nearly as effective. The other very significant issue with this regimen is that it allows sex partners to not use condoms and therefore all the other sexually transmitted diseases (STDs) have been on the rise since this regimen was developed. Patients on PreP are counseled to get STDs checked every few months. The rise in cases of syphilis and gonorrhea has been alarming and is particularly worrisome for gonorrhea where significant antibiotic resistance has developed. Also, the medication regimen cost is $7-10,000 per year excluding all the testing and doctor visits.

The big elephant in the room with HIV is still the lack of an effective vaccine after nearly 40 years. Researchers have been frustrated and hampered as the virus continually mutates in important regions that render vaccines only partially or minimally effective, but work continues in this field. Currently there are no publicly available vaccines.

The horribleness of the AIDS epidemic of the '80s to the mid-'90s has mostly faded into history but is far from gone.

CHAPTER 24

Obesity

Since starting medical school in 1978, Americans were beginning to get fat and have continued getting fatter since. Everyone uses the BMI or *body mass index* as the metric to classify individuals as fat. A BMI greater than 30 gets you into the fat club. Greater than 40 puts you in the "Morbid Obese" club. BMI is simply the ratio of your weight to your height so it adjusts for those that are tall versus those that are small. Height is used as a general approximation of one's body surface area which is the more accurate way to get this ratio. Like everything, there may be some inaccuracy in this ratio in people that have more muscle, like bodybuilders, as muscle weighs more than fat. Also, there may be an issue with some Asian populations where they are naturally of more slender build and less muscle mass and smaller in stature where a BMI above 25 could actually mean higher levels of adipose tissue.

This epidemic has been quite democratic in that rises in obesity have occurred equally in all age groups and in both men and women and in all ethnic/racial groups over this 45-year period. However, it has affected minorities and lower socio-economic folks to a larger degree due to easier available, cheap, poorly nutritious food with high calories, e.g. fast food.

The reasons for this unprecedented continual rise have been copiously studied. Often people have assumed that Americans have become *much less* physically active during this period to account for the increase in weight. However, in large data analysis this appears to be a *minor* factor in the obesity epidemic. The evidence for this is that manual labor jobs have not changed greatly and much obesity has occurred before people started working (adolescence) and there actually was a rise in certain leisure physical activities such as jogging through the late 1970s into the millennium. There is some controversy whether children are less active than previous generations as a set-up to later life obesity but this may be true.

However, it is clear that the significant and predominant factor is simply consuming too many calories in comparison to what is burned off by daily activity and metabolism. The difference is quite significant in that on average Americans consumed about two thousand calories per day in 1975 and this increased to 2500 calories by 2010. An increase of 25% per day! A pound of fat is calculated to have 3500 calories of stored energy. By simple arithmetic, one could gain a pound of fat per week by this constant excess of intake. However, bodily metabolism is complex and not all consumed calories are absorbed and other metabolic factors are at play to help regulate weight. Most people gain weight slowly over their adult life. The average for Americans is to gain 1-2 pounds per year from age 20 to 50, so 30-60 pounds is typical weight gain during those adult years. The specific factors that promote weight gain include eating processed foods and sugar, reducing physical activity after obtaining full time work, a slight slowing of metabolism leading to less calories burned, hormonal changes, chronic stress and lack of sleep.

The difference in caloric intake has been traced to increased sugar and "ultra processed foods (UPF)" which have very little nutritional value per calorie. UPFs include soda, salty snacks, cakes, white bread, ice cream, sweetened breakfast cereals, processed meats, pizza, french fries, and fast food. There was a combination of factors to bring this increase in calories to Americans from the 1970s. Agricultural production of corn increased dramatically due to improving production technologies along with farm subsidies causing prices to drop significantly. The costs for materials and manufacturing UPF came down along with the price of sugar. A significant corporate expansion of the fast-food industry made these high calorie, low nutrient UPF widely available at prices much lower than for healthier foods such as vegetables, fruits, whole grain breads and lean meat. Americans tripled their consumption of meals outside the home from the mid-1970s (9%) to (27%) by the late 1990s, mostly at fast food restaurants. It has been estimated that the 500 extra calories per day noted above can all be attributed to UPFs.

A new industrially produced sugar was introduced into the US in the 1970s, high fructose corn syrup (HFCS). It was quickly added to nearly all processed foods. HFCS is cheaper to produce than traditional sugar (cane or beet) and has a sweeter taste. This makes it economically advantageous to add to a variety of foods such as soda, crackers, cereal, breads, baked products, canned fruits and vegetables as well as a variety foods that are traditionally savory such as ketchup, prepared meats and even cheese. Also, HFCS was found to prolong the shelf life of food. Its introduction has been a significant boon to the food industry over the last 50 years. The data is not clear how much of the increase of 500 calories per day over the last 45 years is due to HFCS but it is likely a significant factor. From the medical standpoint HFCS has several serious negative metabolic effects in the body that promote weight gain and disease. For one, its increased "sweetness" promotes more appeal and increases ingestion of food or liquids and helps lead to sugar addiction. Also, they do not produce a natural satiety, especially in liquids and can easily lead to higher amounts ingested at one sitting. Ingestion of significant fructose at one time has serious metabolic consequences such as promoting fat storage in the liver and insulin resistance which can incite or worsen the development of type 2 diabetes and enhance weight gain. Fatty liver is a common occurrence in many patients who are overweight and is a marker for various metabolic disorders and is related to HFCS intake.

A significant factor in getting people to eat more calories has been the "supersize it" phenomenon promoted in fast food establishments as increased portion size has been instituted in nearly all chain restaurants. This successful economic ploy works as cheaper products such as HFCS allow the food industry to sell larger portions with almost no increase in production costs while increasing cost and profit margins easier.

So, there is not a lot of mystery as to why over 40% of Americans are currently obese. We are all victims of the perfect storm of cheap, available, poorly nutritional foods that promote weight gain. As a species that evolved during prolonged periods of scarcity of food, humans are engineered to ingest more calories than needed in times of plenty. The problem is that the modern world is always in a "time of plenty" and never in scarcity in terms of available calories. The rate of rise has been alarming as the obesity rate in 1980 was 15% and has steadily risen nearly three times that and continues to rise today. While most obesity occurs during adulthood, the US has seen a worrisome rise in childhood obesity. Currently, one in eight children aged 2 to 5 and one in five children (20%) aged six to nineteen are obese, forecasting a continuous epidemic of gargantuan proportions in generations to come. This portends an enormous medical care burden as obesity has a variety of health effects besides those mentioned above. The increased medical complications include: gallbladder disease requiring surgery; cardiovascular diseases such as heart attacks, strokes, high blood pressure and heart failure; respiratory problems of sleep apnea; early and disabling osteoarthritis of knees and hips requiring joint replacement surgery; increase risk of cancers of breast, colon, pancreas and kidney; hormonal and infertility issues; gastrointestinal issues such as acid reflux; and mental health issues of depression, anxiety, social stigmata and body image disturbances. The increased medical costs related to obesity are currently estimated to be greater than *three hundred billion dollars per year* and will only rise with time.

So, are we just destined to become fatter as society progresses and more calories become easily available? Will we end up similar to the world depicted in the movie *WALL-E?* What has been done to combat this epidemic and has it had any benefit? What are the current medical treatments and do they work? The insidiousness of this epidemic evolving slowly has mostly kept it as a side topic for public health. Unlike AIDS which was attacked furiously from the get go, seeing a society getting heavier has mostly seemed like a natural, inevitable event and has become so common that there really is not much publicity or outcry. Unlike AIDS, nobody sees fat people falling over dead in the street. Obesity is a slow-moving glacier of medical complications. Also, it is mostly viewed as an issue of "willpower" and "weakness" that folks just let themselves become obese. The issue of allowing humans to be manipulated by the food and fast-food industry is taken as a societal "right" because people are believed to have a choice to eat less or eat differently. This, of course, is a nice rationalization for using any and all tactics to get folks to eat stuff that is not good for them. A look at the "science of manipulation" of what snacks work the best to entice consumption is telling. It is well known and exploited by those in the food industry that people with little choice particularly (e.g. in urban "food deserts") where the cheapest and least healthy foods are the only ones available and when impulse choices work perfectly (such as occurs every time someone stops for gas) easily makes "bad choices" the only choice.

What has been done to try to stem the tide of obesity? From a public health and government policy standpoint it's largely been passive messaging such as public awareness campaigns and nutritional labeling. There have been some attempts to institute healthier meals in schools. The most significant efforts have been to try to tax sugary beverages but all these proposals have been met with extremely stiff opposition from the sugar and soda industry and only a few cities (and no states) in the US have been able to implement them. In other countries that have been successful in taxing sugary beverages, it has been found to reduce intake. None of the passive programs have been shown to reduce the incidence of obesity or change eating/choice habits.

Recommending very low calories diets are common but suffer from the problem of continuing to adhere to them after a short time. Also, there can be "metabolic adaptation" where one's normal metabolic rate is reduced with less calories taken in. Also, it can result in a disproportionate loss of muscle mass and the famous "yo-yo effect" of going on and off severe diets with an end result of higher weight gain.

What about medical treatment for obesity? Doctors in general are terrible about counseling patients about obesity and mostly focus on the secondary effects such as hypertension, diabetes and osteoarthritis. To be honest, very little didactic and instructional information is given to medical students and residents on addressing this issue. The result has been that treatment has come either from the pharmaceutical industry or from surgical intervention. The history of weight loss medications has mostly come from drugs that stimulate metabolism to increase and to reduce appetite. These medications initially came from the class of medications related to amphetamines. While these medications gained popularity for weight control starting in the 1950s, most doctors remained concerned over their addictive potential and they were prescribed somewhat rarely by small numbers of physicians. In the early 1990s, a successful combination of medications came to market, fenfluramine/phentermine commonly known as *fen-phen*. This was a unique combination that powerfully suppressed working in different ways from amphetamines and were not considered addictive. The expansion of the use of these medications was significant until it was found to have the dangerous side effects of heart valve damage and pulmonary hypertension which caused its withdrawal in 1997. Subsequent similar medications were suspected to also cause similar effects and never gained a foothold in this huge, potential market. While there have been various medications approved by the FDA for treatment of obesity since that time, they remain only occasionally prescribed predominantly because they just don't help much for weight loss, are expensive, and are needed to be taken for long periods of time (2 years or more). The data on their benefits are so modest that it seems silly from a primary care perspective to ever prescribe them. The scientific studies of all these medications results in an approximate weight loss of about 4 pounds in comparison with a placebo after 2 years of taking a daily pill. Really? Is that worth it? It never seemed so to me and most of my colleagues.

Bariatric surgery has been performed for morbid obesity for nearly 70 years but gained prominence in the 1990s as an acceptable, safer and effective procedure for morbidly obese patients with metabolic complications because the procedures became less complicated and more surgeons were doing them. While there are many different procedures that have been done, currently, the most popular fall into the category of reducing the size of the stomach by either removing a large portion of it or placing an adjustable band at the proximal end to reduce the effective size. The effects of these bariatric surgeries are twofold. Firstly, by restricting the size of the stomach reservoir there is a limit to the amount of food that can be taken in without regurgitation. This serves as giving the patient the sensation of being full with a small amount of food and therefore reducing the amount of calories at one time. Patients are instructed to eat only small portions to reduce the risk of vomiting and pain from stretching the remaining stomach pouch. In addition and unknown until somewhat recently, it has been found that bariatric surgery causes hormonal changes that are produced by the stomach. Specifically, the hormone *ghrelin* secreted by the stomach produces a sensation of hunger and is reduced after bariatric surgery which causes patients to feel less hunger overall and maintain lower calorie intake without cravings. The combination of these effects can often result in weight loss of 30 percent in morbidly obese patients. This is much greater than medications or diets can achieve. Simply, this can be a 100-pound weight loss in a 300-pound individual which is quite impressive. However, like any surgery there can be complications and failures. Surgical complications can include leakage at the surgery site, infections, severe esophageal reflux and blood clots. Fortunately, the rate of severe complications are quite low. Metabolic complications can include poor intake of sufficient protein and various vitamin deficiencies. However, the health and metabolic *benefits* of significant weight loss include normalizing blood pressure after being hypertensive, reducing and eliminating type 2 diabetes, improving cholesterol levels, reducing stress on arthritic joints, improving physical exercise capabilities, improved body image and self-confidence and less social stigmata of being obese. Unfortunately, some patients gain back some or all the weight they lost after a period of 2 years. Some patients learn to "get around" their intake restrictions by continually ingesting small amounts of high caloric foods such as soda. I had one patient gain back the 100 pounds she lost and admitted that she took overcooked pasta and made it into a liquid slurry that she drank throughout the day and night.

An important caveat of weight loss is that all that is lost is not fat! Yet most folks assume that when you lose a pound as measured on the scale that it must be by reducing a pound of fat. Unfortunately, the body's metabolic adjustment to lower calorie intake does not automatically shift to only "fat burning". Our bodies use a complex mixture of fuels for energy that include carbohydrates, fat and protein. A consistent level of glucose for proper brain function and energy for muscle metabolism causes sugar to be released by the liver but is also supplemented with the breakdown of protein from muscle sources. While muscles can use fats as energy, the brain is reliant on glucose. The reality is that a pound of weight loss results in a third to a half from muscle breakdown. Muscle metabolism is an important driver of basal metabolic rate which is the number of calories the body uses every day. So, less muscle means less calories needed. This is an important factor in the increased weight gain of "yo-yo dieting". In this scenario, losing a significant amount of weight and then putting it back on means that one has lost a significant amount of muscle but has mostly put back on only fat if one is not doing significant exercise to preserve muscle mass all resulting in lower basal caloric expenditure.

I admit that my handling of obese patients was like most of my colleagues. While I didn't intentionally avoid discussing and counseling patients about the elephant in the room, I didn't routinely bring it up for review either. Of course, patients know they are obese and often readily admit their difficulty with losing weight. "I've always been heavy, just like my parents" was commonly stated. "I have tried every diet and none of them worked and then I gained even more weight" was also typically voiced. Or even the cryptic and suspicious declaration that "I eat so little and still gain weight." Resignation and embarrassment of their obesity was often expressed without me needing to bring it up. While I discussed various strategies, I mostly took a gradual and gentle approach of looking at the long term and to try to make small changes that can translate to more permanent results. Of course, recommending reducing those types of foods that most likely put weight on such as the ubiquitous amounts of processed carbohydrates and sugars was at the top of the list. For individuals who do little exercise, the body can function perfectly well with a very small amount of carbs while having a balance of other nutrients including protein and vegetables. I always try to coax patients to be even a little more active. Simple walking or any type of movement that one can fit into one's day if done regularly can have huge health benefits that extend beyond weight loss. Many folks assume that exercise means going to a gym every day which easily discourages many who are busy and embarrassed by their body and is not practical for all. But anything that one can do and fit into a busy schedule is valuable. Fitting in and doable are key. A simple 15-minute walk after lunch or dinner or even anytime increases one's metabolism while allowing food processing on a healthier level (lowering blood sugar after meals). In the end, being obese is the result of many factors. Culturally, parents that are overweight commonly have overweight children. Our advanced society, where snacks, fast food, convenience stores and having an abundance of calories in the house makes it easy to eat too many. An exploitive food industry makes cheap, high calorie, low nutrient intake a business model for profit. A complete lack of regulation of foods that leads to obesity and disease adds to the difficulty. Finally, we are evolved creatures naturally inclined to overeat at least a bit and occasionally a lot more than needed. Now that most work does not involve physically moving or doing hard work all day such as during the agrarian economy of one hundred years ago, gaining weight is a natural phenomenon of being human in today's world. Attempting to treat severe obesity against all these odds stacked against the patient is extremely difficult. The route of surgery which is becoming more popular every year.

While many patients would like and ask for a pill to solve their obesity problem, from an objective scientific and safety standpoint I never was convinced that the medications previously approved offered much benefit to patients (some were extremely harmful) and strongly discouraged their use and never promoted them. Of those few patients that insisted on trying them and agreed to close monitoring, the results were uniformly disappointing for the long term.

What has been proven to work to reverse obesity from a non-surgical scientific standpoint? Well, from those who have lost a significant amount of weight and kept it off permanently we have learned a lot. Universally for those, it has meant a radical and complete change of life habits. And habit is the key here. The common threads to long-term, significant weight loss include incorporating the following into one's life: 1. Eliminating the threat of highly processed foods at home which means no snacks or junk food where one lives, 2. Eating a healthy diet that includes primarily vegetables, lean meats or other protein sources, small amounts of carbs and no sweetened beverages, 3. Limiting alcohol intake to 1-2 drinks per week, 4. Being physically active or exercising every day, 5. Patience that changing one's life is a long term project and that results will sometimes take years. Literally, this needs to be a life transforming process to be successful, but it is doable and has been done by many and their stories are available online for those to seek encouragement and guidance.

As of this writing in 2024, I need to include a potential medication treatment that is emerging with the distinct possibility of having a significant impact to help both obesity and type 2 diabetes. This new class of medications, the GLP-1 agonists (Glucagon-like peptide-1 receptor agonists), are named for the cell receptor that is found in various tissues of the body including the pancreas (where insulin is made), stomach, kidney, lung, heart, skin, immune cells and in the hypothalamus of the brain. In its natural state, GLP-1 is a protein hormone made in the small intestine. Its main action is to help regulate blood sugar after a meal by stimulating insulin release from the pancreas. At the same time it suppresses glucagon, a hormone also produced in the pancreas, that works in the opposite way of insulin by increasing glucose levels. While drug development and approval on this class of medications started 20 years ago, the latest versions are much more potent and long-lasting. Most of these drugs are given by injection once a week. One of the remarkable beneficial side effects noted in the recent versions is significant weight loss. In comparison to the other feeble weight loss drugs on the market (~2% weight loss), these medications commonly cause 10% or greater weight loss. Currently one of these drugs are now approved for weight loss in non-diabetics. The other significant finding with these drugs are that they are proven to reduce the adverse cardiovascular effects of diabetes such as heart attacks. This is a remarkable triple effect of one medication. The various mechanisms of how these drugs reduce weight initially were thought to mainly have an effect on slowing down the emptying of the stomach giving patients a sense of fullness and therefore reducing food intake. Recently, it has been revealed that these medications also have a powerful effect on the brain to reduce food cravings and to increase the sense of satiety after a small amount of food intake. Of course, no drugs are without potential negative side effects and these drugs can cause nausea, vomiting, abdominal pain and diarrhea in some patients which occasionally can be severe. The jury is still out on the long-term effects of these medications on the body. Social media and general media exposure have put these medications in the spotlight as very desirable and sought after even by celebrities. This rush by the public has caused shortages of the medications for diabetics. Of course, these new medications are expensive (currently >$15,000 per year) and are often not covered by health insurance for obesity or even type 2 diabetes.

CHAPTER 25

Type 2 Diabetes Mellitus

The Type 2 Diabetes Mellitus (T2DM) epidemic evolved in tandem to the obesity epidemic. Understanding diabetes involves complex physiology although many equate it only with an abnormal elevation of blood glucose and with eating too much sugar in the diet. Diabetes can also be easily confusing because there are two forms. The form known as Type 1 is due to complete lack of insulin due to autoimmune destruction of islet (insulin making) cells in the pancreas. The cause of this is still not completely known but genetic, environmental and possible viral infection play an important role in triggering off the permanent damage and loss of insulin production. Type 1 diabetes is actually not very common, causing only 10% of the total patients with diabetes and mostly occurs in children or young adults who seem to be susceptible often dramatically and suddenly. Untreated it rapidly causes severe metabolic derangement and death from complications of ketosis and dehydration. The introduction of purified cow and porcine insulin injections for humans in the 1920s led to saving the lives of countless patients in the century since the start of insulin replacement therapy. The first synthetic, genetically engineered, commercially produced *human* insulin became available in 1982 after the human gene was successfully put into a bacteria to manufacture it. It has made treatment more accurate without any of the adverse effects of animal insulin (allergic reactions).

In contrast, Type 2 Diabetes (90% of all diabetics) has an entirely different onset and physiology. T2DM is caused by a combination of *resistance* (diminished effect) to insulin and a sluggish response of insulin release by the pancreas. Also, an additional hormonal mechanism uncovered over the last 20 years is an increased release of the hormone *glucagon* which essentially works opposite to insulin by increasing glucose release into the bloodstream. These dysregulated processes result in rising glucose levels that stay significantly elevated or take a prolonged period of time to return to normal levels (~100 mg/dl in the bloodstream). Insulin is a protein hormone made by specific cells in the pancreas known as islet cells. It has many actions in the body in various tissues and is released by the glucose monitoring islet cells. Insulin's action on cells helps drive glucose into tissue where energy is needed and therefore lowers the circulation of glucose down to levels that are safe for the body. The main tissue that absorbs glucose are muscles that can either use it directly to produce energy for making muscles work or it can be stored in muscles as glycogen which the muscles can rapidly use when needed. Adipose tissue also absorbs glucose under insulin's action which guides fat storage for future use. One of the crucial organs for regulating glucose is the liver and actions of insulin on the liver are intimately tied to the control of blood sugar and the development of T2DM. It's important to understand that the liver can be looked at as the central processing unit (CPU) of metabolism in the body. The liver's various important actions include: storing and releasing energy (glucose and lipids); manufacturing various proteins and amino acids the body needs; processing digested nutrients from the gut where it detoxifies and transforms them; breaking down and metabolizing many drugs to active and inactive forms; it has a role in storing various vitamins and minerals that the body needs; and it produces blood clotting proteins. In glucose metabolism, the liver has many functions under the direction of insulin while also responding to energy needs by muscles and the brain. Directly, insulin promotes storing glucose as glycogen in the liver and decreases the liver's manufacturing of glucose both helping to regulate and reduce blood glucose.

In T2DM these regulatory mechanisms become less precise and less responsive especially in the liver. Besides having a lower rate of absorbing glucose to store it and remove it from the bloodstream particularly after a meal, the liver's abnormal response to continue to manufacture and release glucose into the bloodstream after a meal contributes greatly to rising glucose levels in the bloodstream. Glucose levels can easily go to twice the normal level, for example, from 100 to 200. Normal blood sugar levels after a meal usually stay under 140 and go back to 100 after a few hours. Since insulin is not working as well to drive glucose into muscle or fat cells in T2DM, it has nowhere to go but to stay in the bloodstream.

Elevated glucose in the bloodstream for periods of time is toxic to the body and causes specific damage to various tissues and organs. Blood vessels can be injured and become clogged leading to heart attacks, strokes and circulation problems. The retina in the eye can be damaged, leading to loss of eyesight and blindness. The kidneys' specific filtering mechanisms become slowly and permanently injured. T2DM is the leading cause of kidney failure and need for dialysis in the US. Prolonged high blood sugar levels damage nerves throughout the body and can cause numbness, weakness and pain commonly in the legs and hands. Also, toxic injury to the skin, brain, feet and even to the pancreas where insulin is produced is responsible for many of the severe medical complications. The complex metabolic effects of T2DM can directly cause high blood pressure and hyperlipidemia/hypercholesterolemia. This triad is called the "metabolic syndrome" which is particularly dangerous for causing cardiovascular complications.

Genetic predisposition plays a significant role in getting type 2 diabetes along with diet, exercise and weight gain. Certain ethnic groups have a much higher prevalence and risk including Native Americans, Asia-Americans, Black-Americans and Hispanic-Americans. The exact risk has been variably reported at 10-25% range but I suspect this is lower than the actual rate.

In Daly City, where I spent the majority of my professional life, the population includes a significant number of Filipinos of first and second generation descent, and also various Pacific Rim immigrants such as those from Fiji, Tonga, Samoa, Japan, China, and Korea. All these groups have an elevated risk of developing T2DM when exposed to the western lifestyle of fast food and less active physical work. My practice had a large number of these ethnicities with diabetes of varying degrees of severity. The typical time someone is diagnosed with T2DM is in their mid 40s although the development from "pre-diabetes" usually takes many years and could even slowly evolve over decades. It is common to diagnose patients with diabetes on routine lab testing who came in for a "physical" at age 40 or higher. With the advancement of the obesity epidemic, more patients in their 20s and 30s are being discovered to have it. Interestingly, one reason the diagnosis is often delayed is because there are no symptoms in the early stages (sometimes for many years). Occasionally early on, there is a vague feeling of numbness in the feet from mild neuropathy or general feeling of thirst. Sometimes they have an ulcer on their leg that is not healing. Others may have some visual difficulties due to very high glucose levels causing swelling in the retina but most feel "perfectly normal".

As a medical student doing a clinical rotation on the Hopi/Navajo reservations in Arizona in the mid-1980s, I was exposed to one of the extreme but telltale signs of severely uncontrolled type 2 diabetes—a perirectal abscess. On several occasions, I accompanied one of the Indian reservation doctors on an evening or nighttime house call where the poor patient had been suffering with increasing pain and swelling deep in one buttocks for several days that then ruptured into a pool of pus and blood. The doctors knew it was diabetes and we brought along materials to clean out the infection, pack the wound, check the glucose level which was usually over 500, give antibiotics and insulin and because most of these patients refused to come to the hospital, arranged a follow-up appointment in a day or so. Over the course of my professional life, I saw a few of these same presentations in both diagnosed and undiagnosed diabetics. This dramatic and painful occurrence definitively convinces patients of the diagnosis and gives them motivation to accept treatment which usually keeps future episodes of this complication away.

As most newly diagnosed T2DM feel "fine", the lack of symptoms often leads to unacceptance or disbelief that such a serious medical problem is present. Usually several visits are needed to have the diagnosis sink in while educating the patient what they have and what's in store for them. Making the diagnosis of diabetes means that both patient and physician are entering into a lifelong relationship of complex interaction. There are many components to evaluate including the severity but also the other metabolic consequences, the complications of their disease, their response to treatment and the progressive nature of the problem which tends to worsen with age.

I found myself accumulating an increasing number of uncomplicated and complicated diabetic patients that needed a range of treatments including some who needed insulin injections and some who had various complications. Most of us in primary care refer complicated diabetic patients to endocrinologists, those experts in diabetes and other hormonal disease, to help figure out what is the best treatment and ongoing monitoring especially in severe cases. Locally, we found there were only a couple of these specialists. Paradoxically when we referred to them, the patients' care was completely appropriated instead of just being consulted on what to do. It didn't take long to realize that the primary care physicians needed to be at the front line of treatment or else we would lose many patients. It was an odd scenario as the endocrinologists were already overloaded and were resorting to hiring inferior nurse practitioners to manage these complex patients.

There is nothing like "on the job" training to become an expert in a particular field of medicine. As I took on managing more of my diabetic patients, the skill and knowledge followed quickly. The ubiquitousness of diabetes where I was practicing gave me all the exposure one needed. After a couple of years in private practice I had more diabetic patients in my practice than most endocrinologists have in most other parts of the US. At times, it seemed that nearly every Filipino or Pacific Islander had diabetes or was soon to be discovered. Fascinatingly, no two diabetics are exactly alike although there were several patterns. The easiest patients were those who embraced the need to pay attention to their life in a real way and take their prescribed medications every day. Some patients were extremely easy when they improved their diet and were then well controlled with one simple pill per day which really meant that their metabolic disorder was not yet so advanced. Many of these fortunate diabetics could be well controlled like this for many years. Other patients were on the opposite spectrum where they remained uncontrolled on a complex regimen of 10 pills per day and insulin injections while developing many of its complications including heart disease, renal failure and nerve damage with some needing amputations due to vascular blockages. Diabetes is a disease where education of the patient is crucial in order to control it. Complex patients need to know what their blood sugar readings mean, what their medications are doing in their bodies and to understand what the results of various tests mean and take in account how their life habits interact with what is happening. It helps to have outside help in this education process and most hospitals and health care organizations have recognized the importance of a diabetic nurse educator to assist the patients in the community. We were lucky to have these excellent local resources for patients to visit and gain understanding and control of their condition and to help us manage them better.

The evolution of the treatment of T2DM parallels the advances in the understanding of underlying pathophysiology. Insulin was the only treatment for all diabetics until the mid-1950s when an insulin stimulating group of medications were discovered accidentally when newly developed sulfur-based antibiotics were found to cause hypoglycemia (low blood sugar). These medications named *sulfonylureas* allowed patients to take pills instead of injections and was a huge breakthrough in treating less severe forms of T2DM particularly patients reluctant to take insulin. By directly boosting insulin levels, these medications helped to bypass the effects of insulin resistance and slow insulin response after meals.

The next group of medications found useful were also discovered accidentally researching drugs for malaria and influenza in the 1940s causing a side effect of low blood sugar. This class of drugs named *biguanides* were effective but tricky in that they could cause a severe metabolic acidosis and death. They were initially rarely used but finally a safe derivative, metformin, was developed in the early 1990s after nearly forty years of only sulfonylureas as the main oral medication. A landmark study of metformin in 1998 in the UK made it standard treatment by demonstrating good glucose control while reducing cardiovascular complications. It has been used in initial treatment of T2DM since and has the added benefit of not causing hypoglycemia (side effects of insulin and sulfonylureas) and can promote weight loss. Metformin works in a unique way in the body by significantly reducing glucose production in the liver and therefore less release into the bloodstream. The side effects of abdominal discomfort and diarrhea are occasionally significant but often can be managed with lower doses.

Also in the early 1990s, another completely different medication was introduced, *acarbose*. This medication was found to inhibit the breakdown of carbohydrates in the intestine after a meal and therefore decrease absorption of glucose and consequently lowering the natural increase of blood sugar after meals, especially those rich in carbs. This seemed like an excellent alternative pathway to lower glucose intake and improve T2DM. However, while it is still on the market, it has remained a little used medication due to its only modest effects in controlling blood sugar and its significant side effects of intestinal gas, bloating, discomfort and diarrhea.

Over the last 25 years, there has been the development of several different types of medications that work entirely differently from each other. One group of medications came and went after a 10-year run starting in the late 1990s, the *thiazolidinediones*. Yes, very difficult to pronounce making its disappearance even more of a joy. This group had an unusual mechanism of action by activating certain genes in various tissues that lower blood sugar and cholesterol levels. Initially, they seemed like a truly new "smart" pill. However, these were found after several years to paradoxically increase heart attacks and strokes and thus have been taken off the market and abandoned. I distinctly remember disliking these medications as in some patients they caused severe body swelling from fluid retention but were a darling of the endocrinologists at the time because they were new and "cutting edge". Even with these severe side effects, they often insisted patients continue to take them, causing primary care physicians to shake their heads.

The last 3 groups of medications for T2DM developed over the last 20 years are an alphabet soup of drugs that work in interesting and different ways to control the metabolic dysregulations that cause high glucose levels. The first group, the *DPP4 inhibitors*, are oral medications that stop the body from breaking down small hormones called incretins that enhance various mechanisms the body uses to control blood sugar. They are used as "add-on" drugs, not first line treatment, and have moderate effects on diabetic control. A newer, different class of medications, the *SGLT2 inhibitors*, work in an interesting and unique way causing the kidneys to excrete glucose into the urine instead of keeping it in the bloodstream. By literally peeing out sugar, patients have lower glucose levels and lose weight as well. This seemingly simple mechanism has a significant impact to control T2DM and has additional benefits of helping to control blood pressure while reducing the risk of kidney damage and heart failure. They are mostly used as secondary medications in the armamentarium against diabetes. Being newer and expensive, insurance company coverage has been limited. Downsides can be from causing urinary or vaginal infections although they are mostly safe except in patients with kidney disease. The last group of new medications are the *GLP-1 agonists* that I discussed above in the obesity section. These have evolved to become powerful for T2DM control and weight loss and there is accumulating evidence that they protect the heart from disease related to diabetes. These are given mostly as weekly injections which is acceptable to most patients but newer oral formulations are starting to be available.

Occasionally, T2DM patients need insulin too. Because there are many modern medications, insulin is usually added later in the course to help those who remain significantly uncontrolled on a combination of the above medications. As there are long-acting preparations, many patients need only a single daily dose per day.

How does one know that treatment is working? It is commonly assumed that all diabetics need to check their blood sugar by poking their fingers many times a day but for most this is not true. For the majority of patients, daily blood sugar testing is not needed because doctors use an analytic blood marker, the *A1C* or *HbA1c* (short for the hemoglobin A1c molecule). This is an important tool that gives a measurement of average blood sugar over the past 3 months and is a standard laboratory blood test done everywhere. It formerly was known as the "glycohemoglobin" level which actually describes it better. What is being measured by this test is the amount of glucose that is attaching itself to hemoglobin and therefore reflects the amount circulating in the bloodstream. Hemoglobin is the oxygen carrying molecule in red cells. Because red cells "live" in the body for 3 months before being recycled, a percentage level of this molecule that has glucose on it can be compared to a normal level in the blood. Glucose can also attach to various proteins, cells and molecules in the body. A normal A1C level is 6% or less in non-diabetics. The goal for T2DM patients is ideally less than 7% but recent outcome studies have shown that a level less than 8% is just as good for preventing the complications of T2DM. Checking blood sugar daily or several times a day by a finger stick glucometer reading can sometimes be confusing and may not add much to the medication management that patients take every day regardless of the instant blood sugar reading. What doctors are looking for are patterns of the high glucose readings when testing is done at home and this can vary depending on the time of day. Some patients have higher "fasting" glucose (before breakfast) and others can have much higher readings after meals. It's common to ask patients to check a "2 hour postprandial" glucose usually after dinner as it is usually the biggest meal and therefore the peak sugar level of the day. The patterns of different peaks throughout the day helps guide medication use. Getting a pattern over a few months is best to evaluate how things are going and so I often ask patients to check a few times a week at different times e.g. morning vs after dinner and then review with their 3-month A1C lab test. The occasional very high glucose reading is generally not very meaningful and no cause for alarm or change in medications. For stable patients a regular A1C check is the most important information. However, patients need to be aware and check home glucose readings if hypoglycemia (low blood sugar) happens or if they are at risk. Low blood sugars (always from medications) is particularly dangerous for the elderly and frequently causes disorientation, unresponsiveness, passing out and falling down. These events require an urgent change in medication regimen and possibly eliminating the specific ones that can cause this e.g. sulfonylureas. In addition to the A1C, diabetics need to be monitored with regular blood pressure checks, kidney tests, lipid levels (treatment of which are very important for prevention of heart attacks and strokes), nerve and feet examinations along with eye examinations on a yearly basis.

Patients often ask: "Can I cure or get rid of my diabetes somehow?" While possible for some, it's not easy or necessarily permanent. Many bariatric surgery patients have been able to go off all the medications and then have normal blood parameters. We have all had a few very motivated patients who have lost a significant amount of weight, started exercising, reduced starchy food in their diet and were able to successfully go off all their medications. This life change can work but is a big ask in today's modern world especially in one's middle years. I've also had a few patients that defiantly refused medications while they purposely eliminated all carbs in their diet and then normalized their glucose. A rare but admirable behavior.

In human evolution, obesity and type 2 diabetes developed as part of our physiology. Obesity being adaptive to starvation while T2DM was physiologically maladaptive and serving no survival purpose. However, T2DM remained insignificant in the history of humanity as the average lifespan had been around 40 years, well before the devastating effects usually take effect. With current life expectancy double that, the full effects of this maladaptation and response to modernity are with us front and center.

CHAPTER 26

Dementia

This epidemic may be more attributable to an aging population as to other factors. The first baby boomers reached age 65 in 2010 and has resulted in the largest increase of seniors since then. Over the last 30 years the percentage of the US population over age 65 has increased nearly 50% from 11.5% to 16.8% according to the 2020 census. More significantly the absolute numbers of the elderly have nearly doubled in that time period from 30 million to 55.5 million. Dementia of all causes is the result of deteriorating cognitive capacity and memory of the aging brain. Alzheimer's disease (aka "old timer's disease" used by many of my senior patient jokesters) is the most common form and is marked by specific brain changes and a continual downward course. The loss of mental abilities can be quite variable in how quickly it progresses. The incidence rises from 5% at age 65 to over 30% for those over 85. For unknown reasons, women are twice as affected as men. This turns out to be a cruel irony as around the world it is mostly women who care for demented patients (70% by women). Currently (2023), there are 6.5 million Americans living with dementia. Other than aging, the increased risk factors for getting Alzheimer's include: smoking, diabetes, high blood pressure, traumatic brain injuries, excessive alcohol intake, being overweight, physical inactivity, social isolation, depression, and also genetics but only to a fairly minor degree.

While some patients come in worried about their memory ("I can't remember things/names/places like I used to"), no one ever sees the doctor with the complaint of "I feel demented". It is always a family member or someone close to the patient who brings them in for concerns of forgetting basic stuff like one's address, wandering behavior, repeatedly asking the same questions or doing something dangerous like leaving the stove on several times. Many family members have claimed that "mom was normal just last week" and are worried about a brain tumor or stroke. I found this an interesting phenomenon and largely related to patients' unique abilities to subtly hide their declining mental functions until it became obvious. Physicians do standard cognitive and neurologic examinations, lab tests, medication review and usually a brain imaging study (CT or MRI) to make sure there is nothing other than Alzheimer's to consider. The vast majority of time we don't find any other reasons and then give the patient and the family the unfortunate clinical diagnosis. While there is research on finding a specific blood or spinal fluid test to definitively make the diagnosis, these are still not ready for prime time just yet.

It is common for concerned family members to have done their homework on medication treatments for Alzheimer's and to request prescriptions "to help dad get back to normal". The sad and honest truth is that there are no such treatments available currently. Donepezil aka Aricept (name brand) was approved in 1996 by the FDA as a novel specific medication in the class known as anticholinesterases. One of the disturbed brain mechanisms found in Alzheimer's is reduction of a neurotransmitter, acetylcholine, and therefore finding medications that can increase the level could theoretically have a positive effect. This medication was greeted with great fanfare and promotion and led to two other similar drugs being approved afterward. In 2003 an entirely different type of medication named memantine or Namenda was introduced that helps regulate glutamate, a different neurotransmitter found to be overactive in Alzheimer's. Both of these medicines have been used and studied extensively over the past 20+ years and have resulted in one big "meh" as far as effectiveness is concerned and in my direct experience are incredibly annoying as far as their frequent side effects. The extensive science on these shows very little effect at preserving cognitive abilities after being started. They have absolutely no effect on reversing any of the effects of

Alzheimer's and any limited benefits have a short time period (at most 18 months). Honestly, these medications are somewhat a joke and take advantage of the desire to "do something". Typically, it's impossible for families to notice any beneficial effects while complaining about all the side effects. Aricept is particularly disturbing by causing dizziness, loss of appetite, drowsiness, weakness, difficulty sleeping, tremors and muscle cramps which makes a demented person's life much worse. Namenda has its own unique side effects of increased agitation and hallucinations. To make matters worse, these drugs have been combined in a single pill. No scientific studies have found these medications to lessen the need for nursing care, progression of dementia or death. While researchers have tried very hard to find something that these drugs may improve, the fact is they do nearly nothing or cause side effects for the vast majority or, at most, have a small, short term stabilizing effect for a minority (~20%). Did I prescribe these? Of course, family members demanded them frequently and wanted to try "anything that might help". I was careful in getting detailed follow up from families and caregivers to determine if continuing the medication was worthwhile which was rare. These medications made billions for the pharmaceutical companies and now are all generic drugs. It upset me to see wasted financial resources when end stage Alzheimer's patients stayed on these unnecessary medicines for years particularly those at end stage confined to nursing homes.

Treating Alzheimer's patients largely means educating the family on the natural course of this devastating neurodegenerative disease. Due to effects on the brain, patients often lose some of their "natural filters" that we all have in regard to behavior and expression. This can manifest in different ways. I have seen "nice" demented patients become more placid and quiet and easy going. On the other hand, and seemingly more common, an uncovering of someone's negative side is revealed. Critical, sarcastic, and cruel verbal and physical behavior can come to the forefront and cause havoc. This is particularly difficult for the caretaker who often is the daughter of one's progressively demented and mean mom. I've spent countless visits advising and counseling family members to "not take it personally" when a demented parent is constantly verbally and/or physically abusing them. Trying to help a guilt-ridden daughter get perspective on her mom's disease induced cruelty is not easy. This loss of control of being able to constrain one's thoughts is a commonly overlooked effect of dementia causing severe psychological pain to the caregivers.

The progression of Alzheimer's is impossible to predict. Some patients manifest mostly memory and confusion which seems stable for several years. Others seem to fall off a cliff and quickly are unable to perform simple self-care, e.g. eating, dressing or bathing, and in 6 months are wheelchair bound, mute and stop eating without being fed. It's always a difficult decision to decide when a loved one needs institutionalization or round-the-clock supervision. Families want their parents to be able to live at home independently as long as they can due to various reasons including and often, economic ones. The boom in residential facilities for dementia has been one of the biggest growth areas of healthcare over the past 20 years. In general, I have advised families to "be safe rather than sorry". It doesn't take much for a tenuous situation to turn into a disaster. A seemingly OK, moderately demented elderly patient can easily fall and get seriously injured carrying stuff up and down stairs; or forget a burner is on and cause a fire; or forget to take needed medications; or wander out at nighttime or an unlimited number of other scenarios that result in deep regret by the family for not intervening earlier.

I am reminded of one particular unusual but tender story of an end stage Alzheimer's patient who was taken care of at home by her husband and who I used to do home visits with. She was in her early 80s when she became bed bound and mute and needed to be hand fed. They were an elderly Italian couple, Maria and Donatello, who emigrated to the US after WW2 and lived in a modest but tidy house in South San Francisco and had a couple of elderly children. As a favor to one of their daughters, Vera, who also was my patient, I began to check in on Maria at their home. It was one of the highlights of my month to stop by after my regular clinic on my way home to their house as I was warmly greeted by Vera and Donatello. Maria lived in a hospital bed with rails up to keep her safe. She couldn't talk and was mostly in a physically contracted state with arms and legs folded up. She couldn't hold anything. Donatello was incredibly dedicated to turning her frequently in bed to prevent bed sores and had a sense of when she wasn't feeling well. She was on a limited number of medications which I regularly reviewed and stopped when she no longer could benefit from them. I would check her blood pressure, examine her and go over any concerns. Incredibly, she would eat when hand fed by either Donatello or Vera and swallowed without choking which is often a big problem in patients in this state. On one occasion, when they thought she was having difficulty, I diagnosed pneumonia and at other times UTI's. At the end of each visit, of which they were greatly appreciative, we often sat together in the kitchen and had a coffee and biscotti while I listened to Donatello tell me stories of their lives and 67-year marriage. Most patients in Maria's late stage of Alzheimer's rarely last more than a year before they die. However, for nearly nine years she lived at home with the care and love of her husband. Donatello told me he knew what his wife needed and wanted and he could feel her love in return in caring for her. She died peacefully in her sleep at the age of 89.

One fascinating trend about dementia is that while absolute numbers continue to rise due to increasing numbers of the elderly, the actual rates of dementia for various age groups are seen to be decreasing! No-one knows quite why this is happening and it's against all previous predictions but it may be due to better cardiovascular health now compared to 20-30 years ago and this could be reflected in better brain reserve. Research on Alzheimer's dementia is regarded still in its infancy and new concepts about what is happening in the brain as a cause are emerging and in some are in contrast with previous assumptions. It appears to be the result from a combination of an accumulation of injurious proteins along with inflammatory injury. The real issue is that by the time someone is diagnosed the brain degenerative process has been active for likely 10 years, so trying to treat Alzheimer's can almost be looked at as similar to treating an advanced cancer, nearly impossible to cure. Recent research on drug development has focused on reducing a buildup of damaging proteins in the brain by using monoclonal antibodies. One very expensive drug in this category has been approved for early onset disease but the obvious limitations of requiring intravenous infusions and cost have essentially made it inaccessible for general use.

CHAPTER 27

The Opioid Epidemic

Note: I'm going to use the terms "opioid" and "narcotic" interchangeably here as they mean the same class of medications, although in the layperson's literature sometimes "narcotic" means a bunch of different drugs that are not opioids. Strict speaking in medical parlance they are in the same class of pain medicines related to the prototype drug morphine.

This tragic, horrible, ongoing, devastating medically induced epidemic can bizarrely be traced to a letter published in the *New England Journal of Medicine* in 1980. This section will be mostly about the development of *prescription* narcotic addiction and will not be as detailed about street drugs such as heroin and now fentanyl. For an extensive and insightful view of the societal, corporate, governmental and medical aspects of this topic I recommend the book *Dreamland: The True Tale of America's Opiate Epidemic* by Sam Quinones.

But what about this letter and how did it spur an epidemic? Since it's such a short letter, let's read it in its entirety by its author, Dr. Herschel Jick:

Recently, we examined our current files to determine the incidence of narcotic addiction in 39,946 hospitalized medical patients who were monitored consecutively. Although there were 11,882 patients who received at least one narcotic preparation, there were only four cases of reasonably well documented addiction in patients who had no history of addiction. The addiction was considered major in only one instance. The drugs implicated were meperidine in two patients, Percodan in one, and hydromorphone in one. We conclude that despite widespread use of narcotic drugs in hospitals, the development of addiction is rare in medical patients with no history of addiction.

At the time, the author thought of this as a simple survey of medical charts of *only* hospitalized patients. It's important to note it was done at a time before electronic records or advanced computerized database analysis and certainly was lacking data about patients *after* they left the hospital. Today, this sort of "letter" or study would not be accepted by any journal without more detailed data analysis and procedure protocols and extensive peer review. However, because it contained a very large number of nearly 40,000 patients and was printed in the most revered medical journal in the world, it began to get more and more attention each passing year. It was severely deficient from a scientific research standpoint in that it did not include any of the methods for data gathering or analysis and its intent was not to be a true deeply researched scientific study as it was a simple report in the form of a letter. It took nearly a decade of citations and twisted interpretations to transform this letter into a "major study" that experts in the field of addiction and opioid treatment took and propelled as gospel. The transformation of this letter seems similar to the old game of whispering a phrase to a group of people in a circle and seeing how it changes after going around the room. Starting in the 1990s and for the next decade or so, researchers, scholars, the media and crucially the pharmaceutical industry misconstrued this letter while blatantly and incorrectly touting it as a "seminal", "landmark" and "important" *study* on the safety of treating outpatients with chronic narcotics. This brief, superficial report says nothing about the real-life incidence of developing medically induced addiction after hospitalization as there was no follow up. Even the methods of determining true addiction are not clear. Certainly, this letter says absolutely nothing about the risk of addiction in outpatients getting narcotic prescriptions.

It's important to go back before all this got going in the early 1990s to the prior period where *all* doctors were very aware and concerned about the addictive nature of prescription narcotics. We had all seen various types of manipulative, addicted patients and didn't want to contribute to their numbers. For example, the middle-aged woman with migraines that could "only be treated with Demerol injections" or back pain patients that cried to us on the weekends that "someone stole my vicodin" or "the dog ate my pain pills" or "I left my pills at the hotel" as lame excuses for trying to get more from any doctor they could. It was common sense and good medicine to prescribe the lowest doses for the shortest times for specific pain situations such as surgery or acute injuries to mitigate the risk of abuse. Patients with cancer were looked at differently and a much more compassionate and logical need was seen but these patients were mostly handled by oncologists. Chronic benign pain (not cancer related) has always been a bug-a-boo for physicians as it is unclear how much pain a patient is having and the fear of the nasty rabbit hole the physician and patient can go down prescribing addictive medications. The muddiness of trying to help a suffering soul versus getting a susceptible person hooked never escapes the decision-making process. Unfortunately, there are no blood tests, X-rays or scans that tell how much pain an individual is in so it's all the doctor's judgment at the moment of prescribing.

Working at a spine center from the early to mid-1990s, I was front and center to a non-stop parade of patients in pain. Some had ruptured discs, some had four, five, or even six back surgeries under their belts and wanted more, some were severely depressed, some were angry, some were just strange. Many had terrible lives and a good percentage were taking narcotics for their pain. In retrospect, this was the most difficult period of my career in figuring out what to do with these patients. The surgeons I worked with were always looking to cut on these poor souls. For a large number their treatments had been failures and many of these patients were just "taking the edge off" by popping daily narcotics.

My hyperactive, gregarious senior colleague, Jerome Schofferman, prided himself on being on the "cutting edge" of current treatment and medical advances in the evolving field of pain management. In fact,

Jerome changed his title as an internist and referred to himself as a "pain specialist". The field of "pain management" up to that point included almost exclusively anesthesiologists who had done special training in injections for pain problems and were not skilled or delved into medication management and certainly not opioid therapy. So Jerome's leap to being a specialist in medication management was somewhat unique at that time. This preceded the explosion of "pain centers" that came into existence around the country over the next 2 decades. Jerome was hip to all the emerging new ideas that chronic pain could be safely and successfully treated with chronic opioids. He was an expert on the pharmacology of each narcotic on the market and had read every issue of the journal *Pain* and every available book (of which there were only a few in 1991). He also went to pain conferences where the nation's experts discussed the latest research and treatment recommendations for pain patients. He was one of the first to become certified in the new discipline of *Pain Management* for non-anesthesiologists. Always eager to share his knowledge at our work conferences, he would talk about this new way of thinking about the treatment of chronic pain with opioids. He seemed quite convinced that this new method was correct. It essentially meant making sure the patient always had adequate blood levels of opioids so that pain would not be allowed to rise to significant levels. This new method required that patients take medications around the clock to assure that their pain was always suppressed. This concept actually was borrowed from post operative protocols that had been in place for many years. After surgery, patients in the hospital could self-administer a small dose of an IV opioid regularly before their pain got severe in order to "keep up with the pain". This works extremely well in situations where acute pain has a predictable time course, such as a few days after surgery. But what about when someone's pain was indefinite?

Jerome was quick to assure everyone in our group that there was good "science" to back up this new hypothesis and I distinctly recall him summarizing the "large study from the *NEJM*" that showed a miniscule number of patients got addicted to narcotics. Of course, he was referring to *that* letter from 1980. Certainly, there were a lot of our spine patients who complained that their pain was poorly controlled with taking their pain pills *prn* (as needed). Jerome started prescribing his chronic pain patients daily scheduled doses of opioids and began to use longer acting formulations. The problem with nearly all the opioid pain pills on the market then is that they were all relatively short acting, lasting only up to about 4 hours. The longest acting opioid is methadone. It is as powerful as morphine and lasts in the body for 24 hours. So once a day dosing can work, it's the reason for giving heroin addicts this medication in clinics around the world as it suppresses withdrawal. Its other benefit is that it doesn't give an opioid "high" like heroin. Prior to the 1990s no-one was using it to actually treat pain. It can be dangerous because high levels could build up in a patient's blood stream leading to a respiratory arrest and death. All of those who overdose and die from narcotics is due to this mechanism. So slow increases in dosage are crucial as well as frequent monitoring. I remember Jerome telling how he was getting good success by prescribing methadone to his chronic pain patients and encouraged me to use it as well. He would quote a report on using long-acting opioids by one the nation's pain experts at the time, Russell Portenoy. This neurologist built a career advising and writing about pain treatments through the 1990s and 2000s. He was known as the "King of Pain" and was director of Pain and Palliative Care at the prestigious Beth Israel Hospital in NYC. Portenoy greatly helped propagate the false conclusions of the famous *letter* to the American medical community and even scared physicians that they could be under threat of malpractice "for not treating pain adequately".

Things were moving swiftly from many directions to push this along. In California where I was practicing, a law was passed in 1994 requiring physicians to take a mandatory 12 hours of continuing education on pain treatment to renew their license which focused primarily on treatment with narcotics. This went along with legislation to limit the liability of physicians prescribing "adequate" amounts of pain medicine with the "Intractable Pain Act". The American Pain Society with support from the opioid pharmaceutical company, Purdue, put forth the concept of pain being the *fifth vital sign* adding it to the other conventional vital signs used for a century: the patient's pulse, blood pressure, temperature and respiratory rate. The Veterans Health administration adopted this 5th vital sign in 1999 and then it gained widespread acceptance when in 2001 the regulatory agency for all hospitals implemented its use.

In 1995, Purdue pharmaceuticals received FDA approval for its long-acting opioid preparation, Oxycontin and was also permitted for unknown reasons and with no research backing it to legally market it as "less risky to create dependence". This was assumedly based on its formulation that the drug would be slowly released in the body. The difference in this new formulation is that because it could be taken twice a day, the amount of medication in each pill was up to sixteen times higher than previously standard dosing (80 mg versus 5 mg). However, because it did not contain any other ingredients like acetaminophen, it was quickly discovered it could be crushed or melted down and safely snorted or injected by addicts. This single drug would transform the pain medication market and make billions for this company over the next two decades. After its release, Purdue aggressively began pushing doctors to prescribe it as a "safe, efficient and compassionate" medication, falsely claiming that only 1 in 10,000 would become addicted (again misconstruing *that letter*). At around the same time, there emerged a brand-new metric for evaluating treatment "success", namely, patient satisfaction surveys. This new method included measuring patients' *pain relief* in hospitals, ERs, and outpatient clinics as an important marker of determining *quality of care*. This assumption was not based on any scientific research but was pushed forward by medical advisory institutions and was subsequently adopted by the national regulatory agency responsible for certifying payments to hospitals. The pressure of patient satisfaction surveys began to be felt by all doctors as large medical groups and even insurance companies adopted this simple and simplistic way of ranking physicians. Of course, this infuriated many who knew that if a patient was happy with their treatment (especially those getting copious narcotics), it did not equate to having received good treatment.

All these events had a dramatic effect on prescribing narcotics in the US. In parallel, there developed a dramatic rise in the number of pain clinics which focused mainly on prescribing narcotics for chronic non cancer related pains such as low back pain. From 1990 to 1995, opioid prescriptions rose by 2 million per year and continued to rise until the peak in 2010 in the US. The increase in prescriptions was seen in all three scenarios: acute pain from surgery or injury, cancer pain and chronic benign pain. This rise correlated exactly with the increasing number of addicted patients, overdose events and deaths that ensued.

What evolved over the next 20 years is a gruesome story revealed in the statistics. Overall, the amount opioids prescribed increased by 500% from 1992 to their peak in 2010. The greatest growth came from oxycontin and hydrocodone especially when longer acting formulations were approved. The other opioids (codeine, morphine, methadone, fentanyl, etc.) grew also but less than the other two during this period. Prescription overdose deaths rose steadily, reaching a peak in 2017 of 17,000 deaths. From 1999 to 2015 over 180,000 Americans died from prescription opioids.

What happens when someone gets addicted to opioids? Medically we break down three phenomena which can overlap with each other, namely: opioid tolerance, physical dependence and addiction. Opioid tolerance is due to the diminishing pain-relieving effect of a specific dose of narcotic after using it continuously for some time. Narcotics work primarily in the brain to suppress pain and enhance pleasure through the dopamine pathway. The brain naturally adapts to decrease these effects after a relatively short period of time of continuous opioid intake. Humans manufacture in their brains natural opioids, named endorphins, that are secreted in times of stress and pain but only do so in small, discrete amounts as needed and determined by the body. Opioid medications act at exactly the same places in the brain but are in concentrations much higher than the brain produces. Since most systems in our body are in a constant vigilance and balance of monitoring *over activation* versus *under activation*, the pain fighting mechanisms self-modulate to become less responsive to more exposure to powerful narcotics. This is called *downregulation* or tolerance. For narcotic pain medications this simply means that the person will need to take more of the same medication to get the same pain fighting effect. After a couple of weeks, patients can commonly report "I need 2 pills now instead of one to kill my pain." This is a somewhat expected effect after taking narcotics every day for a period of time. This is not universal for all patients, however. Some continue to get good pain relief with the same dose for a long time. Tolerance can be mitigated by taking less of the medicine or stopping for a short period of time to restore natural responses as the body compensates relatively quickly.

Physical dependence which causes a *withdrawal reaction* can also develop after a period (usually a few weeks) of taking daily opioids. Withdrawal occurs after abruptly stopping opioids and is characterized by anxiety, sweating, shaking, abdominal pain and increased pain. This is a normal physiological reaction and should not be confused with addiction. The management of physical dependence is simply to slowly taper off the dosage so that the body can adjust physiologically. Withdrawal reactions can be very dramatic but are not in themselves medically dangerous. Many addicts go through withdrawal via "cold turkey" when they are sent to prison and are suddenly cut off from their daily narcotics. It is important to note that while *tolerance* and *physical dependence* are physiological components to addiction, they are not equivalent.

Addiction to narcotics is a brain disorder that has a significant genetic predisposition. It results in compulsive drug seeking, cravings and disregard for the negative health, life and relationship consequences. The genetic or inherited component of opioid addiction is complicated as it involves many different genes but is currently estimated to be responsible for at least 50% of factors that lead someone to be addicted. It is estimated that about 20% of patients exposed to chronic opioids can become addicted. The other factors that can help induce addiction are environmental (constant exposure), social and psychological factors (including developmental). Successful treatment usually requires several modalities including drug treatment (opioid substitution with methadone or buprenorphine) or weaning off, along with counseling and support such as financial and housing assistance. One lesser known but important aspect of opioid addiction is that due to the tolerance and physical dependency components addicts no longer take these drugs to get "high". The euphoric effects of initially taking narcotics are adjusted down relatively quickly and are replaced by the addicted person taking drugs only to "feel somewhat normal again" and prevent withdrawal.

The cracks in the wall of this tsunami of opioids and its destructive force started around 2007. Drug related deaths were rapidly approaching motor vehicle accidents and surpassed them the following year. In a criminal and civil lawsuit, twenty-five states sued the drug company Purdue Pharma (the maker of Oxycontin) who pleaded guilty to criminal charges that they misled regulators, doctors and patients about the drug's risk of addiction and its potential to be abused and were forced to pay $600 million in damages. By this time, America had been overrun with Oxycontin addicts for many years fueled by the proliferation of pain treatment centers that were prescribing enormous amounts of narcotics to everyone who came in asking for them. Florida became the epicenter of the prescription epidemic as "pill mills" proliferated faster than McDonald's. Florida doctors were prescribing 10 times more Oxycontin than all the other states combined by 2010! Patients were driving down the "Oxy Express" highway, route I-75, from all over the south to go and stock up in Florida. Finally, the DEA, federal, state and local officials started cracking down on the big business of pain prescriptions in 2011 in Florida. Importantly, Florida had refused to put in place a prescription monitoring system, allowing "patients" to go to many clinics and procure vast amounts of prescription narcotics. Much of this turned into *diversion* which means the pills were being given to others or more commonly sold on the street. The street price of Oxycontin made this procurement quite lucrative.

This was less of an issue in California which had previously initiated a *triplicate prescription* format for controlled substances many decades ago but still there was not a simple, direct way for doctors to know if their patients were getting narcotics from several sources and abusing and/or selling them, but it was difficult to forge or steal the prescriptions. On a rare occasion, I would get an alert call from a pharmacy that a certain patient had gotten the same controlled medication from several doctors. Then in 2014, California required physicians to check an online database, CURES, to monitor patients' controlled substance prescriptions. Unexpectedly after starting to use this online database, I uncovered several "under the radar" addicts in my practice. The odd part was that most of these were unassuming, seemingly honest middle-aged women who I was prescribing a regular but not excessive amount of opioids for a chronic pain condition on a scheduled basis. In monitoring these medications, the patients were required to come in for a check-up every 4 months. I was astonished to find these "housewife addicts" were getting various controlled medications from several doctors at the same time and for a long period of time! After discovery, my approach was to have an honest, in-person confrontation explaining their condition at a follow-up appointment. Their responses were varied. A small number denied having the problem outright but most sat in my office seemingly unfazed of my discovery with their small children in attendance while I told them they were caught, what they needed to do (enter a drug treatment program) and the consequences (which were to stop all future prescriptions and inform the other prescribing physicians). These women listened until I was finished and then mostly just got up and left my office without a word. There were a few who were embarrassed, regretful and crying when confronted. CURES put the clamp down on patients shopping for unrestrictive and secretly procured opioids and tranquilizers.

By 2015, the medical profession and the world was on to this prescription scam and the tide had turned against this wave of incorrect and corrupt professionally supported prescription addiction. The world of wily-nily opioid prescription was coming to an end, fortunately. However, along the way, some of the collateral damage included patients getting way too much medication for simple things like a knee surgery. Several patients and even acquaintances of mine became dependent on narcotics because their orthopedic surgeons prescribed an enormous amount of pain medication after surgery in order to: keep the patient happy, not be bothered for renewal phone calls, and to be "up to date" with current pain practices. This resulted in patients and friends needing counseling and help in slowly weaning off their opioids after unnecessarily taking way too much for several months.

Various patch work legislation and practice guidelines were subsequently put in place to try to correct the disaster. This included mandatory continuing education detailing the *dangers* of overprescribing narcotics (as compared to previously encouraging overprescribing 10 years before); guidelines on establishing contracts with patients who were deemed in need of long-term opioids; regulation of pain clinics; and strict oversight and discipline by the California medical board monitoring physicians found to be overprescribing controlled medications.

While there was general recognition and response to the opioid crisis and a resultant flattening of the number of opioid prescriptions by 2015, they still remained much higher than before the epidemic.

The medical profession thought they were doing much better by 2015 with the awareness and controls that took place. Unfortunately, there had already appeared a new threat with the introduction of cheap and widely available street heroin starting about 2010. The significant influx of black and powdered heroin from the Afghanistan-African route brought to prescription addicts a powerful and very cheap alternative to the Oxycontin they were having trouble getting. The beginning of the second wave of the opioid crisis saw the death rates from overdose beginning to soar. These overdose rates would become even greater with the arrival of synthetic fentanyl by 2014, the third wave of this epidemic. Overdose deaths went from 50,000 in 2014 to 70,000 in 2017. Fentanyl became the game changer. Being about 100 times more potent than Oxycontin and fairly easy to manufacture, its import from the Mexican cartels has spelled disaster and death. Fentanyl has been around for a long time, it is used mostly by anesthesiologists to assist with analgesia during surgery. A transdermal formulation became available in the early 1990s and has been used primarily for cancer pain as it delivers a steady amount of pain relief continuously for 3 days. Its use during the early phase of the opioid epidemic was actually fairly limited by pain specialists. Its pharmacology is favorable for anesthesia in that it starts working nearly immediately after injection and has less side effects than other opioids. I gratefully recall these pleasant effects when given it prior to a shoulder surgery. However, there have been huge problems with its introduction as a street drug. First, because it is so powerful it is difficult for addicts to know how much to use. Also, because it has been commonly mixed with heroin (simply because it is cheaper), many have overdosed and died without knowing what they were taking.

Overdose deaths have kept increasing every year and totaled 109,000 in 2022. About 75% of these involve use of an opioid. A significant change is that now these deaths frequently involve more than one drug such as methamphetamine or cocaine. Today fentanyl is blatantly sold without heroin as a simple matter of economics as heroin is more difficult and expensive to import. Many experts are now changing the name of this crisis to the "fentanyl epidemic". While there are some minor regional differences in deaths, they are nearly equal in urban and rural America. More men than women die from overdose in a ratio of two to one. However, recently, slightly more women than men are dying from overdoses in rural areas reversing that trend. The evolution and expansion of these three waves rolls on without an end in sight while getting worse each year. The main societal response has been to supply police and users with naloxone, a medication that reverses the effect of pulmonary arrest preventing overdose death. The increasing distribution of this medication has already saved thousands of lives but the root issues of importation, supply and distribution of opiates across America have not been addressed. With the receding Covid pandemic, opioid related deaths are poised to take over as a major health issue in the country.

In their studies of *Deaths of Despair* from 2015 and 2017, Princeton University economists Anne Case and Angus Deaton clearly reveal the details and causes of falling life expectancy from 2012-2017. Their expansive work describes precisely the factors responsible and include the triad of drug overdoses, suicides and alcohol related deaths as directly causing this extremely unusual downturn unseen during the previous hundred years. They document the rise of these *Deaths of Despair* accelerating from 1999 onward and are directly related to the rise of opioid use. What is most revealing are the differences in the demographics and age groups. The most significantly affected are middle-aged whites with only a high school education aged 40-60. Men were significantly more affected than women. The mortality rate increased nearly *three* times its previous rate during this 20-year period resulting in a steep decline in life expectancy which then affected the US life expectancy as a whole. In contrast, white, college educated folks continued to have *increased* life expectancy and falling mortality rates as did Blacks, Hispanics and

Asians in the US. In comparing international death rates and life expectancy, only the US experienced a decline. In looking at other medical causes of mortality such as cancer and heart disease there was no increase in mortality during this period with any age or demographic. This study definitively demonstrated the hollowing out of the middle class in America over the past two generations resulting in early deaths of the less educated white population. Whites without a college degree suffering from less job opportunities, falling wages, increasing disability and social disconnection fall by the wayside to succumb to these *Deaths of Despair* by drugs, alcohol and suicide (predominately by firearms). This continued loss of a significant portion of middle-aged Americans has not been addressed in any meaningful way and has continued through the Covid pandemic with the escalation of easily available street opioids and other drugs resulting in increasing overdose deaths every year. Truly a depressing, persistent failure in our country.

So, what role did I play in this epidemic? As mentioned, I was involved with many chronic pain patients and was somewhat convinced that "proper" treatment could help many of them. Many of these patients were placed on a long-acting opioid preparation and monitored for their response and, importantly, to determine their ability to live and function better on treatment. Some actually did better on scheduled dosing. Many, however, were not able to "live a normal life" and return to work. Some did worse and experienced worse pain! Yes, there are a small percentage of patients on chronic opioids that experience a paradoxical *increase* of pain. These are, obviously, some of the most difficult but are in most need of weaning off.

I left the spine group to start my private practice in 1995 and most of my chronic spine patients decided to keep their treatment in that clinic. In general medicine these patients make up a small percentage of one's practice, so it was easier to deal with from a numbers standpoint and was in the context of treating a variety of medical illnesses. While I treated all the patients who wished to continue to have me treat their chronic pain along with their other medical problems, I no longer wished to be in the "business" of chronic pain treatment. There were now several pain centers around that I could refer to, especially the academic centers, UCSF and Stanford, that were closeby. Interestingly, these university pain centers, staffed with anesthesiologists, were mostly interested in doing various injections and were unwilling to take on these chronic opioid patients. After referrals, I quickly found them back in my office with a "recommendation" to prescribe various combinations of opioids and other medications. My approach was to keep a close watch on those whom I was prescribing daily opioids by having them come in every few months for new prescriptions and monitor if they were abusing. I was vigilant in keeping them clear from other addictive meds such as benzodiazepines (tranquilizers). Still, there were many in my practice taking chronic opioids and some died along the way. Typically, I would find out about their death by getting a call from the coroner's office of a patient of mine being found dead and being asked to sign the death certificate. Most of the time the cause of these deaths were not apparent, most were middle aged patients, some had other medical problems but not a clear reason for sudden death. I always requested an autopsy to try to determine if the patient overdosed. However, the county coroner's offices vigorously put up a big fuss and generally refused which I suspect was for economic reasons. Many of these deaths were unresolved but, of course, many had to be overdoses, either accidentally or intentionally. As mentioned earlier, with the initiation of the California database of prescribed controlled medications available, I was able to accurately monitor what my patients were taking and could discover those who were abusing. As this epidemic unfolded, it became clear the movement of overprescribing opioids was just wrong and it was clear that limiting access along with close supervision was the best practice. While I was swept up in the early nonsense of this epidemic, fortunately, I was mostly able to keep away from being a big part of the problem.

And what about the players in this fiasco? Dr. Portenoy, the "king of pain", finally in 2016 recanted his initial recommendations and admitted he was mistaken after being paid handsomely by big pharma. However, he was able to keep his prestigious chairmanship position in New York. Purdue Pharmaceuticals, privately held by the Sackler family, after copious lawsuits from every level of government and individuals, filed for bankruptcy in 2019 being unable to pay the many billions in fines and facing hundreds of lawsuits. Their most recent deal has been to agree to pay 6 billion dollars but be shielded from any personal lawsuits. This compromise is currently under review as possibly not being legal. Many other opioid pharmaceutical companies have settled lawsuits totaling in the billions. And what about the infamous letter that set this disaster off? In 2017, for the first time in its history, the *New England Journal of Medicine* printed a retraction of it and presented a study of how that letter was misquoted and how often. The authors of the letter had repeatedly stated it was never their intention to have it misinterpreted and used so wrongly and have stated it was their worst research project in their careers.

While this epidemic has evolved past its origins of prescription narcotics, its continued growth in the US sees no foreseeable end and spells ongoing tragedy for the foreseeable future. A hopeful and recent downward trend in opioid overdose deaths occurred in the year prior to April 2024, as numbers declined by 10 percent in the US (from 110,000 to 100,000), although they continued to rise in the west of the country with increasing distribution of synthetic fentanyl. This decrease may be due to the more widespread availability and use of the naloxone, which reverses the respiratory arrest effect quickly and can be given as a nose spray with newer over the counter formulations although the exact reasons for the decrease are as of yet unclear. One can only hope this trend will continue.

CHAPTER 28

The Covid 19 Pandemic

May 15, 2003. Right before noon I got a call from the ER that a patient needs admission who doesn't have a primary physician on staff and being on-call requires me to check her into the hospital. The ER doc gives me the low down on this 25-year-old Asian woman with pneumonia who has low oxygen levels and needs to be admitted to the general medical floor for oxygen therapy, antibiotics and IV fluids. He tells me that she just returned from a trip to Hong Kong visiting family for a couple of weeks and got sick before she left. *Huh?… What?* I say to myself and then to the ER doc. "Don't you think this woman could have this deadly new flu from China recently named *SARS-1?*" "Did you guys put her in isolation, and have you called the infectious disease specialist to consult yet?", I asked in a confrontational tone. "We didn't think of that, but you have a point" is answered and *no* and *no* to the other questions. Now my clinical and personal anxiety is beginning to rise dramatically. The recent reports of this new viral illness being very contagious in medical situations with a high mortality rate are blinking red in my mind. "Please," I said, "call Dr. Rumack, and you guys all put on protective gowns, gloves and masks and get some ready for me," and hung up and went on-line to find any recent info I could on this disease. Now my concern was possibly contracting a deadly virus and giving it to my 3-year-old at home. Yikes! In a very unusual twist of being a doctor, I suddenly found that disease can take on a very personal paranoia when it can directly kill you and your family. I made it over to the ER after Dr. Rumack, who assured me that this case was *not* SARS-1 but he sent off some studies to the CDC and we kept her in an isolated unit for 2 days after which all the tests came back negative and at which time she was much better and was discharged home with a "regular" pneumonia. *Whew!*

Fast forward to February 8, 2020. I'm working in the outpatient clinic at PAMF (Palo Alto Medical Foundation) in Daly City, California and the front desk informs me that they have just added a new patient onto my schedule. She is a 36-year-old woman who just got off the plane at SFO from China and is sick with a flu. "*Huh?... What?...*", somehow reflexively repeating to myself and the front staff the same disbelief from 17 years prior. "Are you not aware of this deadly virus from China now in the US?" "How could you let her sit there waiting with all the other patients?" "Did you put her in the isolation room?" "Did you put a mask on the patient and tell the nurse to do so as well?" All the answers came back *no*. Oh jeez, I sigh to myself and wonder if we all are going to be infected with this new SARS-2 coronavirus that has been given the name COVID-19 (as a contraction of its long scientific name and year it was discovered, 2019). So starts the early days of the pandemic. I am shaking my head and wondering if there is some pattern here that medical personnel behave as ostriches oblivious to a possible life-threatening illness landing on their doorstep albeit many years apart.

My first Covid-19 patient was sick but far from critically ill. She had just returned from central China visiting her family for the Chinese New Year. Her illness started a few days before with a cold-like illness (sore throat, fever, cough) but she was not having trouble breathing and her vital signs were normal. She even saw a Chinese doctor before she left and was given a penicillin injection for obscure reasons (her symptoms were not at all consistent with a strep throat). A good deal of my afternoon that day was spent dealing with this woman, our fumbling clinic, the county health department and her Covid diagnosis. No one in our clinic had dealt with a case as of yet. After donning all the protective coverings we had (gown, mask, face shield, gloves and booties), I examined her after having spoken with the county health department. Since this was one of the early suspect cases, they were recommending an extensive amount of testing including several throat and nasal swabs, sputum and blood samples for a complete battery of various tests that *could* include testing for Covid. This case demonstrates how terribly unprepared and incompetent the US was through the first several months of the pandemic. At the time, only the CDC had the available tests for Covid which were under lock and key and used only at their discretion. In their hubris, the CDC had decided to reject the well-developed tests from Germany and elsewhere to "do it themselves" in January. However, their tests were cumbersome to perform and there was a limited supply and their early versions were inaccurate. Samples had to be sent to Atlanta *if* they approved of doing them. All the details of each case were relayed from the various county health departments to the CDC. I had no direct access to anyone at CDC. Due to their strict protocol and limited testing ability it turned out that the CDC was testing *no-one* who was not in the ICU and severely ill at that time. After many back and forth calls that afternoon with the county health department, I was told that the CDC refused to test this patient but we sent all the samples to our county health department anyway. Since there was no specific treatment back then, she was told to quarantine at home for 14 days with no direct contact with anyone including her husband and family. I called her everyday to check up on her at home and had told her if she developed difficulty breathing she would need to go to the ER. She was ill for about a week before feeling better and didn't progress to serious lung involvement, fortunately. This was a typical course for a younger person.

Quarantine is an interesting word that gets tossed around during pandemics. It comes from the Italian for 40 days (*quaranta giorni*) and its practice was first used during the mid-14th century bubonic plague that killed one-third of the population of Europe. As the *black death* was spreading from the middle east via shipping routes to Europe, Venice smartly required boats to remain in port for 40 days before their cargo or crew could come ashore as a preventative measure from the plague and it worked!

SARS-1 and *SARS-2* had remarkable initial similarities but they developed drastic differences. Strikingly, both outbreaks emanated from food markets in China and spread to health care workers who were caring for those ill. In both, initially, the Chinese government suppressed all news about the outbreaks and delayed informing the World Health Organization (WHO) and prevented any WHO investigation for weeks after recognizing the pandemics. And, of course, they were both coronaviruses and were related genetically but were not identical. They likely both started in live "wet" animal markets sold for food and have been likely traced to wild bats as the original source, although for Covid 19 there remains suspicion of a possible lab leak close to the area where the first outbreak began in Wuhan. Both of these viruses spread quickly worldwide within a month of their initial outbreaks. Here is where the similarities end, however. SARS-1 did not have the infectivity to the general public and was largely spread with direct contact from infected persons. This led to much fewer infections and faded quickly after 8 months with a total number of documented cases only about 8,000. However, unlike SARS-2 the mortality rate was nearly 10%, much higher than the ~1% of Covid. Fortunately, no further SARS-1 outbreaks occurred after one year and have not returned. No-one in the US died from SARS-1. A cousin of both viruses emerged in 2012 in the Middle East after mutations caused camels to carry the MERS (Middle East respiratory syndrome) coronavirus. This was frightening because of its mortality rate, 34%, but was also a short-lived event.

Quickly, our clinic developed a "respiratory protocol" on any patient requesting an appointment with any symptoms related to Covid, including cough, fever, sore throat, headache, diarrhea and abdominal pain, the emerging symptom complex, and did not give patients an appointment in person. They were referred to receive nursing advice initially but if found to be developing severe disease they were referred to the ER for evaluation. Essentially, we stopped seeing in person *any* patient in the office who might have Covid and isolated anyone who had any suspicious symptoms while being checked into the clinic. With no ability to test anyone, we had no choice.

There are several important sequential and intertwined stories about how the pandemic evolved. Due to modern genetic sequencing the virus was discovered, identified and its genome completed by Chinese researchers in early January 2020. However, because the Chinese government was downplaying infections and suppressing news and scientific information to the world, their sequencing was not available to the rest of the world for several weeks. Covid 19 was found to have nearly 80% of the same genetic makeup as SARS-1. Sequencing the genetic code of this new coronavirus commenced around the world as cases spread globally. By continually updating its genetic makeup in real time, scientists have determined any differences or strains that emerged as the pandemic progressed which has proved invaluable in monitoring the developments of mutations throughout the pandemic.

The rapid development of testing for the virus is also one of the incredible advances of modern science in the current age. While many tests for the virus have emerged and are available, the first one used exclusively relied on previous genetic technology developed in the US in the 1980s. The use of *polymerase chain reaction* (PCR) which is the ability to amplify a small area of DNA in order to analyze and study its specific components has revolutionized the study of genomics since its invention in 1983 by the eccentric American Nobel prize winner, Kary Mullis, who claimed that the process came to him during an LSD trip! PCR has a very broad range of applications in genomic and medical science and its specific modification for the RNA virus of Covid quickly made it the standard for worldwide testing. Unfortunately, due to the hubris of the CDC, who could have used the very capable test developed by the World Health Organization (WHO) by mid-January, its decision to develop their own was to the detriment of the US by creating a test that was cumbersome, inaccurate and exclusively available to the CDC. My colleagues and I were shaking our heads over this bungling. There was nothing more important in the early phase than being able to know who was infected with Covid. Remember that January, February and March are peak cold and influenza seasons in the US and being able to identify and isolate infected Covid individuals early in the course of a spreading infection would have been crucial to containing it. It took nearly 2 months before commercial labs were allowed to develop their own version and become widely available which was well into March. Importantly, these tests had to be performed by a health care person and sent to a specific lab to obtain a result which, fortunately, the technology could complete quickly (within a few hours). The medical community was stunned by the lack of clear leadership by the CDC throughout the first year of the pandemic. We were all used to being "overalerted" by bulletins and emails of any possible threat to public health in the past and were now being largely left in the dark and unable to properly care for patients. Importantly due to such limited testing, no-one knew the extent of this rapidly expanding worldwide pandemic during the first year.

For the first time in 50 years, on January 31st, 2000, the US placed an international travel ban. This ban was initially for non-citizens coming from China but expanded as the pandemic spread quickly to Europe. In early February, 49 senators sent a letter to the head of the CDC requesting to allow states to develop and use their own tests. At the same time, it was revealed that the US had a serious shortage of protective equipment (masks, gloves, gowns, etc.) and were reliant on China for supplying them as nearly none were made in the US any longer. The spread around the world continued unimpeded even though China started its lockdown efforts on January 23rd. The cat was already out of the bag after nearly half a million travelers from China had visited the US and nearly as many had gone to Europe by the end of January 2020.

While it was originally assumed that all infections were due to contact from Chinese visitors, it became increasingly apparent through month two, February, that outbreaks were being discovered that were not directly related to any contact with Chinese or American travelers from China indicating that community spread had begun. Also, news from a Princess cruise ship held in port in Japan that many of the passengers were testing positive *without any symptoms* started the concern of asymptomatic carriers and transmission.

In our clinic, we kept seeing non respiratory patients as *if* there was not any threat of getting sick. We were not wearing masks, although we discussed the idea. There were three times a week updates from our senior medical directors on the progress of hospitalized and ER Covid patients and death counts. In retrospect, it seemed odd that we went to work unprotected but there was the concern that there was a limited amount of protective equipment to go around. The prevailing view and recommendation at that time were based on previous infectious disease data and assumptions that the infection was spread by "droplets" and/ or direct contact and therefore was preventable by "social distancing" of 6 feet and cleaning surfaces with bleach. These assumptions were completely upended within a few months.

On March 19, California became the first state to "shelter in place" and everyone was directed to stay home except for "essential workers" and to limit medical care to only the sickest patients as mandated by Governor Gavin Newsom. Suddenly, there were no patients to see in the clinics, all elective surgery was canceled and the only patients seen were those in the ER and those needing in-hospital care. All the doctors and staff were sent home, and we began the difficult process of starting a never done style of medical care—remote visits via phone and internet. Sutter Health (the parent company where I worked) had absolutely no experience and no infrastructure to transition to this method of medical care but rapidly put in place phone visits and then video visits via computer applications for patients to use. The problem, of course, is that while we all quickly learned how to use the technology, the patients didn't and were mostly in the dark, ill-equipped, confused, frustrated and fearful of using the technology (except for phone calls) and mostly gave up initially. This meant that for over a month, there was bare bones medical care given everywhere, except for Kaiser! Interestingly, the Kaiser system was the most advanced in having set up video visits and electronic communication for their patients many years before the pandemic. They seamlessly shifted to remote video visits and their patients were able to continue to get medical treatment with much less disruption.

New rapid PCR testing became available from commercial laboratories in late March. Sutter set up drive-thru testing centers in the parking lots of some of its hospitals for patients with respiratory symptoms or contacts of Covid positive patients to get tested. This well-organized assembly line operation consisted of patients in their cars with an appointment wearing a mask getting checked in, performing self-nasal swabbing under observation with the windows closed and passing the enclosed swab to gowned, gloved, and masked health professionals to have it sent to the lab for processing. Since the encounters were staffed by doctors and nurses, we got to evaluate the symptoms the patients were having and offer advice. This type of drive-thru testing was done all over America and was the standard for over the next 6 months.

After a couple of positive preliminary studies were published, the FDA gave an "emergency use authorization" (EUA) to the malaria drugs, hydroxychloroquine and chloroquine for treatment of Covid-19 at the end of March. There was a significant amount of medical controversy from the get-go on the study results and even the rationality of considering these medications. While these older medications still had some effect on treating mild forms of malaria (a parasite) in the world, there was no scientific data on a mechanism where they would suppress a virus. Also, in unscientific fashion, these were proposed to be an effective cocktail with the antibiotic azithromycin. Within 2 months, the data in these studies were found to be faulty and the authorization and the published studies were withdrawn but there remained unscientific and misleading proponents including a person in the White House.

Around the same time in March, a study from China portended a brand-new way this infection was able to be transmitted. Ophthalmologists found patients infected via the eye even though the Covid virus is minimally present in tears. This began to open up the concept of airborne transmission which has turned out to be one of the major revelations of viral infections discovered in this pandemic.

Within a few days of that study, a new vaccine company, Moderna, was one of two companies (the other being Pfizer) who were developing the untested technique of *mRNA vaccines* and beginning its first clinical trial on humans. Remarkably, this was just 2 months into the pandemic by scientists who had started work on the vaccine immediately after the Covid virus genome was sequenced! This technology had been in development in the aftermath of SARS-1 but lost momentum and funding as that epidemic faded in 2004. It was quickly resurrected and pushed forward by urgent necessity. Vaccine development had never before seen such a speedy advancement. Vaccines had traditionally taken a decade or more before they were available to the public.

The "shelter-in-place" order remained until June 18th in California at which time Governor Newsom instituted a masking order for all individuals in any public space. Putting a mask on became the first but not the only *militant* controversy of the pandemic. It quickly became a symbol of "freedom" by those opposed who expressed: "If I choose to get Covid, it's my right!", ignoring common sense, international practices (where in China it was simply done routinely) and the science. Those opposed openly defied the ruling helping spread contagion to the surprise and disgust of most of us in the medical profession. One glaringly missing element in educating the public about masking was the lack of public service announcements. Messages were absent on radio, TV, the internet, print news, billboards, or anywhere! In contrast, in Italy and France, every 15 minutes there was a short announcement explaining the benefits of masking and social distancing in preventing spread. Here in the US it was a silent, brooding, misinformation landscape that had no connection to the societal threat that had descended on the world. While one could possibly sympathize with an individual's decision to take the "personal risk" of getting infected and accepting the consequences including dying, this stance took only a one-sided, narcissistic view. What had emerged early was the understanding that asymptomatic, minimally symptomatic and presymptomatic infections were a large percentage of the total number of infections and a significant component to the pandemic's spread. Does one have the "right" to spread infection and therefore kill fellow citizens during a pandemic? To me, that is morally indefensible. The science was very clear that wearing a mask prevented *infected* persons from spreading contagion. The whole masking issue was also made confusing by another CDC fumble. Because there was a limited supply of surgical and N95 masks in the country, it was thought that the supply should be conserved for medical personnel and they initially told the public to not wear a mask against evidence while "not thinking" of recommending the public use a cloth mask for protection, which later became standard advice and were easily made.

After doing telemedicine for 6 weeks, we went back to the office in mid-June after the lockdown was opened up in California. For those few months, I was also confronting a personal dilemma. As I was approaching age 65, I had planned a year ago to retire from practicing full time medicine after 35 years! It seemed like an appropriate time to explore life outside of work. However, as the pandemic took over everything in life, I increasingly felt enormous guilt and a sense of deserting my duty by quitting in the middle of this mess. Especially, since so many of my long-term patients were stressing out over all that was going on! I decided to postpone my retirement to the end of the year and see how things were then and got back to work with a clearer mindset.

Back at work, we were all wearing masks and were seeing very few patients in the office mostly due to patients' reluctance. Most of my patient care was done via video or phone visits. There was mounting evidence that the virus was spread via airborne methods, especially indoors. This meant that 6 feet social distancing recommendations were doing very little as a preventive method as microscopic aerosolized virus particles remained floating in the air for many hours, especially indoors. On July 6th, 2020, over 100 scientists wrote a request demanding that WHO revise their recommendations for preventing Covid by including airborne transmission as a significant component of contagion. By early July in the US cases were spiking significantly in many states that were considering reopening their economy completely. California put their reopening on pause in mid-July. It's crucial to emphasize the importance of this new finding on transmission via airborne pathway. The new science also discovered that *all* colds, flu, respiratory viruses, bacteria pneumonias and even TB (tuberculosis) can become aerosolized and airborne and be particularly infectious in indoor spaces without sophisticated ventilation. These diseases are sent into the air easily by just talking and breathing from an infected person!! This upended all the previous assumptions that persisted over the past 100 hundred years.

With increasing concern, I began to ask at work to consider routine testing of all the personnel in our clinic on a weekly basis to keep our work environment as safe as possible. Our medical directors brushed this off as unnecessary and too expensive and claimed there was still a shortage of testing abilities. Then in late July, we found one of the medical assistants who had come to work for 2 days "with a mild cold" had Covid. I then asked that we all be tested to see if there were some of us with asymptomatic infections which were increasingly found to represent at least 25% of all cases of Covid. Again, this request was denied.

I tried to rally my colleagues to petition for more extensive testing but there was little support to challenge the administration. I began to feel that some thought of me as a troublemaker. At this time, I decided to wear clear goggles as well as an N95 mask (all of which were easily available by that time) at work knowing that transmission of airborne virus to the eyes was a real thing as increasing data showed that those who wore glasses or eyewear had lower chances of infections. Then in August, another medical assistant was found to have Covid after being at work for several days before getting tested. I was getting progressively worried that protective measures were not being instituted for those at the front lines of health care. We needed regular testing and strict protocols for indoor work that were not being attended to. Personally, I was concerned about being in the age category that had a much higher rate of mortality than others and I didn't want to end my career dying from getting a virus at work. I changed my plan and took a vacation in September and negotiated to work only remotely until the end of the year at which time I would officially retire. The vaccines were still months away at that point.

Testing was advancing, while blood antibody testing had been available for many months that could prove if one had a previous Covid infection (at least 2 weeks previously), commercial labs developed a rapid home nasal swab test that used an antigen-antibody reaction that could give a result in 5 minutes and became authorized by the FDA by the end of the summer. The beauty of this type of testing was its simplicity and its interpretation as it was similar to a home pregnancy test: 1 line (control)—negative; 2 lines—positive. While there were issues with some of the initially produced tests that gave more *false positives* than it should, this type of testing evolved to be the best and simplest way for individuals to check their status. Eventually, the US government sent several of these to anyone who requested them for free! If there was doubt about the accuracy, one could still have a PCR test. However, there was an issue that arose with PCR testing which was the result could remain *positive* for a prolonged period after one was infected with Covid. This was due to the extreme sensitivity of detecting fragments of the viral DNA that could remain in the nose after the infection was cleared. There was a period where employers were demanding that workers submit a negative PCR test before allowing them to return to work. We saw many patients that were perfectly well and recovered yet tested positive for several weeks after their infection. These patients were not infectious. It was decided to not test patients after 2 weeks from their initial test because of these possible confusing results. Fortunately, post Covid infection does *not* have a residual carrier state where patients can infect others after about 2 weeks from the initial infection.

Several other important medical advances came out by the end of the summer, 2020. A previously approved intravenous medication, remdesivir, was found, after several months of use, to essentially have no benefit in preventing or reducing severe Covid infections. This was after the company had decided to gouge everyone by charging up to ten thousand dollars to treat one patient! More importantly, it was found that a common and extremely inexpensive form of cortisone, dexamethasone, reduced the risk of dying from Covid in sick hospitalized patients by a whopping one-third! Truly a fantastic lifesaving finding and became the standard of care in all hospitalized Covid patients. Also on a positive side, the development of monoclonal antibody infusion improved recovery and reduced infections in patients at higher risk, mostly the elderly. This was given mostly as a preventative measure. However, ominously, a report from Houston on September 23rd, 2020, that a more contagious strain of Covid was identified led to discovery that this pandemic could and would be changing and for the worse.

The evolution of the Covid-19 virus strains gave us all a nice review of the Greek alphabet. It's important to point out that all viruses develop mutations on a continuous basis and are part of their normal machinery for reproduction in that a small change in their genetic code occurs easily and naturally as they make new copies of themselves *inside* other cells. Viruses depend on entering and using a living cell's internal physiology to accomplish its only goal—make more of itself and then break out to go find other living cells it can use. They cannot reproduce on their own and because of this limitation biologic science does not classify viruses as living organisms. Changes in the genetic makeup of viruses can possibly have many results including: doing nothing, making it easier to enter certain cells, make its reproduction increase (or decrease), make it more or less adaptable to its environment, or a combination of these and other effects. At a basic biological level, viruses carry out the process of evolution in real time. The vast majority of viruses in the world cause no harm to humans, animals or other living organisms and there are vast quantities and varieties in the world floating in the air, swimming and hanging around our world. It is likely that the Covid-19 virus was initially hiding out in bats for some time before it developed enough mutations to be able to infect humans. Bats are fascinating because of their immune system tolerance. They can harbor many viruses that in other animals cause disease. This novel coronavirus of which there are a total of seven types has been known for a long time and has mostly caused mild cold-like infections. The shape of the virus gives it its name. It is a ball shaped virus coated with protein spikes (a corona of spikes) that attach and enter a susceptible cell via the specific binding capabilities of those spikes.

The first variant of Covid-19, the Alpha variant, was discovered in Great Britain in November 2020 and quickly spread worldwide to become the dominant variant infecting humans. The reason this and many of the following variants quickly became the *only* variant in the world was due to its increased ability to infect humans. It was estimated that Alpha was nearly 50% more infectious that the original strain of Covid-19 and unfortunately also caused more severe disease. The Beta variant was found in South Africa at the end of 2020 and was found to be even more infectious than Alpha. However, for unknown reasons it did not spread much beyond Africa. This pattern of increased infectability has been traced to changes in the spike protein that attaches to cells in the respiratory system (nose, sinuses, lungs). Several mutations favoring attachment allow more of the new variant to infect and subsequently spread to others.

The Delta variant was found in India in late 2020 and turned out to be much worse from a standpoint of infectivity and causing more severe disease. It was estimated to be nearly twice as able to infect someone than the Alpha variant while resulting in worse infections, hospitalizations and death. Delta progressed to be the dominant worldwide strain and remained the predominant strain for nearly a year until Omicron took over in November 2021. Omicron and its children (subtypes) have been around for over 2 years as of this writing. It has been a prodigious spreader of Covid infections with greater than a million per day in late 2021 due to acquiring over 20 mutations in its spike protein. Interestingly, it causes significantly *less* severe illness and rates of death. Its increased infectivity is due to its affinity for the upper part of the airways, sinuses and nose and less so deep in the lungs.

What exactly does Covid-19 do in the body and how does it kill people? Initially, it acts very similar to other respiratory viruses by attaching to the mucosa of the nose, sinuses or lungs, entering those cells, replicating, then bursts out to repeat the process to nearby cells until the person's immune system mounts a response and begins neutralizing the viruses with antibodies and certain immune cells. This process typically takes many days before it is slowed down then stopped completely. Illness is caused by *both* local damage to the tissues and from the immunological response which induces increased mucus production, local tissue inflammation, and circulating inflammatory proteins (cytokines). These cause the infected person to be congested, coughing, feverish and a general feeling of "being sick". After a week or so, the infected person begins to feel better as the virus and inflammation are cleared from the body. A process we all are familiar with. However, in some individuals the bodies' immunologic responses get way out of whack due to overstimulation and over responding. What has been found with severe Covid-19 are two immunologic processes that lead to serious lung and other organ damage. The first is that making *interferons* (specific proteins that prevent viruses from entering cells) is suppressed by Covid-19. The second is the extreme production of very high levels of inflammatory proteins called cytokines in a process known as *cytokine storm*. These two events lead to huge amounts of virus and inflammation throughout the body. In creating so much inflammation, injury and damage can occur in the lungs and other organs such as the heart, liver and kidneys known as *multi-organ failure*. Often, dying from Covid-19 is due to drowning in one's own inflamed fluids in the lungs. This excessive inflammatory response prevents the lungs from getting oxygen to the blood. It's a brutal thing to see as patients on mechanical ventilators and 100% oxygen still unable to get enough oxygen in their bloodstream to allow the heart and brain to work. It seems somewhat odd that these deaths are due to the secondary effects of the virus on the immune system and not directly from the virus itself. This is not a unique phenomenon, however. People who die of the flu have a similar mechanism, but Covid-19 induced this hyper-inflammatory response at a rate 10 times higher especially in older populations, those with diabetes, severe obesity or a compromised immune system.

For the last few months of 2020, the first year of the pandemic, I was working in a similar fashion to millions of others, remotely from home. I had a regular schedule of video visits of various patients that included some of my long-term patients but a significant number of Covid patients, probably about half of all those visits. These included the variety of the different ways Covid affected folks. Some were seen regularly after having survived a terrible bout in the hospital being on a ventilator and in the ICU for a long period before recovering well enough to be at home. These patients remained debilitated usually for months before regaining a semblance of decent health. The ravages of lung damage, severe weakness, brain fog and slow recovery particularly in those with pre-existing medical problems such as diabetes portended a very long, slow road back to their former lives after severe illness with Covid. However, most had a relatively minor event after being slightly ill, testing positive and recovering completely in 1-2 weeks. The early strains of Covid were famous for patients losing their sense of smell and taste. For most patients this came back but often it took months of the very strange sensation of all food being tasteless due to the virus attacking and damaging those specific parts of the nervous system. Many patients, due to confinement, limited activity, stress, loss of work and social isolation succumbed to gaining significant weight and many developed anxiety and depressive symptoms. Ten, twenty or even forty pounds were put on during that long first year although it seemed most were in the range of gaining the "Covid 19 pounds".

In a telling and ironic representation of the first year of Covid, as I was preparing for real retirement in December, with the Christmas holidays nearing, my 94-year-old dad underwent emergency surgery for an intestinal blockage. He was being treated at Thomas Jefferson Hospital in Philadelphia which is the main teaching facility of the medical school I had graduated from 40 years prior! After undergoing a second surgery, he was slowly recovering after being in the ICU for several days. I received a call that he had developed a cough and tested positive for Covid-19 and then quickly died 24 hours later. He had, unfortunately, contracted Covid from a health care worker in the hospital. While there has been well documented studies of transmission to health care workers from infected patients, the opposite phenomenon has received no study or reports even though I have heard many stories of this occurring throughout the time of the pandemic. It was not surprising that this would happen. With over a quarter of infections being asymptomatic and the time of someone being contagious extending to several days before being ill and after being ill, many don't know they are contagious. With the close, continuous contact in the small indoor environment of hospital rooms with the same personnel—doctors, nurses and staff, there is the formula for contagion easily spreading. After my dad's death, I didn't hear any follow-up on any of his caregivers being tested. In fact, in all hospitals (and in clinics such as ours) in the US there *never* developed protocols to routinely test hospital (or medical clinic) workers and so there was ample opportunity for this to occur.

The amazing initial clinical reports of 3 vaccines being 90% or greater effective in preventing infections were released in mid-November 2020 and surprised everyone in the medical world. These studies were completed on tens of thousands of patients, allowing the FDA to fast-track emergency use approval (EUA) by the middle of December. This meant that in less than a year several extremely effective vaccines were going to be available for the public. An incredible event that no-one would have predicted at the start of the year. As an initial rollout, the vaccines were available to healthcare personnel by the end of the year. Then it was deemed important to start vaccinating the most vulnerable, the elderly, and those with qualifying medical conditions.

As the first year of pandemic closed, the devastating effects and profound changes in every area of society were truly unprecedented and touched everyone. Economically, the US went on a downward spiral for the first six months with GDP plummeting 31.4% in the second quarter while 21 million Americans lost their jobs with an unemployment rate of nearly 15%. Large job losses were seen in the service sectors of restaurants, bars, hotels, entertainment, airlines, tourism, retail and manufacturing. This decline was reflected in the S&P 500 losing 34% of its value. However, in an almost equally incredible turnaround, GDP rose by 33% in the third quarter and by year end the stock market had recouped all its early loss and had a positive return of 16%! The rapid shift to remote work with high-tech infrastructure allowed office jobs (and even medical care) to use video conferencing and other digital tools as never before as companies adopted the "new normal" of flexible work policies. Ordering everything online became the standard way to shop. Of course, live entertainment, sports, the arts and even the Tokyo Olympics were put on hold. In my field of work, I discovered that several primary care colleagues in the area decided to just roll up their shingle and retire early. These were doctors near the end of their careers like myself and could not easily transform their small business into a high-tech video conferencing office overnight and after a few months of no income closed shop. I would have likely been in the same boat if I had not shifted to a large organization 2 years prior. In our medical group, there was intense debate about the needed adjustment in compensation with the abrupt and severe drop in revenue from not really seeing many patients for several months. Fortunately, I was shielded from these issues being a contracted employee of the medical group until my retirement.

The social and psychological impact of that first year was enormous and had devastating effects on many. Seniors were largely isolated from their families and when hospitalized could not have visitors. Folks shifting to remote work at home encountered an isolated world and extremely limited in-person contact due to confinements and social distancing. Working parents struggled enormously with the concept that not only did they need to work but also provide all day childcare and help their school aged children adapt to online schooling. I observed this directly with several of my female colleagues with young children at home. Their stress level went through the roof and they ended up cutting back their work hours to attempt to accommodate all the new demands of life. Teaching young children with video classrooms did not go well and along with their loss of direct contact with other students, teachers and the world has left a large proportion behind the benchmarks for their level. We all experienced the new Zoom-infused world of mostly screen connections. In our household, my wife and myself were working remotely, one son was sent home from the college dorms doing online classwork and a daughter was working remotely in her hi-tech job. It became a dance of spreading out and finding a comfortable quiet spot to work in the house and then convening for meals and chats. As empty nesters, we actually relished having our adult children at home as an extended family experience while they grumbled continuously about their "loss of my life". A fascinating neighborhood experience took effect as everyone was cooped up all day—the late afternoon/evening walk. Suddenly, everyone was just out walking around to get some fresh air and be outside. I've never seen so many of my neighbors so regularly, although most of them wore masks and simply waved as getting to know new people was not part of the formula. Some actually organized social distanced street "parties" with cocktails and the kids running around. My favorite was this fabulous group of elderly women who gathered for happy hour often on the driveway of one of their townhouses, complete with fold out chairs, *high balls* in hand, chatting, laughing, playing music and cards while saying "hello" to everyone who passed by! For a significant number, however, the social isolation and contraction of life drove many to experience severe anxiety, some to deep depression and some turned to alcohol or drug use and some to suicide. I encountered many patients on video visits that were experiencing new and intense anxieties about life that they never had previously. While there was an effort to get these patients counseling, many had a tough time seeing their life turn into a prison with economic hardship on top of it. As a reactive measure, all of us on the front lines found ourselves prescribing antidepressants and anti-anxiety medicines frequently.

Medical care basically came to a standstill after the first lockdown in March and remained limited throughout the rest of the year. Elective surgeries stopped, no-one went to the doctor for routine follow-ups or preventative care or for any minor problems. We were basically trying to keep our patients on chronic treatments going and attempting to monitor them as best we could. We treated patients over the phone and video without any benefit of examination or testing. Patients usually refused to go for labs or X-rays anyway. This meant we used our best judgements on various problems such as chest, abdominal and pelvic pains, injuries, neurologic complaints, and all the other what-have-you problems under the sun. Actually, we were encountering only about a quarter of patients than before the lockdowns while those who were significantly sick had to be referred to the ER. Treating patients online after they had survived a severe bout of Covid in the hospital enlightened us to how debilitated, weak and fragile they were after battling the disease for sometimes many weeks in the hospital and/or ICU. Of course, some of our patients died. We had a weekly count from the hospital about how many Covid patients were in the ICU, the number of deaths and total numbers admitted. This was our real time way to see what this pandemic was doing locally. Another new effect of social distancing was that funerals were also run online via a Zoom call as social gatherings were prohibited. The life of a doctor was similar to the rest of society, filled with uncertainty, restriction, vulnerability, new stresses and an entirely new way of interacting with the world. As hospitals began to fill up with Covid patients, there was growing concern that all of us that had been strictly outpatient physicians for many years were going to be needed to help care for the growing storm of critically ill pandemic patients. This created another area of potential stress as the rigors, changes and urgency of caring for ICU patients was no longer at our fingertips. Various possible scenarios emerged and were discussed and we began to review in detail hospital care protocols in anticipation of returning to hospital work. While our hospital and most hospitals had an increasing number of Covid patients, all the other types of patients decreased significantly allowing the hospital based physicians to continue to care for everyone and, fortunately, for us in primary care to not have to go back to intensive hospital care. Northern California never got to the breakpoint that hospitals in New York got to, where all beds were taken and patients were backed up in the ERs for days or weeks. As a stopgap, my former hospital, Seton, was designated as a "pandemic" hospital and received special funding from the state which actually helped its bleak economic picture improve for over a year.

The bizarre political machinations that occurred in that first year of the pandemic created a governmental and societal nightmare equally unseen in the US previously. The person in the white house at the time was a major factor in expanding misinformation, denying the science surrounding the pandemic and directly caused at least 100,000 (by conservative estimates) of the deaths from Covid (out of 350,000) in 2020. The pronouncements against mask wearing, testing, social distancing, interference of accurate scientific information from the CDC and promotion of unproven and dangerous treatments fueled his supporters to avoid preventative measures and resulted in a death rate 3 times higher in those counties that voted for him. Diffuse and persistent misinformation rampant on social media and conservative media increased the risk of death and the subsequent movement to not be vaccinated in his followers accelerated deaths in the following years. Of course, there was a presidential election in November 2020 that changed the administration and party in the White House which also dramatically changed the direction of public health policy. It is important to note that an extremely important result of vaccine development was spurred on by *Operation Warp Speed* (OWS) (in a reference to the TV show *Star Trek*). Interestingly (in contrast to the denial of the seriousness of the pandemic from the administration in place at that time), OWS was included in the aid package approved by Congress, CARES, and was implemented in May 2020 as a joint venture of private-public development, manufacturing and distribution of vaccines and other therapeutics for Covid. Clearly, without this early support vaccines would never have been developed so quickly.

In January 2021, starting my new retirement life, I immediately signed up and got the two Moderna vaccines spaced 4 weeks apart of this remarkable new vaccine technology. Unlike previous vaccines like influenza that used eggs to produce inactivated viruses, these new vaccines from Moderna and Pfizer incorporated genetic material, *messenger RNA* (mRNA), to induce the body to directly produce specific proteins of the virus that would then produce an immunological response. In this case, the encoded genetic material was for the spike proteins of the Covid-19 virus circulating in 2020. While the vaccine was complicated to produce as mRNA is not stable in a pure form, requiring a special coating and refrigeration for mass distribution, its efficacy was extraordinary and unique in being nearly 95% in preventing infections. This technology followed up the initial work on developing vaccines for SARS-1. In comparison, the annual flu vaccine is between 40-60% effective. Like most folks (~90%), I had some side effects which for me included "flu-like" feelings for 24 hours and a sore arm for a couple of days. The second shot caused much less of a reaction to me. In contrast, my wife got the red swollen "Covid arm" that continued for several days after her second shot.

From the medical standpoint, this was a miracle with the ability to halt an advancing worldwide infectious disease. However, the demons of misinformation quickly capitalized to spread doubt and falsehoods and enhance the conspiracy theories floating on social media, causing reluctance and further loss of life to those susceptible to the nonsense. Not only was this protection against a potentially deadly disease, it was free! Something Americans also were not used to in regards to medical care.

With a new administration in place in the Federal government, the change was rapid from altering and discounting scientific information to a more honest, realistic appraisal of the pandemic. While there was a somewhat slow roll out to distribute the vaccines, by the end January 2021 over 24 million Americans had received at least one vaccine dose and this number went to 100 million by the end of March. Testing was vastly expanded and a new rule that all travelers entering the US had to demonstrate a negative test was appropriately initiated. However, the pandemic was in full swing with daily deaths in the US approaching 3,000 by the end February when over half a million in total had died from Covid-19. It became the leading cause of death in the country. In a stark turnaround from the previous year, the US government started shipping home rapid test kits to all Americans, also for free so that appropriate measures can be taken by individuals.

In March 2021 guidelines began to change to allow fully vaccinated individuals to not have to mask in indoor public places. Also,
the administration passed a nearly 2-trillion-dollar rescue plan for extended unemployment benefits, rental assistance, child tax credits and
direct financial aid of $1400 to eligible Americans helping a significant
portion of the population weather the severe economic hardship of
the first year of the pandemic. In April, travel restrictions for the fully
vaccinated were loosened and follow up studies on the two mRNA
vaccines show protection for those over 65 from hospitalization at
an incredible 95% rate and in May the vaccines are shown to protect
against getting infected by 94%.

With all this good news of the decreasing number of cases, hospitalizations and deaths, there was a sense of relief that maybe this pandemic
was going to be beat back and life would return to "normal" in the reasonably near future. Then the Delta variant migrated from India to the
US and quickly became the dominant strain in June 2021, starting the
third wave of Covid infections. The Delta variant demonstrated natural evolution at work. Simply because it was nearly twice as contagious
as the previous variant, Alpha, it took over quickly worldwide. Along
with this increased infectivity it also caused more severe disease than
previous variants particularly in those unvaccinated. The current vaccines did demonstrate continued good protection against Delta. By the
end of July due to the Delta surge, masking and social contact restrictions were re-instituted appropriately. However, the trajectory of the
pandemic began a sharp demarcation between the vaccinated and the
unvaccinated. Vaccinated folks were largely protected from severe disease and deaths even though there were some breakthrough infections.
The unvaccinated took the full force of repeat infections, easy transmission through the community, severe disease, hospitalizations and a
sharp rise in deaths that continued unabated. Much has been written
about this divide that reflected political affiliations. Blue states and communities did much better than red ones due to the pervasive resistance
to vaccination from misinformation. Many experts have projected that
a fully vaccinated population would have been able to limit the damage of Delta and subsequent variants as the concept of "herd immunity"

became discussed. For an effective herd immunity, an 80% vaccination or prior infection rate needs to be attained to halt the spread of contagion. Unfortunately, the vaccination rate of Republicans at the start of the Delta wave was only about 50% and most of those had only received one of the two shots needed, setting up the rapid spread of a more infectious and deadly version of Covid-19 and possibly the development of new more deadly variants. Also, the unvaccinated were found to be five times as likely to get *reinfected* by Delta. In October, the first booster vaccine was approved to try to provide additional protection against infections. The struggle with Covid was far from over and with regional differences in infection rates and changing recommendations for social interaction, the public was becoming weary, frustrated and confused as we approached the end of the second year of the pandemic.

Then just in time for the end of the year holidays, the Omicron variant arrived on our shores from its origin in South Africa in early December 2021 and spread rapidly worldwide within a few weeks pushing all other variants aside. Again, virus evolution was in play here but was super charged this time. The Omicron variant was significantly different from previous strains with more than 30 mutations on its spike protein; it was able to gain entry into the upper respiratory tract much easier. This, of course, is what one would expect with a "survival of the fittest" strategy as all the other variants quickly faded away. The body count in the US for 2021 after the first year of vaccines becoming available was not very encouraging with over 500,000 Americans having officially died from Covid-19 during 2021. It is likely that this figure was below the actual number of Covid deaths due to misreporting such as other causes being listed on death certificates like "pneumonia" or "respiratory illness".

Right before Christmas, 2021, a new oral medication was given emergency use authorization by the FDA, Paxlovid. Building on the pharmacologic advances against HIV viruses, this new drug was a combination of two antiviral medications that were shown to halt Covid from reproducing. This drug was approved to treat mild to moderate positive Covid-19 and was shown to prevent infections from becoming serious. It needed to be given within a few days of symptom onset. While it generally worked well to shorten infection times, it had in some patients an unfortunate limitation in that some developed *rebound* symptoms after stopping the five-day course. It could not be given a second time and so patients just had to wait out their second bout of Covid after thinking they were done with it. Fortunately, this rebound effect was in a small percentage of patients, but I had 3 friends who had this happen, and boy, were they not happy about it!

Thus began the fourth wave of Covid-19 to start the third year of the pandemic and it was ferocious! On January 3rd 2022 the number of new cases topped 1 million *per day* in the US. This number was likely lower than the actual incidence as by this time many infections were diagnosed with the home rapid antigen kit and not reported or required to health agencies. The medical world was bracing for the worst after 2 years of several peaks and valleys. Additional booster vaccines were recommended to those more susceptible immediately. There was more bad news from studies using the previously approved monoclonal antibody infusions for those at risk in that they were *ineffective* against Omicron. An additional 100,000 Americans died of Covid by early February. Again, those most vulnerable to severe disease and death were the unvaccinated even if they had previous Covid infections. Fortunately, it quickly became apparent that Omicron, while highly contagious, caused, in general, less severe disease. There were several plausible factors for this. In March, the WHO (World Health Organization) estimated that nearly 90% of the world's population had antibodies from Covid from either infections or vaccinations which gave some immunological protection to most. Also, Omicron was different from previous strains in that it predominantly infected the upper respiratory airways, the nose and sinuses, and did not go deep into the lungs where severe disease happens. These factors meant that the vast majority of infections were similar to the common cold or asymptomatic. Remember that it has been estimated that about one-quarter of all Covid infections produced no symptoms. We were all lucky that the new variant strain did not also cause worse infections with its increased infectivity! However, all the previous vaccines only had partial effectiveness to Omicron as it was found to cleverly develop "immunologic escape" due to all its mutations preventing antibodies and immune cells to neutralize it quickly. Studies gave reassurance that those who had full vaccination status (2 doses and a booster) had 94% protection against severe disease and death with Omicron infection. Still, the US crossed the 1 million dead from Covid mark in May.

I discovered the latest Omicron variant personally on a family trip to Italy in June 2021. Getting an additional booster shot a week before departure did not prevent me from getting Covid a few days after landing. A bit of a sore throat and runny nose which I first chalked up to a possible allergy was shown to be the real thing with a two lines positive home antigen test. I tried to isolate but subsequently everyone tested positive even my wife's 79-year-old mother. I had mild symptoms for 5 days and everyone else had even less symptoms or none. Everyone tested negative by day 7. I was the unlucky one who remained with some positional dizziness and fatigue for an additional month while everyone else was fine. Fortunately, I didn't get the dreaded "Long Covid" syndrome.

While Long Covid is a recognized malady resulting after infection, it remains mysterious to its exact pathologic process, ambiguous in that it can include up to nearly 200 different symptoms, that there are no specific blood or imaging tests that confirm it and frustrating as there are no specific treatments that have been proven as treatments. Long Covid is simply defined as any collection of the many identified symptoms that persist 3 months after initial infection, impacting the patient's life and cannot be attributed to any other disease state. Some of the common symptoms include: fatigue, headache, "brain fog", fever, cough, dizziness, sleep disturbance, joint or muscle pains, abdominal pains, tingling of hands or feet, chest pains, fast heart rates, depression and anxiety.

Long Covid should not be confused with patients who have significant residual problems after a severe bout of Covid. For example, patients recovering from significant lung or heart damage from a Covid infection can have chronic difficulty with breathing, cough, limited activity or chest pain. If the damage is permanent, these difficulties can be lifelong.

Long Covid shares many of the symptoms and difficulty of treatment with other chronic syndromes such *fibromyalgia, chronic fatigue syndrome* and *chronic Lyme disease.* Also, many patients can have profound fatigue and brain fog after *any* serious illness such as sepsis where they spent a significant amount of time in the ICU getting treatment. Many of these patients can take years to recover and some remain significantly disabled. The incidence of Long Covid after an acute infection has been very difficult to accurately determine but most experts put it at about 1% incidence. That still makes a lot of folks with Long Covid in the world. The best prevention against Long Covid has been shown to be fully vaccinated. The time course of recovery is unpredictable and can be quite variable. Some patients improve after several months but many have daily symptoms years after. It is likely that Long Covid represents many different processes that involve immune function dysregulation and chronic inflammation as causes. Physicians are stuck trying to manage the most prominent symptoms as best as can be helped but symptoms such as chronic brain fog remain without a specific effective treatment.

Even with the surges and high hospitalization rates and deaths from Omicron throughout 2022, the public and the government had developed pandemic fatigue and were no longer able or willing to institute lockdowns, school closings, mandated masking as the world and US began to accept Covid as a part of life. The virus was less deadly while it was more transmissible. Even China, which had maintained a "Zero-Covid" policy through most of 2022, succumbed to public pressure against lockdowns in November. However, this change did unleash a huge wave of new infections almost immediately due to its rapid spread and lack of previous public exposure. Omicron continued to evolve and develop more mutations allowing it to further escape the immune system but humans and science struck back with a new Omicron booster in September 2022. The battle against Covid for protective immunity was full on! It had been assumed but not proven that many of these immune avoiding mutations developed in patients with impaired immune systems where the virus could freely mutate and even combine with other Omicron strains to form new variants.

By December 31st, 2022, the end of the third year of the pandemic, an additional 250,000 Americans had died from Covid-19 (which was fortunately half the number of deaths in 2021) bringing the total number to 1.1 million.

As of this writing at the conclusion of the fourth year of the pandemic, life on earth has returned nearly to its "normal" state during

2023. There are no longer mask mandates (but recommendations on prolonged indoor crowd gatherings remain), there are no travel restrictions or requirements, the vast majority of remote work has returned, at least in part, back to the office. The Omicron variants have continued to mutate but have not become significantly more infectious but instead have been able to further avoid prior exposure immunity. Some experts have claimed that the new variants should be called something new other than Omicron. An updated booster vaccine was developed against new variants in September 2023. Second, third, fourth or more re-infections are not uncommon, even in those fully vaccinated but the vast majority are minor annoyances. The medical world has accepted an "endemic" state of Covid, meaning that it is likely it will remain circulating in the world indefinitely and that future booster vaccines will be developed yearly, like the influenza vaccine. Less and less folks are dying or hospitalized from Covid, but it is still a presence in hospitals around the country. No new medications have become available in the past 2 years. While it is reassuring that the currently less virulent strains are killing less people, we cannot be sure this will be the case going forward although it makes sense from an evolutionary point of view.

What have we learned from this one? Well, modern life tells us that any new emerging infectious disease will not remain local and will spread worldwide and quickly. Modern science can jump right on new infections, especially viruses, immediately with identifying, developing tests and likely vaccines at an extraordinarily rapid pace. We learned that *all* respiratory diseases can be spread easily, at long distance and for long periods via aerosol/airborne routes especially indoors. We, unfortunately, learned that misinformation and poorly directed public health measures can lead to a huge number of unnecessary illnesses, hospitalizations and deaths. We also learned that there is a limit to the general public being tolerant of having to "behave" differently for their own and others' health.

Comparing this pandemic to the 1918 Influenza pandemic, the public response was remarkably similar. Then, the H1N1 influenza virus spread worldwide in the aftermath of the First World War by soldiers and workers returning and traveling. Initial reports of the flu's spread and seriousness were suppressed in the northern European countries it was hitting the hardest. This was due to a combination of political and economic reasons. However, in Spain the press reported on it openly which led to that pandemic being inaccurately labeled the "Spanish Flu" as many assumed that is where it started and was most prevalent. The 1918 pandemic was marked by a significantly worse 2nd wave after the virus mutated to become more virulent, killing a significantly high percentage of young people. This was in contrast to the more deadly Delta second wave of Covid which continued to have a higher death rate in the elderly. Then, after the second wave of the influenza pandemic, when everyone was tired of social distancing, quarantining and masking, many cities abandoned any preventative measures which prolonged the misery and death for an additional year. The impact on the world was much greater in 1918-1920 as conservative estimates calculated that over 50 million lives were lost in comparison to 10 million from Covid-19. Importantly, back then there were no medications, tests or vaccines available during the influenza pandemic but still it completely died out after 3 years.

Covid-19 remains throughout the world after 5 years. The new variants seem to be able to acquire mutations that can further avoid prior immunity but it is largely fading into the background as are many of the aforementioned epidemics of the past 30 years. One common ground message for humanity is that for the first time, nearly all have experienced the same infection demonstrating that new diseases easily cross all national and cultural barriers. While there have been some admirable cooperative efforts in this pandemic, it certainly would be prudent to complete a process for world-wide surveillance, detection, evaluation and treatment of future global health threats instead of the current fragmented system based on nations and resources.

PART 5

Then and Now

CHAPTER 29

A Brief History of Medicine

To be clear, this section will only follow the course of Western medicine and will not include other ancient and still practiced forms of medicine, for example, Ayurvedic from India or traditional Chinese medicine. Of course, there are numerous medical practices that have occurred around the world since ancient times including local folk medicine, various religious based spiritual healing, acupuncture, and many others. However, I have chosen to focus on the story of medicine in western civilization as it is the one I have spent a lifetime learning, using and seeing its modern development. It's also a great story of how we got here.

Our starting point is Hippocrates, the "Father of Medicine" (~460-370 BC), who was born on the Greek island of Kos in the eastern Mediterranean. He was a contemporary of the ancient philosophers Socrates, Plato and Aristotle but likely had no direct contact with them although he was mentioned in some of their works. He revolutionized the ancient healing arts into an organized discipline with the concepts of disease categorization, clinical observation, prognosis of diseases and developing the concept of *humoral theory*. This describes the four bodily fluids as crucial to health: *blood, phlegm, yellow bile,* and *black bile.* These bodily *humors* were conceptually connected to the then accepted four basic elements: air (*blood*), water (*phlegm*), fire (*yellow bile*), and *black bile* (*earth*). Each was linked with specific physical *and* mental state and were expanded to connect to the seasons of the year and extended to the stages of life to encompass a system that integrated all aspects of life and the world. In this system an excess or deficiency of any of the *humors* put the body out of balance and was the cause of disease. Examples of these integrated concepts include: one having an extremely sanguine (calm) temperament or excessive cheerfulness was linked to a *blood* (*air*) imbalance. An imbalance of *yellow bile* (*fire*) could cause fevers, anger and a choleric temperament. While not much is known of his life, his teachings were collected by his followers in the *Hippocratic Corpus*. Hippocrates was the first who took illness out of the realm of religions and gods and placed disease in the body as part of nature. His treatments were usually gentle and passive and were generally guided by the principle of self healing. His concepts of disease and *humorism* were used for nearly 2 millennia until the scientific revolution of the 16th century! A modernized *Hippocratic Oath* (which was unlikely written by him) is still taken by all graduates of medical schools promising high standards of professionalism and ethics. The famous medical dictum "First, do no harm" likely was added in the 17th century to the *Oath*.

It's important to put into context just how revolutionary the ideas of Hippocrates and his followers were. At that time, disease was thought to result from evil spirits or from angry gods and that sacrifice and prayers, especially to the god Asclepius, would cure illness. In Greek mythology, Asclepius, the son of Apollo, was the god of healing and he was portrayed as carrying a staff wrapped in a snake which remains the symbol of the medical profession today. However, the exact meaning of these symbols remains obscure and is still in dispute. Certain mythologies have included Hippocrates as a descendent of Asclepius. Even after Hippocrates' teachings and medical school became well known, much of the populace continued to worship and pray for healing at the temples of Asclepius of which there were several scattered around ancient Greece. Mystical and religious healers persisted throughout the ancient world despite this new natural early scientific thinking. Hippocrates proposed strict observation, examination and experience to diagnose and prognose the course of diseases. The concept of opposites in consort with his *humoral theory* was crucial to the development of treatments and included the four basic qualities of wet, dry, hot and cold which were associated with the four humors. His view of disease took into account the whole person and included the psychological as well as the physical state. He was an early proponent of the mind-body connection. In this context, one can see the logic of using various treatments such as emetics, bowel stimulants and blood letting to purge the body of excessive humors and bring the body back into harmony. Along with advice on diets, rest, exercise, massage, and sea bathing, he recommended various herbs, minerals, and animal products be used individually or in combination as treatments. Hippocrates was a proponent of the concept of building up the body to resist disease which was incorporated into treatments for this holistic approach. One simple example used a liquid diet for fevers in order to cool the inner fire. Of course, this medical construct was rudimentary with incomplete knowledge of human anatomy and physiology. Dissections were prohibited and no scientific studies were done to evaluate treatments but close observation and experience drove the recommended treatment regimens. Knowledge of the exact functions of organ systems was at a primitive or incorrect level. It is unclear which treatments had any true beneficial effects or were the result of the natural course of a disease and/or placebo effects.

It is personally fascinating to read the *Hippocratic Corpus* as the first detailed collection of medical knowledge, treatments and thoughts (all written by his followers over the century or more after his death). The topics are similarly organized as in modern textbooks on medicine. They include discussions on the history of ancient treatments, specific organs (the heart or bladder for example), sections on women's health and childbirth, ethics of proper treatment of patients and the art of medicine. One section, the *Epidemics,* includes 40 specific case studies of diseases such as pneumonia, cholera and skin infections in which most patients died. It is impressive to read the detailed and accurate descriptions of common diseases that still affect mankind today. Anatomy knowledge at that time was often obtained by physicians examining injuries after a war battle. Fascinatingly, there are significant discussions of the struggles of physicians in trying to make the correct diagnosis, provide good treatments and understand the problems. All of which are still present for doctors today! Hippocratic schools of medicine were established throughout the ancient Greek and subsequent Roman empires and were considered the highest standards of medical treatments.

The search, use and belief in medicinal plants is as old as mankind himself. The *Hippocratic Corpus* contains hundreds of plants used as herbal treatments. The most comprehensive collection of medicinal plants, their preparation, storage and use was compiled several centuries after Hippocrates when Pedanius Dioscorides wrote *De materia medica* (On medical material) over a 20-year period from 50-70 AD. This expansive 5 volume work includes over 600 plants and 1000 medicinals collected and categorized around the ancient world by the Greeks, Romans, Egyptians and other cultures. Copies of this work spread to the Arab world becoming the authoritative source for plant pharmacology through the Middle Ages in the Middle East. This work was discovered in the west during the Renaissance spurring its use into the modern age up to the 19th century. Dioscorides was a Greek physician in the Roman army and traveled extensively collecting, documenting, and observing the use of various plants, minerals and animal products. He was meticulous in documenting which part of the plant was to be used, how and when it should be collected, how it should be stored and for what ailments it was best used for. He did not just take for granted local folklore but relied on a more scientific approach by testing remedies himself and collecting the experiences of local experts before including them in his writing. He used the *empirical method* which was largely by trial and error. The book is divided into five sections: Volume 1, *Aromatics*, which included oils and ointments derived from plants; Volume 2, *Animals and Herbs*, which included even sea creatures like seahorses and crabs and various herbs such as garlic; Volume 3 & 4, *Roots, seeds and herbs*, included common items such as parsley, cumin, fennel, licorice and daffodils; Volume 5, *Vines, Wines and Minerals*, included various recipes for boiling vines, using wine as remedies and minerals such as zinc and iron oxide. The list of pharmacopeia included many common plants, animals and minerals found at that time. The book evolved over time and included beautiful illustrations set in a natural setting to help identify many of the plants and animals. Clearly, this work was following the Hippocratic aphorism: "Let food be your medicine, and medicine be your food." Unlike many works from the ancient world, this was translated and used in Arab speaking countries until rediscovered in the West and translated into Latin in the Renaissance. Its continued use for 2 millennia is testament to its world influence. Many of the formulations were recommended for several conditions and it was common to use them in combination. Some have been proven to have medicinal effects such as *willow bark* which contains a form of aspirin, *colchicum* containing a compound useful for gout and *opium poppy* containing narcotic pain-relieving compounds such as morphine. In one modern scientific analysis, herbs recommended as diuretics were accurate about 60% of time in containing a naturally occurring diuretic.

Interestingly, at about the same time and not too far away, Pliny the Elder was putting together his magnum opus, *Naturalis Historia* (Natural History), which most consider the world's first encyclopedia and is the largest single written work from ancient Roman times. Pliny was a polymath, naturalist, philosopher, writer and an officer in the Roman Empire in the first century AD (24-79). He died trying to rescue a friend from the eruption of Mount Vesuvius at age 56. His work consisted of 37 books and was composed in the last years of his life. It was intended to include all known knowledge at the time and is still used today as a resource to understand the ancient world. It includes various topics such as astronomy, mathematics, geography, agriculture, zoology and botany, mineralogy and art. There are several sections of his book that deal with over 1,000 medicinal plants, animal products and minerals. In general, there is overlap of many of the common medicinals used at that time with those described in Dioscorides' *De Materia Medica* but the later work was more scientific in the descriptions and use. The two men did not know of each other and never met.

There is yet a third work of medical writing from this time by the Roman writer, Aulas Cornelius Celsus, whose only surviving work was *De Medicina* (Of Medicine) published around 47 AD. Nothing is known of his life, but this book includes the three components of medical treatments of the time: diet, pharmacology and surgery. He is the first person to accurately describe the four cardinal signs of inflammation:

calor (warmth), *dolor* (pain), *tumor* (swelling), and *rubor* (redness). He should not be confused with the term for measuring temperature, the Celsius scale. That came from the 18th century Swedish scientist, Anders Celsius, who proposed the centigrade scale for temperature with freezing being 0 and the boiling point being 100.

The greatest advances in the ancient world came a century later with the Greek physician, researcher, and philosopher Galen, who was born in modern day Bergama, Turkey. He was born into wealth, received an extensive early education including medical studies at the healing temple, the *Aesclepion*, where he was taught by prominent healers and philosophers. He then traveled throughout the Roman Empire learning various medical practices while incorporating the teachings of Hippocrates into his practice. His experience as a physician to the gladiators gave him insights into human anatomy, wound care, severe trauma, fractures and surgery as he was hired by the high priest of Asia for this role. He was renowned for being an excellent surgeon and being able to heal wounds by flushing with clean water, fig leaf dressings and wine to keep infections away. He carried on the teachings of Hippocrates' *humoral theory* and further expanded it, incorporating philosophy and preventative care into his concept of health. He was the first to document anatomy by dissection of apes (human dissection was not permitted) which became the anatomical standard until the Renaissance. He advanced new concepts of physiology including the circulatory system consisting of venous (dark) blood and arterial (bright) blood and neurology by identifying the brain being at the center of the nervous system and with spinal nerves having a separate motor (to muscles) and sensory components.

Galen was a very prolific writer and his collected works include over 20,000 pages of material. He apparently hired dozens of scribes to take down his dictations. His extensive *Corpus* includes sections on anatomy, physiology, hygiene, pharmacology, instruments and therapeutics as well as extensive writings on the nature of man, the soul, philosophy and psychology. It has been estimated that his writings are equal to all the other combined writings from ancient Greece! However, because his work was not translated into Latin it was lost to western civilization after the fall of the Roman Empire but continued in the Greek speaking eastern Byzantine Empire and was subsequently translated into Arabic finding its way into the lexicon of the Middle East.

While Galen's fame brought him to become the personal physician for the emperor Marcus Aurelius, it's hard to truly understand the life of a typical physician in his time. They likely were stationed in various temples, schools or homes where patients would come. Also, while there were some infirmary-like centers that resembled modern hospices, there was nothing that resembled a modern hospital.

During the Middle Ages in the western world, science took a back seat to religious beliefs and faith. The teachings and writings of the ancient physicians were largely lost due to not being translated into Latin. However, the works of Hippocrates and Galen did make it to the Arab world where they were translated from the Greek and were used for a millennia as guideposts to medical care.

Avicenna's monumental work written in Arabic, *The Canon of Medicine* (~1020 AD), was the synthesis of medical knowledge from the ancient Greek, Roman, Persian and Indian worlds including teachings from Hippocrates and Galen. Like many of the ancient physicians, he was also a philosopher and wrote extensively on metaphysics, ethics and logic. Three centuries later his work was translated into Latin bringing the ancient teachings into the Renaissance. Avicenna's teachings brought back rational medical thinking (instead of the belief that disease was inflicted on those who sinned against God) along with systematic classification of diseases. His work was used for medical education in many places until the mid-17th century. It stayed true to the influence of the *humoral theory* described by Hippocrates and expanded by Galen.

As the Renaissance brought ancient writings back for reexamination and use they were also open to scrutiny, new interpretation and criticism. While Galen's work was greatly admired and used for teaching, others questioned his methods and accuracy. One was the German physician later named Paracelsus (1493-1541 AD). He challenged Galen's *Humoral Theory* and many prevailing dogmatic ideas of his time that did not include strict empirical study. His contrarian personality heightened his challenges to any theory that was not supported by evidence. He proposed that disease was caused by chemical imbalances instead of humor imbalances and was an outspoken critic of bloodletting as a treatment. His career was marked by extensive travel and work around Europe including enlisting as an army surgeon during the Venetian wars against the Ottoman Empire. His persistent criticism of unproven medical theory led him to stage a famous book burning of the works of Galen and Avicenna in 1527. He is known as a pioneer on the study of toxicology and antisepsis and wrote on various non-medical topics including astrology, alchemy, chemistry and philosophy. He achieved a somewhat cult status in Europe after his death as the posthumous leader of the medical movement named *Paracelsism* which persisted for over a century. This approach was based on balancing the body's microcosm (internal bodily functions) with the macrocosm (external world). The movement faded in the late 17th century with the rise of the scientific revolution. In his time, Paracelsus was compared to his religious contemporary, Martin Luther, as a revolutionary reformer.

The 16th century also saw the direction of medical study and methodology change drastically due initially to Andreas Vesalius' detailed exploration of human anatomy. This brilliant young physician from Brussels was given an academic professorship in anatomy at the prestigious Padua University in Italy at the age of 23. Having extensive knowledge of Galen's work based on animal anatomy, Vesalius compared his findings dissecting human corpses and discovered monumental differences. His masterpiece *De Humani Corporis Fabrica Libri Septem* (On the fabric of the human body in seven books) included sections on each anatomical system of the body (e.g. muscles, skin, nerves, intestines, reproduction, etc.). This magnum opus can be seen as combining all the scientific and artistic advances of the Renaissance into this one book. It included an entirely new, complete and accurate way of illustrating and describing human anatomy that set a new standard going forward. The artwork of the illustrations by artists trained under famous painters such Titian are exquisite and gorgeously detailed and reflect all the development of advanced painting techniques of the late Renaissance. Vesalius also completely changed the way dissections and anatomy instruction were done by doing them himself, explaining and showing every detail to his students in a logical, sequential method with tools he designed himself. He is rightly called the "father of anatomy" and forever changed the direction of medical knowledge and inquiry. He dedicated the first edition of the *Fabrica* in 1543 to the Holy Roman Emperor Charles V, which included 250 woodcut artistic illustrations correcting all the mistakes made by Galen. The book was printed at one of finest printing houses in Europe where Vesalius oversaw the process directly in order for it to be done to his high standard.

The dark side of anatomic study during this time was in the procurement of human bodies for dissection. While it was legal to perform human dissection, it was limited to using condemned, executed criminals as subjects. There apparently was an extensive black market from other sources as well to fill the needs of universities and anatomists to obtain sufficient numbers for study.

Hundreds of copies of Vesalius' book have survived today to still be marveled at as the culmination of art and science during the Renaissance. By offering a definitive roadmap of human anatomy, the *Fabrica* then spurred others to discover *how* the body worked i.e. *human physiology*.

It is notable that the University of Padua produced several important figures of medical science in the years following Vesalius from the late 16th century into the early 17th century. Gabrielle Fallopio (1522-1562 AD) was a student of Vesalius who advanced the detailed anatomy of the ear and studied women's reproductive organs for which are named the fallopian tubes. Girolamo Fabrizio (1533-1619 AD) was taught by Fallopio and is famous for discovering the valves in veins that keep blood flowing in one direction. He also extensively studied animal and human fetuses and became known as the "Father of Embryology".

On the heels of these men came the advances from yet another alumni of Padua University, William Harvey (1578-1657 AD) from England, who accurately described the human circulatory system. Until his time, it was thought that blood was "consumed" in the tissues and was then produced in the liver, veins and right ventricle and that the heart's primary function was to produce heat and to act as a "sucking" device to bring blood back from the body. Harvey's work included examining various live animals' hearts and following Vesalius' human descriptions. He determined by measuring blood flow and the mechanics of the beating heart that the circulatory system was a closed connected system forming a continuous flow of blood pumped by the heart. He correctly observed the beating of both ventricles in synchrony and traced blood vessels from the large arteries down to tiny capillaries that flowed to the veins and back to the right ventricle. He was able to scientifically measure the amount of blood flowing through the heart and that it was not being consumed. He was the first to connect the one-way flow of the circulation. Blood is pumped through the body back to the heart (right ventricle), out to the lungs (to become oxygenated) then back to the heart (left ventricle) and out to the body as a continuous circuit. The world of cardiovascular physiology was born with Harvey's studies published in 1628.

The combination of technologic innovations, original thought and scientific inquiry produces the formula that leads to major advances in medicine. The first great technological advance in the study of medicine came from the development of the microscope. After the wide dissemination of the printing press, invented in 1443, there came a huge need for eyeglasses leading to the expanded industry of glass lens making. Although the exact inventor is not truly known, somewhere in the 1590s in Holland, the first microscope was invented by aligning two standard convex lenses commonly used for glasses to produce a significantly magnified image. Magnification levels were on the order of two to ten times the actual size of small objects. Within a couple of decades the telescope was also invented using different focal lengths to magnify distant objects. It took until 1665 when the English polymath, Robert Hooke, published his illustrated book *Micrographia* that the use of microscopes could visualize and define small biologic objects such as a fly's eye, small insects and a bee's honeycomb. Hooke would be the first to use the word *cell* looking at plants close-up. However, it took Antonie van Leeuwenhoek in the following decades to invent his own secretively developed single lens microscope which had a magnification power a hundred times stronger than Hooke's to really start seeing microscopic life. He extensively studied simple pond water where he saw single celled animals, paramecia, amoeba and bacteria calling them *animalcules* leading to his history title as the "Father of Microbiology". He accurately described red blood cells and spermatozoa which led to a more accurate understanding of human reproduction of joining sperm and egg. Interestingly, he never published a book but sent his findings in the form of letters to the Royal Society of London, the leading scientific organization in Europe which was headed by Hooke himself. His findings were initially met with criticism but with substantiated and reproducible visual proof he became the leading expert in the new world of microscopy. Van Leeuwenhoek (1632-1723) came from Delft, a small town in Holland, and was born in the same year and same town as the famous Dutch painter Johannes Vermeer. In their lifetimes they were both celebrity citizens and knew each other. It had been speculated that van Leeuwenhoek's figure was used in a couple of Vermeer's paintings. He even presided over Vermeer's will when he died at age 53. His mysterious way of making a spherical glass bead as the lens for his very powerful small hand-held microscope was never revealed. Early microscopes suffered from impurities and irregularities in the lenses until improved manufacturing in the 19th century. Today all medical students still need to rent or purchase one for personal use in order to understand the cellular microscopic world of the body and its invasive organisms. Microscopes have gone through vast development and transformation especially over the past century and now include electron scanning microscopes that can magnify an object up to 1 million times its size giving extraordinary detail to extremely tiny components of the cell leading to an expansive understanding of how the body works down to the basic chemical level!

These advances set up the next phase of early scientific study of the body. The shift to begin to understand disease better from a scientific standpoint and then start making inroads into specific treatments. The scourge of scurvy was known for millennia especially in sailors on long trips. Scurvy occurs uncommonly these days but as a deficiency of Vitamin C, it can cause devastating health effects such as anemia, bleeding, infection and death. In 1753, a Scottish surgeon, James Lind, proved that it could be prevented by eating citrus fruits. This led to the nickname of British sailors being called "limeys" as then all navy ships stocked lemons (or limes) on their voyages.

Many have never heard of English physician Edward Jenner, the "Father of Immunology" who developed the first vaccine against the deadly smallpox virus. Likely no physicians practicing today have ever seen a case after the successful global eradication campaign was completed in 1980. The scourge of smallpox is likely the greatest infectious disease killer ever encountered by humanity, estimated killing hundreds of millions over the past few millennia. Infection with the severe form kills one in three while causing blindness, deformity, infertility and disability in survivors. It was a gruesome disease to observe, causing high fevers, vomiting, and fluid filled sores that could cover the entire body often ending in death 2 weeks after it began. The newly evolving scientific method in medicine is emblematically demonstrated when Jenner developed and proved his technique of vaccination. Building on the observations of others in the 18th century that initially saw that *variolation*, a technique developed in Asia and Middle East as a somewhat dangerous method of taking infected smallpox scabs and rubbing them into scratched skin of an unaffected individual could impart immunization in some people. This technique was brought back to England in 1721 by Lady Mary Wortley Montagu from Istanbul. However, many would contract a full form of the disease and die. In 1768, reports that individuals who had a "cowpox" infection (a milder related form of smallpox affecting mostly cows causing a mild infection in humans seen often in milkmaids) were protected against future smallpox infections. This led to the concept of cross immunization which attracted Jenner to try to use it in a clinical trial. Jenner's method proved the process of inoculation and protective immunity scientifically. He took scrapings of cowpox infected milkmaids and inoculated the arms of young men, many of which developed a mild infection but recovered fully. Jenner then challenged those with direct inoculation of smallpox and showed that none developed smallpox infection or died, proving his theory. His initial published study included 23 cases including his 11-month-old son. Subsequent studies of a similar nature proved that vaccination worked and eventually became standard and mandatory practice over the next several decades. It has been estimated that Jenner's vaccine has saved more lives in the world than any other known medical treatment in history. The science of developing a treatment and validating its effectiveness finally pushed the scientific study of medical treatments in the correct direction. However, it would take over a century later to discover that smallpox was caused by a highly contagious virus.

In contrast, the real practice of medicine at the turn of the 19th century consisted largely of unproven therapies and a continued modified belief of Hippocrates' *humoral theory* from two and half millennia previously. One stark example is from the advice that Benjamin Rush, a prominent Philadelphia physician, signer of the Declaration of Independence and friend of Thomas Jefferson, gave to Merriwether Lewis before embarking on the Lewis and Clark Expedition in 1803. He instructed Lewis on bloodletting for nearly any illness and gave a supply of emetics and his famous *Thunderclapper* pills that caused severe diarrhea as primary medical treatments for nearly every malady.

In a reaction to the aggressiveness and unreliable results of medical treatments there emerged alternative theories of disease and their treatments. Several of these pseudoscientific but pleasant-sounding theories took hold in the 19th century. *Homeopathy* conceived in 1796 by Samuel Hahnemann, a German physician who was very critical of bloodletting, purported the concept that "like cures likes" with the odd twist of logic assuming that something that causes symptoms of disease in a healthy person can cure a sick one in tiny doses. This led to diluting small quantities of a substance so much that it was indistinguishable from water! The "cures" of homeopathy were all due to the placebo effect or the natural course of a disease resolving itself. No valid scientific study has ever shown any value in their remedies. But, at least it causes no harm! *Homeopathy* grew to become a significant movement through the 19th century and then faded. It made a significant comeback during the *New Age* movement of the 1970s but today has been relegated as a non-covered entity by insurance treatment by most Western governments, fortunately!

Mary Baker Eddy, frustrated with her own long-term, untreatable somatic symptoms, developed the movement of *Christian Science* in the late 19th century. Her personal experience developed the view that disease was a mental error and not a physical disorder and could be treated with certain prayers and attracted a significant following by returning healing to the religious realm instead of scientific proof. She was sharply criticized by Mark Twain at the turn of the 20th century. The church she founded grew cultishly and substantially after her death in 1910 and peaked around 1960 but has declined substantially since. However, well publicized legal battles have been noted of parent followers of her church and their refusal to have standard medical care provided for their children sometimes resulting in death.

Mary Eddy was influenced by another form of alternative healing/ hocus pocus that developed in the late 18th century, *Mesmerism*, from another German physician, Franz Mesmer, who came up with the idea that energy can be transferred between living and inanimate objects naming it "animal magnetism". Its concept evolved to include hypnotism and was fairly popular during the first half of the 19th century before fading badly after being public proved a hoax on many occasions.

Scientific medical thinking and teaching began ushering in real advances through the 19th century assisted by using the scientific method and new technology. Academic physicians expanding the understanding of the physical signs of disease and the art of physical examination became an important skill taught to medical students. Medical education itself expanded into formal schools that granted degrees after completion of classroom and clinical instruction in the early 19th century. The invention of the stethoscope by the French physician Rene Laennec in 1816 opened up listening to the heart, lungs and abdomen to give direct clues of illness. In the first half of the 19th century, Paris became the focal point of the highest level of medical education. Students came from all over the world to study under such luminaries as Pierre Louis who developed bedside teaching methods at the new hospitals often dedicated to caring for certain diseases. Medical teaching began to correlate symptoms and physical signs of disease into what became known as the "differential diagnosis". This crucial modern concept means that one needs to include all the diseases that *could* be present given the set of data and then to narrow down the diagnosis as more data and the disease progresses. The development of autopsies to determine the cause of death became an important tool of expanding understanding and teaching while advancing basic knowledge significantly. These new scientifically oriented methods of teaching and of public health soon spread throughout Europe and then later to the US as graduates returned to their home countries after studying in Paris. Along with the development of large teaching hospitals, physicians started to become "specialized" in certain areas of medical care. Surgery, the separate disciplines of women's care and child delivery, neurology, cardiology and other organ systems began to have their organized followers and disciplines.

The remarkable development of two anesthetic agents in the 1840s led to the greatest change in the world of surgery and patient comfort up to that time. The use of inhaled ether or nitrous oxide rapidly became the standard for allowing painless surgery to finally be performed.

Along with the use of morphine for postoperative pain, patients could get through an operation without excessive suffering which allowed the expansion of surgery as a standard acceptable procedure. Still, antisepsis and germ theory were decades away so there remained significant morbidity and death after surgery from infections as well as overdoses from the new anesthetics.

Extensive use of the improving lenses of the microscope made examining blood and tissues advance the understanding of pathologic processes enormously. Rudolf Virchow, a German physician and polymath (1821-1902), led the way. He is known as the "Father of Pathology" with his seminal work *Cellular Pathology* (1858). Studying and writing over 2000 scientific articles, he described the modern methods of autopsy and detailed the pathology of various diseases such leukemia and thrombosis (blood clots in a vein or artery). He is famous for his dictum of cell physiology (although he plagiarized it): "all cells come from cells" helping to dispel the continuing myth of spontaneous generation. He developed the initial concept of cancer developing from normal cells by associating the transformation due to inflammation.

In Vienna in 1847, Ignaz Semmelweis observed and developed the concept of anti-sepsis by hand washing and used a chlorinated solution to prevent infections after childbirth. His study showed a reduction of maternal mortality from 18% to 2%! However, his ideas were met with great resistance in established medical teaching centers causing him to be ostracized and even imprisoned for his scientifically accurate views.

The next two monumental figures in our story completely abolished the concept of spontaneous generation and pushed medical science to a new level. The work of Louis Pasteur and Robert Koch transformed the medical world by proving the existence and development of the *germ theory of diseases* in the second half of the 19th century. The brilliance of Pasteur (1822-1895) figuring out the several thousand-year-old conundrum of fermentation of wine and beer by determining that living yeast produces alcohol by consuming sugar anaerobically. He proved his theory with the counterpunctual technique of sterilizing the process with heat providing a shining example of scientific deduction and experimentation. Famously, by showing that spoiled milk, wine and beer were caused by organisms not involved with fermentation and then preventing spoilage by heat treatment developed the process we all know as *pasteurization*. In addition, he also developed vaccines for chicken cholera by using "attenuated" or weakened bacteria to inoculate and immunize chickens following up on the work of Jenner nearly a century earlier. He developed the first vaccines against anthrax and rabies. A colleague and competitor of Pasteur, Robert Koch (1843-1910) fully established the science of microbiology and bacteriology. Koch's accomplishments would include not only discovering the bacteria anthrax, but proving its cause of the disease in 1876 as well as developing laboratory techniques for growing cultures of bacteria. By developing the microscopic technique of using a drop of oil between the lower lens and his slide, specimen examinations were greatly enhanced by the magnification and resolution. His additional discovery of the cause of tuberculosis by the slow growing bacteria *Mycobacterium tuberculosis* solved a medical mystery to this ancient disease and was nicknamed "Koch's bacillus". There had never before been proof of a bacteria causing disease. With these revolutionary discoveries, Koch developed a scientific method to determine if an infection was caused by a specific organism known as *Koch's Postulates*. They include the following conditions: 1) the microorganism should be found in those suffering from the disease and not in those who are healthy, 2) the microorganism is able to be isolated and grown in a culture, 3) the cultured microorganism *should* (but not necessarily always) reproduce the disease when inoculated into a healthy individual, and 4) that those inoculated experimentally will have the identical microorganism that can be shown with re-culturing. These postulates pushed the science of bacteriology into a reality. While eventually it was shown that these postulates do not apply to viruses, they were helpful for studying bacterial infections well into the 20th century. Later, he abandoned the first postulate after discovering that both cholera and typhoid could exist in a carrier state, namely, not causing an active infection in every case. From Koch's laboratory emerged the definitive way to culture bacteria using the culture medium *agar* in a closed sterile glass dish known as a *Petri dish* named after the technician who developed it. Petri dishes and agar are still used today in labs around the world for the study and culturing of bacteria nearly 150 years later! Koch received the fourth Nobel Prize in medicine in 1905 for his work on tuberculosis.

An intense interest in infectious diseases followed and is highlighted in the discovery of the parasite of the genus *Plasmodium* that causes malaria, another ancient scourge of the world whose naming came from the term in Medieval Italian for bad air—*"mala aria"*. Interestingly, malaria was one of very few diseases for which existed an effective treatment. The bark of the Cinchona tree, which contains the active ingredient quinine, was found by ancient Peruvians to cure the severe fever producing disease and was brought to the new world in the 17th century. Several key investigators by 1897 were able to put the complicated life cycle of malaria parasites together following its course from the salivary glands of mosquitos to inside the red cells of infected patients and back to mosquitos. In a controversial decision the Nobel prize for malaria discovery was given to the British doctor Ronald Ross in 1902. The race was on to discover a whole host of parasitic diseases that fall under the rubric "Tropical Medicine".

The English surgeon Joseph Lister (1827-1912) was very familiar with traumatic and post-operative wound infections, gangrene and the need for amputation. He was critical of the prevailing thinking in the mid-19th century that infections were caused by *miasma* (bad air) and that *pus* was beneficial for wound healing. His interest in microscopy and inflammation led him to discover the work of Pasteur and the *germ theory of disease* which led him to advance the new revolutionary techniques of *antisepsis*. This included using carbolic acid to kill germs on wounds and to sterilize surgical equipment and use hand washing to keep microbes from infecting wounds. As with any major change of paradigm in medicine, his ideas were met with great resistance and criticism but after publishing several well designed and written studies on his antiseptic techniques starting in 1867, he became the spokesperson for this advance in medical understanding.

At the start of the 20th century, medicine had leaped forward into being an actual science with proven and accurate concepts of disease, explanations and a system for understanding what symptoms and physical signs could translate into what was going on inside the body although from a biochemical basis very little was known. Doctors were equipped with stethoscopes, powerful microscopes, the ability to culture bacteria, anesthesia for comfortable surgery, and with the discovery of X-rays in 1895 were about to obtain a powerful tool for examining the internal parts of the body not previously imagined.

The accidental discovery of mysterious radiation dubbed X-rays in 1895 by physicist Wilhelm Roentgen seeing energetic waves from a cathode cause a glow on a fluorescent screen caused an immediate sensation in the scientific world. He quickly discovered that it could pass through many materials including human tissue like skin and muscle but were absorbed by dense tissue like bone and could produce a photographic imprint behind the source. One of his early X-ray photos was of his wife's hand which showed bones for the first time. This technology was quickly adapted for medical use due to its obvious practical applicability. The demonstration of broken bones and foreign objects such as bullets or other metal objects in the body greatly advanced treatment of those problems. The expansion of its unrestricted use continued well into the middle of the 20th century. Another famous physicist, Marie Curie, put a portable X-ray machine on a mobile truck during WWI and personally assisted evaluating injured soldiers on the front lines. The dangers of excessive radiation were only slowly recognized. Even up until the 1950s shoe stores were offering X-rays of customers' feet as a marketing tool. Roentgen received the Nobel Prize in Physics in 1901 for his work.

In 1901, building on the work of others in electrical detection of the beating of the heart, Willem Einthoven in Holland developed an accurate galvanometer that could record the electrical deflections occurring during individual heartbeats. He specifically named each deflection P, Q, R, S and T, which is still used in today's nomenclature, and described various abnormalities of electrical activity in his studies of the first EKG (electrocardiogram) machine. He was the first electrocardiologist and received the Nobel Prize in 1924. This important diagnostic technology remains a mainstay of medical evaluation 120 years later using 12 leads to record the heart's electrical activity in 2 planes. It took until the mid-1920s before a portable machine was developed which then led to its widespread use in medical offices and hospitals. Starting my private practice in 1995, I bought an excellent used EKG machine from a retiring primary care internist. It produced perfect tracings by jet ink printing techniques developed in the late 1940s on special graph paper that rolled in timed synchronization when turned on. This machine worked flawlessly on hundreds of patients until I replaced it with a new digital machine 15 years later that was equipped with software that could give an "interpretation" on the printout. I noticed, however, that sometimes the computer reading was not quite correct, requiring that I check every EKG myself anyway!

While elevated blood pressure or "hard pulse" as it was sometimes called was recognized as a possible health hazard that could cause heart or kidney damage in the 19th century, it took until 1905 when the Russian physician, Nikolai Korotkov, used the stethoscope and a mercury sphygmometer on the arm to describe and define an accurate method for measuring both the systolic and diastolic blood pressure. His technique is still the gold standard for properly auscultating blood pressure readings. However, scientific study took another 50 years to clarify the significance and then be able to begin to treat uncontrolled blood pressure with effective medications.

What the medical world was still sorely missing at the turn of the 20th century were specific treatments based on the science of human physiology. Revelations of physiology and biochemistry of disease and subsequent treatments would emerge in an expansive and dramatic way in the 20th century, "the century of breakthroughs".

Various attempts to perfect the technique of blood transfusion to treat severe bleeding or blood loss were developed in the 19th century after the final abandonment of bloodletting by 1830. However, all the techniques were very risky until the discovery and testing of the various blood types A, B, 0 in 1901 by the Austrian Karl Landsteiner. His work detailed how mixing blood types caused an immune reaction and clumping of red cells. Using compatible blood greatly reduced the chance for lethal reactions. However, routine blood transfusion still took a couple of decades to become safe by using a small amount of citrate to prevent clotting and perfecting the techniques of blood collecting, storage and intravenous infusion.

Building on the work of Pasteur and Koch, the concepts and science of *Immunology* developed by observing specific white blood cells "eating" germs but also noticing that serum in blood could destroy bacteria heralding the discovery of antibodies. The "Father of Immunology", Paul Ehrlich (1854-1915) who won the Nobel Prize for his work in 1908 on coming up with the first concepts of antibodies produced by cells in the blood to combat toxins known as his "side-chain theory". He developed the first antibiotic by scientifically experimenting with various chemicals and finding one that could kill the spirochete that causes syphilis. *Arsphenamine* was the first scientifically validated antibiotic and was vastly superior to mercuric compounds tried previously. While it included arsenic in the compound, it was not toxic to humans and was greatly used over the next few decades until penicillin became available 30 years later.

Advancement in laboratory science and observation of specific diseases related to certain dietary deficiencies led to the discoveries of the 13 vitamins needed for human health in the first half of the 20th century. All "*Vital Amines*" as they were first named were discovered between 1913 and 1948. While the prevention of scurvy was known for 150 years, its exact cause due to vitamin C deficiency was not elucidated until 1928 when ascorbic acid was chemically isolated and proven to be the culprit. Beri-beri was a common disease at the turn of the 20th century caused by deficiency of thiamine (vitamin B1) resulting in edema (bodily swelling), abnormal heart rates and neurologic disorders. Causation was linked to "polished rice" consumption (deficient in B1), heavy alcohol intake (causing quick loss from the body) or other restrictive diets and found to be treatable with whole grains and a varied diet of meat and vegetables in 1911. As more essential dietary molecules were discovered, convention drove the naming of each by letters of the alphabet and subsequently were divided into "fat soluble" (Vitamins A, D, E, K) and "water soluble" (all eight B vitamins, and C, there is no F vitamin). In general, fat-soluble vitamins stay in the body much longer (many months) and are often stored in fat tissues but water-soluble vitamins are used and cleared from the body in relatively short periods of time such as days to weeks. Modern public health policies have resulted in fortifying milk with Vitamins A and D and wheat products being fortified with B vitamins to prevent deficiencies. These days vitamin deficiencies are rare in the US. Several Nobel prizes have been awarded in work related to vitamin discovery and supplementation in the first half of the century.

In parallel to the work above, discovery of the body's internal signaling processes by hormones developed into the field of *endocrinology*. Hormones are substances (proteins or compound molecules) that are secreted directly into the bloodstream from their glands to have various metabolic and/or growth effects at areas specific for their action, sometimes in one part of the body or in several areas. In the first part of the 20th century, several discoveries included that the thyroid produces *thyroxine* for regulating energy metabolism, that the testes produce *testosterone* for normal male reproductive development, that the stomach and pancreas secrete proteins that stimulate acid and digestive enzymes, and that the pituitary gland in the brain was found to excrete various regulatory hormones for normal health. One highlight of this period was in the discovery and use of insulin for treating a disease that was universally fatal in young people, Type 1 diabetes mellitus, in which the body loses the ability to make insulin in the pancreas. Two Canadian physicians, Fred Banting and Charles Best, initially did experiments on dogs inducing diabetes by removing the pancreas and then injecting certain cells, the islet cells, back into the dogs which stabilized the glucose levels proving the existence and regulation of insulin. In 1921, they did the first injection of a purified animal insulin into a young boy with diabetes and reversed his terminal disease, starting the first drug revolution for controlling a deadly affliction and were deservedly awarded the Nobel prize soon after. The endocrine system can be understood as monitoring and maintaining the body's metabolic processes in order to stay in balance, called *homeostasis*. In general, the glands that secrete hormones work as both a monitor and responder to different levels and needs in the body by producing more or less of their specific hormones.

In the century since the discovery of insulin, endocrinology has undergone a fascinating and expansive field of understanding how the body's metabolism works. In general, tests that evaluate if an endocrine disorder is present can either measure directly the level of hormone in blood or check its performance by stimulation or suppression of the gland chemically. Due to advances in laboratory analysis, most chemical composition of hormones are known, allowing fabricating replacement therapy of 11 deficiencies including thyroid, adrenal, pituitary and reproductive hormones. One of the great changes of modern societal reproductive choice with the identification and structure of female sex hormones, estrogen and progesterone, led to the introduction of the birth control pill in 1960. Advances in imaging techniques in the last 50 years, especially CT scanning and MRIs have allowed identification of abnormal growths or deficiencies of hormone specific glands as well. Type 1 and Type 2 diabetes mellitus are still the most common problems that endocrinologists treat today. Fascinatingly, the study of hormones continues to expand as in the last 20 years specific hormones have been discovered that were not thought to be glandular organs. For example, *myokines* secreted by skeletal muscle help regulate insulin, weight loss and various metabolic adaptive responses to exercise.

Fat tissue has been shown to excrete *leptin* which controls hunger perceived in the brain.

Of course, the best known and ubiquitous hormone that most know about is *cortisone* which is actually a generic term for a class of hormones produced by the adrenal glands. Cortisone hormones also known as *corticosteroids* are produced from the cholesterol molecule and includes *cortisol*, a glucocorticoid that is secreted in times of stress and reduces inflammation as well as increases glucose. While cholesterol is commonly associated with bad effects in the body such as causing blocked arteries, it is a crucial component in the body for producing all the various *steroid* hormones (cortisol, testosterone, estrogen, progesterone). Cholesterol is an important component in the cell and forms the basis of other important compounds such as vitamin D. Cortisone was discovered in 1929 at the Mayo Clinic and then purified and found to possess powerful anti-inflammatory effects. It was used as a medicine for rheumatoid arthritis in 1948 with a dramatic effect of improving severe joint swelling and pain and was quickly dubbed a "miracle drug" in the 1950s. It found its way to popular culture in the film *Bigger than Life* released in 1956 dramatizing the life of a cortisone abuser! It was initially overused but became part of the treatment of a variety of diseases that caused inflammation. Various synthetic preparations have been developed with different potencies in different mediums such as topical creams, aerosolized nasal and lung sprays, pills and injectable formulations. The myriad diseases for its use include skin conditions like eczema, psoriasis and allergic reactions; pulmonary diseases such as asthma and COPD; rheumatologic diseases such as lupus and rheumatoid arthritis; various inflammatory gastrointestinal conditions such Crohn's disease and hepatitis; neurologic diseases such multiple sclerosis and other nerve inflammations; and also a long list of other inflammatory conditions. Of course, all "miracles" have downsides and long-term use of systemic cortisone weakens the immune system, can induce diabetes, suppresses natural cortisone production and causes various skin and body changes. The complexity of the endocrine system has been greatly elucidated to show that there are hormones that stimulate the production of other hormones. An example of this complex system is how the pituitary gland in the brain produces several hormones that increase or suppress hormone production in the body affecting thyroid, adrenal and sex hormone production.

Advances in the understanding of the nervous system over the last 120 years started with accurately describing nerve cells, the *neuron*. Building on work from the 19th century, the Spanish anatomist, Santiago Ramon y Cajal, refined a special silver stain and accurately described *neurons* as individual cells. He developed the modern concept of the *neuron doctrine* with *neurons* having extensions reaching out from either end called dendrites and axons meeting other neurons at separated junctions called *synapses* (defined by the British physiologist Charles Sherrington). At synapses is where the transfer of electrical stimulus is converted into chemical reactions released and absorbed in the neighboring neuron by chemicals called *neurotransmitters*. Cajal's beautiful illustrations of nerve cells of the brain are still greatly appreciated for their precision and artistic qualities and he was rewarded with a Nobel prize in 1906 for his work. Sequentially, the common and most important neurotransmitters were discovered starting with *acetylcholine* in the 1920s, *norepinephrine, dopamine, serotonin, glutamate* and *GABA*, all with different properties of excitation or inhibition of the nervous system and working in different parts of the brain, spinal cord and nerves. By studying brain and nerve diseases as well as injuries, neurologists were able to accurately identify specific areas of the brain that control various functions such as eyesight, motor control of muscles and the sense organs of touch and smell. The first real brain diagnostic tool was the EEG (electro-encephalograph aka brainwave) machine in 1929 which was able to measure brain waves and to diagnose epilepsy coming from a specific brain region. What neurology lacked, however, were any significant treatments for the major neurologic disease and it remained mostly a "descriptive" science most of the 20th century. For epilepsy, the discovery in 1912 that phenobarbital helped prevent and treat seizures was a great advance in a disease that had in previous eras believed to be caused by demon possession. Phenytoin was a much better medication and discovered by trying various chemicals and using the EEG to determine what suppressed seizures in cats in 1938. It is still commonly used today. However, over the next 40 years only two other seizure medications were approved for use as drug development remained slow. In the past 40 years nearly 20 other anti-seizure medications have come to market without any one being greatly superior to the others making modern treatment still somewhat of a trial and error of finding a good combination of medications for seizure control. Modern imaging techniques over the past 50 years via CT and MRI scanning have transformed neurology and neurosurgery with the ability to non-invasively visualize major problems such as strokes, bleeds and tumors in the brain. Advances in using tiny "coils" to treat brain aneurysms, precision radiotherapy for tumors and deep brain stimulation for various diseases have all been developed in the last 40 years. Medications, biologic immunotherapy and advances in genetics have begun to have an impact in treating neurologic diseases such as Parkinson's, Multiple Sclerosis and Alzheimer's all within the last 50 years. It is still quite apparent that neurologic diseases and treatment still remain today in a very embryonic stage. With the recent international effort of the *Brain Project* starting in 2012 along with other scientific research will likely begin to unravel the immense complexity of our cognitive organ.

It will be an exciting and revealing future for neuroscience.

Wars have always been a good training ground for doctors, especially surgeons, due to its intrinsic nature of being "an epidemic of trauma". The variety of injuries, communal illnesses and infections paved the way for understanding the body due to concentrated exposure. From Hippocrates to Galen and through the Renaissance, physicians interested in understanding the body better have gone to war to help, see, learn and advance the study of human biology and more recently to perform *surgery* to acutely help the gravely injured. During the Civil War, surgeons performed copious amputations (over 30,000) and got fast (2-10 minutes each). They had little skill, however, in repairing damaged tissues. Fortunately, chloroform was available for anesthesia, but a quarter of soldiers died afterward from infections or other complications. Two important observations became truisms: 1) the sooner the amputation, the more likely was survival and 2) the further away from the torso the amputation was done, predicted a higher survival rate. Remember, no sterile techniques were used then.

In the brutal trench warfare of WWI, surgeons were confronted with a myriad of mortal shell injuries which led to an entirely new type of surgical care, reconstructive surgery. This included extensive skin and bone grafts to damaged faces and limbs. Prosthetic limb devices were first developed for amputees then. The technical skills of surgeons treating hand injuries took a big leap forward during WWII creating a new surgical subspecialty, the hand surgeon. Also during WWII, surgeons for the first time were near the front lines in field hospitals with the ability to quickly start treating injuries which drastically reduced mortality. Advances in wound care, new skills in repairing injured blood vessels and nerves along with rapid blood transfusions saved thousands of lives. Surgical advances after WWII were unimaginable a decade earlier, especially when in 1953 John Gibbon, Jr. (an alum of my medical school, Jefferson, in Philadelphia) repaired a heart defect using his newly invented *cardiopulmonary bypass machine* while chemically stopping the heart during the operation. A decade later, the first heart transplant surgery was performed in South Africa by Christian Barnard with help from new medical techniques of immunosuppression to prevent rejection. The world of repairing and replacing damaged heart valves evolved to become a commonplace procedure by the 1970s. The explosion of evaluating blocked coronary arteries with angiography in the mid-1970s led to a rapid expansion of coronary artery bypass surgery by the late 1970s. It seemed that nearly every middle-aged man was getting this new procedure! As a medical student doing my cardiothoracic surgery rotation in 1980, I was amazed and overwhelmed by the seemingly "factory" style schedule of bypass operations. I recall a daily schedule of at least six cases per day at the community hospital where I was stationed! This was the apex of this operation as soon the cardiologists were able to perform angioplasty to the same blocked arteries with good results.

The theme of the advances in all the surgical fields over the past 40 years can be summed up by "smaller, quicker, less trauma, faster healing" operations. Certainly, one can point to the first laparoscopic gallbladder surgery done by Erich Muhe in Germany in 1985 as the tipping point. This heralded in the era of *instead of* using a scalpel cutting into the body, surgeons began "poking" holes with a thin long instrument that was equipped with a camera to see, a maneuverable cutting blade and a holding device that could sew sutures all *inside* the body beginning the revolution of *minimally invasive surgery*. It's notable to mention that initially Dr. Muhe's technique was met with severe criticism as he was ostracized by his surgical colleagues and even faced manslaughter charges when one his patients died (out of several hundred successful operations) only to be honored a few years later as a pioneer in the field! His story is a common one in the history of medicine. This revolution in the use of "scope" surgery has spread to all the surgical disciplines such gynecology, orthopedics, ENT and neurosurgery all resulting in equal or better outcomes and less complications compared to standard scalpel surgery and reducing hospitalization to the point where the majority of surgery done today is via a small scope and as an outpatient. Of course, not all surgery is done this way as scalpels and sutures are still used. Technology advanced at the start of the 21st century which saw the introduction of full robotic surgery for certain procedures, currently used mostly for prostate operations. Orthopedics has seen the introduction of joint replacement surgery greatly expand over the past 40 years.

Before I review the greatest advance of medical treatment in the 20th century, the introduction of antibiotics, it's important to understand the state of medical care prior to this revolution. An accurate portrayal of the pre-antibiotic era comes from the physician author, Lewis Thomas, M.D., in his delightful 1983 book *The Youngest Science* where he describes in detail the state of the art of medicine in the 1930s prior to the introduction of antibiotics, specifically in his essays titled "1933 Medicine" and "1937 Internship". Dr. Lewis was the son of a physician, who accompanied his dad on house calls as a child in the post WWI era where there was only morphine and digitalis in the doctor's bag. He witnessed his father's decision to become a surgeon after several years of general practice because of the severe limitation of medical care outside surgery. Doctors at that time could do very little for patients except for giving an accurate diagnosis and an explanation including a real prognosis of their illnesses and giving supportive care. His 18-month internship in 1937 (these days shortened to 1 year) was an apprenticeship of learning all the technical laboratory and diagnostic skills that were available then in order to come up with an accurate diagnosis. Hospital wards in academic Boston, where he interned, were filled with patients with untreatable terminal infections such as tuberculosis, late-stage syphilis, or other deadly infections and other untreatable diseases such as cancer, strokes or heart attacks. Patients basically received custodial care as the young doctors in training ran around doing various tests to confirm the diagnosis. An exception was in high level academic teaching hospitals where there was an expensive and difficult to produce antibody serum from rabbits that could treat certain pneumonias. Therefore, great effort was made to identify those who might be saved. Dr. Lewis documents the wonder and amazement when the first sulfur-based antibiotics were introduced in the late 1930s. Heralding for the first time a cure for specific deadly infections! His obvious frustration and realistic view of medicine's limitations drove him to later become a medical researcher in immunology and then a dean and administrator for medical schools and institutions. I've often wondered myself, if I would have stayed in the world of bedside medicine watching patients suffer and die with very little effective treatments available if I was in his shoes during that time.

Often scientific breakthroughs are the result of luck, good timing, hard work and even carelessness followed by insightful observation. That is exactly the story of the Scottish physician, Alexander Fleming, and his famous discovery of penicillin. Fleming worked for years during the 1920s observing and documenting that certain proteins of biologic fluids including nasal mucus and tears could suppress bacterial growth. He named the substance *lysozyme*. However, these scientific studies drew little attention and advancement from academic researchers in London in the 1920s and went undeveloped. He continued to research bacteria, however. In the summer of 1928, he was studying the staphylococcus bacteria, growing it on culture media in his lab. He was noted to be a bit nonchalant with his samples, leaving some open on his work bench when he went for a month-long vacation. Returning in September, he noticed that there was mold contamination in one of the culture dishes and that there was a clear one-inch ring around the mold free from the bacteria that were unable to grow there. "That's funny," he famously said to his assistant as he conjectured that the mold had secreted a substance that killed the nearby bacteria. He named the substance *penicillin* after the genus of mold that was growing there. After growing and isolating the substance from the mold, he tested it against various bacteria to see its effects. He found it inhibited and then killed the "gram-positive" bacteria but not the "gram-negative" ones (a different class of bacteria). Again, his initially published reports on penicillin were essentially ignored and thought not to be important by the scientific community. Additionally, there was difficulty with isolating and purifying enough of this substance to try to use it clinically, to see if it worked on human infections. Initially, he could only produce enough to treat a couple of patients with infectious conjunctivitis which worked. While he toiled away for years in his lab, a group of biochemists from Oxford in 1940 (10 years later) elucidated the chemical structure and developed techniques to produce enough penicillin for clinical trials and then they worked together to use it in patients. Definitive proof of its effectiveness was when Fleming treated and cured a normally fatal streptococcal meningitis in 1942. The published report sent the medical world into a frenzy for mass producing this incredible treatment that was desperately needed during the Second World War. A collaboration between British and American scientists ensued and penicillin became available for all the Allied troops by D-Day. Interestingly, penicillin is still produced today, 80 years later, in a similar way by growing the fungus in a large vat and harvesting the product.

While the fanfare of penicillin changed the course of medical treatment and research and ushered in an entirely new age of effective compounds to treat infections and other diseases, it was not actually the first antibiotic. Sulfanilamide was found in the mid-1930s to effectively treat various infections. It was initially derived from testing various dye compounds against bacteria. It was largely used topically but also in pill form and found to have good effects against a range of infections and, interestingly, was responsible for curing Winston Churchill's pneumonia in 1943. The "sulfa" antibiotics, as they eventually were known, underwent many changes in composition over future decades and had a big impact on reducing mortality from infections during WW2. However, they were accompanied by bacterial resistance and side effects and became less important than penicillin by 1945 when Fleming and his collaborators won the Nobel prize for penicillin. The ironic aspect is that the first sulfa antibiotic was developed in Germany in the same year Hitler came to power, 1933, but fortunately was easily manufactured by other companies around Europe so was not limited in supply by the Allies. Various forms of sulfa based antibiotics are still used today.

The success of penicillin spurred medical research to find new antibiotics as infectious diseases were the number one cause of death at that time. Development of new antibiotics evolved over the next 50 years to include a dozen different classes effective for nearly every *bacterial* infection. However, soon after introduction, the issue of antibiotic resistance was met due to natural evolution and from overuse. The development of antibiotics for the ancient disease, tuberculosis, in the 1950s was also an incredible win for medical science. With penicillin exquisitely effective against syphilis, the hospital wards of Dr. Lewis' experience in the 1930s vanished by the end of the 1950s. Since the large armamentaria of antibiotics that developed up to the 1990s, antibiotic development has severely waned in recent decades due to lack of interest and diminished economic opportunities by pharmaceutical companies. While there is concern over resistant strains of bacteria, this has not turned into a crisis at the current time. Overall, in the modern age of medicine and medical training, antibiotic protocols are well-defined and antibiotics are still so effective that deaths from bacterial infections are actually rare unless a patient also has an immunodeficiency. There has also been significant progress in antibiotics against fungal infections and viruses although on a much smaller scale than for bacteria.

From the view of evolution and the story of medicine, antibiotics represent an important understanding of the natural balance of life forces with fungi battling bacteria for a niche in the ecosystem and how evolution swings the balance back and forth with bacteria able to mount a defense by acquiring genetic resistance against poisons produced by fungi. Also important in this story is man's eternal search for medicinal use of plants to treat illness which is truly confirmed with penicillin being a prime example.

Cancer is the most feared word in the medical lexicon. Named and described by Hippocrates who noticed strange tumors that looked like crabs with veins and continued to grow and overtake the person with an early death leading to its name consistent with its appearance. As with most diseases there were essentially no effective cancer treatments for the entire history of mankind until relatively recently. William Halsted, M.D., the pioneer American surgeon who helped found Johns Hopkins Hospital, developed the first surgery and real treatment for any cancer with his *radical mastectomy surgical technique* published in 1894. His concept of cancer surgery was forward thinking in that cancer cells spread to adjacent tissues and lymph nodes and that by removing everything one could downstream gave the patient a better chance of long-term survival. This really was radical in that it removed not only the breast tissue, but all the muscles, skin and any lymph tissue in the area. It did result in a doubling of the 5-year survival rate from 20 to 40%. Surgery has always seemed a good solution to cancer by simply "cutting it out". However, cancer is not simply a lump of rogue tissue. Cancer is also not *one* disease. It can arise from any tissue and is caused by a myriad of factors: genetic mutations and alterations are part of the basic mechanism with inherited forms among the least common direct causes while environmental causes and lifestyle issues the largest inducers.

During WWII, the use of mustard gas as chemical warfare was noted to also cause severe lowering of white blood cells in those exposed. This led two Yale pharmacologists exploring this effect to try a chemotherapeutic drug for a specific cancer of white blood cells, lymphoma, in 1942. This was the first trial of a chemical compound that prolonged a patient's life for many months.

With the growing understanding of cell biology in cancer, the search and trials for potential cancer drugs was on but, unfortunately, was met with many more failures than successes which were mostly short-term remissions rather than cures for the following decades. Breakthroughs came with the rare cancer choriocarcinoma (cancer of the placenta) in 1956 and then with combination therapy for childhood acute leukemia and Hodgkins lymphoma in the mid-1960s. Most chemotherapy is designed to poison cancer cells as they divide quickly. However normal cells are susceptible to actions causing many side effects such as hair loss, nausea and vomiting, low blood counts, nerve damage and others. Most side effects are temporary but make getting through the treatment challenging and difficult. If one is interested, I highly recommend the excellent and extensive history of cancer in the "Emperor of All Maladies" by Siddhartha Mukherjee, M.D. Over the past 50 years, cancer treatment has evolved enormously with treatment options that can include radiation therapy, surgery and chemotherapy for a large variety. In the 21st century the addition of new and powerful immunotherapy drugs (monoclonal antibodies and checkpoint inhibitors) has led the way for treating previously fatal cancer. An incredible example is in the treatment of metastatic melanoma which previously was uniformly fatal and now can be cured!

Along with cancer, cardiovascular diseases have been consistently the two most deadly diseases in the developed world for the past half century. Besides using an EKG to diagnose heart attacks and arrhythmias, nothing was available to treat heart disease until heart defects could be repaired in the early 1950s as noted previously. The Framingham Heart Study funded by Congress started in 1948 has proven that heart health is related to lifestyle, environmental and genetic factors. Although well known today as being important risk factors for cardiovascular disease, in the 1950s it was assumed that high blood pressure and high cholesterol were just normal components of aging and were not treated as medical problems. It was not until the 1960s that cigarette smoking was shown to cause heart attacks, strokes and cancer. Since then, many new different classes of medications have been developed to treat hypertension, high cholesterol, heart rhythm disturbances, strokes, and heart attacks. A powerful "clot busting" injectable medicine introduced 30 years ago is used routinely to treat heart attacks and strokes. A whole variety of diagnostic tools have been developed including echocardiograms to look directly at the heart and valves non-invasively with ultrasound. In the 1970s, cardiologists started accurately documenting coronary blockages with angiograms and soon developed balloon dilation techniques and then metal stents to unclog arteries. A huge advance in the emergency treatment of heart attacks has evolved since the start of the 21st century with patients being rushed to the cath lab to have their blood clots dissolved and blockages opened before damage has taken place. No other medical specialty has as many diagnostic tests available to evaluate patients as cardiology. Medical therapy for active treatment and prevention of heart disease has undergone an incredible expansion over the past 30 years especially with the use of statins to reduce and prevent blockages. In this century, implantable defibrillator devices have been used to prevent sudden death. While seemingly an excellent preventive measure, its practical use has caused controversy in selecting the correct patients for the procedure. Overall, deaths from cardiovascular diseases have decreased greater than 50% in the past 50 years, a remarkable turn-around to a previously untreated set of diseases.

The bizarre spread of the anti-vaxxer movement during the recent Covid pandemic has led to tens of thousands of unnecessary deaths from a preventable illness by an incredibly safe and effective vaccine developed within one year of its start. Some of the reluctance may be due to Covid having only a 0.6% mortality rate overall. In previous eras where smallpox killed a significant portion of those infected, the population was much more eager to get vaccinated after Jenner's inoculation technique became widely available in the early decades of the 19th century. Similarly, I would bet everyone would have signed up for a vaccine against the influenza pandemic of 1918 that killed 50 million worldwide. Vaccine development has largely occurred over the last 100 years and has included immunization against certain viruses and bacteria although predominantly viruses as those are easier to produce and are generally more effective. I also wonder if parents today would be so concerned about childhood vaccinations if diphtheria was still around. In the 1920s prior to the introduction of the vaccine against the toxin produced by the bacteria that infects the throat, 10% of infected children would die a slow, progressive, horrible, untreatable death of suffocation from growth of "pseudo-membranes" causing progressive blocking of their windpipe. This terrible disease went from 200,000 deaths *per year* a century ago to only 14 *total* deaths in this century due to an effective and safe vaccine. Also, I would wonder if anyone would not want to be vaccinated with the polio vaccine if we were seeing children dying from not being able to breath or left paralyzed as was common in the 1950s prior to the Salk and then oral Sabin vaccine. The answer is an obvious and loud no. The absence of these terrible, disabling, fatal diseases has led to forgetting, misthinking and misinformation about how bad these have been for humanity and how absolutely wonderful their prevention has been. Various vaccine types have been developed and include using the "toxoid" (the harmful protein) itself such as with tetanus and diphtheria. Others use inactivated viruses such as influenza, polio, rabies and hepatitis A. Still others have used "attenuated" (weakened, low virulence) viruses such as for measles, mumps, rubella and yellow fever. The most advanced techniques have come recently from Covid-19 with the entirely new technical development of using messenger RNA and DNA in vaccines that cause small harmless components of the virus to be manufactured in the body inducing a natural immunological response. Incredibly, these Covid vaccines have been over 90% in protecting the individual against the specific strains. However, due to mutations in the virus, there has been the need to adapt the vaccines against newer strains with booster shots.

While there has been great interest and research into trying to develop specific vaccines against cancer. This remains in the investigation phase. However, there are available two antiviral vaccines that prevent the cancer caused by them. HPV (human papillomavirus) is a known cause of cervical cancer in women and certain throat cancers and is now preventable with an easily tolerable two shot vaccine now given to teenagers. Chronic hepatitis B infection is a common cause of liver cancer worldwide and a preventable disease with vaccination. All healthcare workers have been required to have this vaccine for decades to prevent transmission from contaminated blood. The Bacillus Calmette-Guerin vaccine (BCG) was initially developed as a vaccine against tuberculosis over a century ago. It is still given to children in endemic countries (not in the US) and prevents serious infections about 40% of the time. It is an attenuated TB strain. However, it has found great use in treating bladder cancer and has been a standard for 50 years by activating the immune system to suppress its growth.

It has only been since the second half of the 20th century that *hospital care* has been for actually treating disease instead of its predominant role previously as a place only for diagnosis and comfort care. The old adage "hospitals are where people go to die" was quite true prior to the modern antibiotic era. Most hospital care prior to 1950 would be largely equivalent to modern day "hospice" care. Starting in the 1960s, hospitals equipped with newly developed technology for clinical care at the bedside, in their laboratories and radiology equipment (such as ultrasound and X-ray fluoroscopy) along with advancing surgical techniques and new medicines began to have specialized departments of care. The *emergency room* (ER) emerged as a specialized area for acutely treating severely ill and injured patients. Laboratory equipment developed automatization to quickly determine results of various samples of body fluids and processed tissue samples overseen by pathology specialists. Improved X-ray and ultrasound equipment overseen by radiologists working all day in the hospital could quickly give an interpretation of a specific study to treating doctors. Surgical care evolved to have multiple operating rooms available at all times of the day for needed emergency and elective surgery. Labor and delivery departments were organized by obstetricians with all the tools and technology to safely deliver complex childbirth. Patients were placed in various departments in the hospital that were particular to different conditions. General medical care, post-surgical care, cardiac monitoring and gynecology were separated into their own departments with nursing care specialized to each area. The most advanced modernization came with *intensive care units* (ICUs) in the mid-1960s. These areas developed as contained spaces equipped with every possible monitoring device and treatment option with patients having constant care by one or two nurses at a time for the sickest patients in the hospital. This system further evolved to include a *surgical intensive care unit* for complicated post-op patients. The *cardiac care unit* became a special unit for the care of heart attacks and other heart diseases. By 1970, most larger hospitals were equipped with intensive medical, cardiac and surgical care units and as a result severely ill patients were finally being saved from dying. The complexity of hospital care continued to advance to the end of the 20th century with advanced radiology (CT scans and MRIs), more sophisticated monitoring equipment, surgical advances of minimally invasive surgeries and short stays, and specialization of hospital based physicians that saw the care of patients by doctors working only in the hospital (hospitalists), along with specialty training and certification of intensive care physicians (intensivists). This has resulted in highly trained physicians in the hospital round the clock to take care of more complex and sicker patients than previously. In the 21st century, hospital care has adopted all advanced technology to assist in every aspect. Electronic records, advanced monitoring systems, integrated and coordinated data systems are the norm. Modern hospitals are becoming "smart" and are at the center of comprehensive medical centers that include doctors' offices, labs, radiology, outpatient treatment and rehabilitation centers. Modern hospitals today have the look and feel of a high-end resort equipped with all the high-tech comforts in well-designed, private, comfortable rooms with gourmet food.

Sir William Osler, M.D. (1849-1919), one of founders of Johns Hopkins Medical School and Hospital, professor emeritus at Oxford late in his career, started modern physician training methods by having young doctors do "residencies" at the hospital for several years and wrote one of the first complete medical texts that became a standard reference for over 40 years, *The Principles and Practice of Medicine* (1892). He was quite critical of most medical care, medications and the so-called "art of medicine" of his time. He was anchored in the belief that medical care should and must be a science not a belief system and taught young doctors this mantra changing the way medical care was evolving at the start of the 20th century. Ironically, he held onto the old belief that bloodletting could be helpful for some conditions. While 20th century medicine is filled with dramatic discoveries and breakthroughs, the science of *how* to treat patients from a true scientific perspective took nearly the entire century to adopt proper ways for medical science to study itself. The "art of medicine" remained the standard which meant that individual doctors would treat diseases with methods they thought, experienced or believed were true. For most of the 20th century, medical literature became filled with thousands of studies that described anecdotal evidence of a particular treatment, sometimes a bit more advanced with studying a group of patients treated in a certain manner that the writer determined successful. The *experts* (usually the highest ranking at respected teaching centers) in each field were deemed to know the proper treatment methods both in medicine and surgery and were highly esteemed and listened to. Osler rightly remained skeptical of medicines except for the use of opium and digitalis and generally recommended "natural" healing. The tug of war against *experts* and proper scientific inquiry continued for most of the 20th century.

In the early 1970s, there developed a forceful movement to bring hard science into play. One of the pioneers of this movement, Archie Cochrane, a Scottish physician, published his book *Effectiveness and Efficiency* (1972) which espoused randomized controlled trials of different treatments in medicine to determine which was best. He went on to establish a medical database of scientific studies which eventually evolved into the Cochrane Collaboration which is active and important today in performing extensive reviews of specific medical topics to give advice and guidance. The concept of a randomized controlled scientific study is crucial to determine if a specific treatment is effective over either: *no treatment* (a control group), *another treatment* (a comparison group) or *placebo* (to determine the placebo effect vs active treatment). Currently, for new drugs to get approval by the FDA, a randomized controlled study is needed.

Serious concern over the quality of medical studies, the methods used and the interpretations were steadily growing by the early 1980s. Also, medical practice data was accumulating that showed large variations of physician treatments and procedures. Of course, the push to have the science and practice of medicine increase to a high standard was met with resistance by many of the "experts" who thought they knew better. Fortunately, by the 1990s the concept and term of *Evidence-based Medicine* (meaning well performed scientific studies supporting the treatment) became the standard and medical journals were rejecting obviously biased or poorly done studies. However, the surgical literature still lagged in the old ways of individual methods and opinions without critical scientific scrutiny until even recent times.

I'll offer an example from my residency days in the early 1980s in Boston. Adopting new scientific data was actually an important part of our learning and teaching process. During that time, an updated yearly pocket manual that everyone had named the *Washington Manual of Medical Therapeutics* was used daily. This wire bound book was a synthesis of the latest medical treatments from a scientific study standpoint even though many of the studies were not of the highest quality. At that time, when a patient came to the ER with an acute heart attack, it was recommended to give everyone an intravenous injection of lidocaine (yes, the same medicine that dentists used to numb teeth) to prevent cardiac arrhythmias and supposedly prevent sudden death. It was often not a pleasant experience for patients as it often caused dizziness, a general tingling and disorientation for a period of time, but we gave it explaining the potential life-saving effects. It turns out that the studies on this drug given for this purpose were small and observational, but everyone thought the conclusion was true as we had all seen patients die suddenly from ventricular tachycardia. By the end of my residency, this particular use was finally studied in a randomized, controlled study with a large group of patients able to determine if it was effective. It turned out that there was *no* benefit from preventing dangerous or deadly arrhythmias and showed a proportion of patients had serious side effects and there was even a slight trend of increased overall mortality. The use of lidocaine preventatively abruptly stopped and rightly so and thankfully due to a well-done study.

While *randomized controlled studies* cannot solve every question and problem, they bring us closer to the best possible treatments for patients and are the gold standard for approving new drugs, medical devices and protocols for treatments. Medicine finally reached into the scientific realm by the 21st century.

Another good example worth mentioning is a recent study on *appendectomies* from 2020. In this randomized study patients were either given a ten-day course of antibiotics or sent to "standard" surgery. The result was that 70% of the antibiotics patients were cured without surgery! It also means that nearly a third needed to eventually have an appendectomy. However, this study was fascinating in countering "old school" thinking that preached that *any* patient with *possible* appendicitis should be taken to surgery immediately to prevent the possibility of "rupture" and death in a treatable "surgical" disease. It was well known that half the patients taken to surgery for possible appendicitis in the past did *not* have appendicitis even though it was suspected. This low accuracy rate was deemed acceptable to avoid a supposed "disastrous" outcome. Appendicitis also became a more certain diagnosis after the routine use of CT scan was introduced leading to less unnecessary surgeries. An equally remarkable aspect about this study is that the surgeons accepted its result and applauded this long overdue needed understanding of what happens in real life to appendicitis patients. This represents a huge shift in understanding the importance of scientific studies that have evolved over the past 40 years.

The youngest of all the medical science disciplines is genetics. Heritable traits have been appreciated for millennia. However, the basic understanding of the passing along specific physical characteristics started with Darwin in his paradigm changing book that first described evolutionary biology in *On the Origin of Species* (1859). Soon afterward Gregor Mendel studied the different modes of inheriting specific *genes* (the word first used in 1909) as being dominantly or recessively passed on in his work on peas (1865). The connection of genetic inheritance and chromosomes took another 50 years to become known. Afterward there developed an interest in discovering specific diseases that were related to altered genes. In 1949, *sickle cell disease* was the first disease shown to be related to a gene inheritance causing abnormal hemoglobins that folded and collapsed in the red cell when oxygen levels became reduced. Sickle cell disease is an awful, disastrous disease that causes severe pain, life threatening anemia and early death but evolutionarily it developed as a response to humans being infected by malaria. The red cells that "sickle" can kill the invasive organism.

An odd and cruel path away from evolution, the *Eugenics* movement, developed from Darwin's cousin who coined the word (1883) and began espousing ways to "improve the human race" by proper inbreeding. This controversial movement grew in the early 20th century in Europe and the US eventually divorcing itself from evolutionary theory and natural selection of Darwinism. In the US, the concepts of trying to improve humans devolved into blatant racist and discriminatory laws that targeted the mentally ill, Blacks, Native Americans and Asians subjected to forced sterilization, prohibition against mixed marriages and limited immigration against "inferior races". Historically, the movement was supported and financed by some of the largest corporations in America, e.g. Rockefeller, Carnegie, Kellog. Its demise in popularity and public policy came after Hitler's blatant use of it in Nazi Germany.

The precise structure of DNA was not unraveled until 1952 when Watson, Crick and Franklin precisely described the elegant double helix that could be unwound revealing its inherent property of self-replication present in all living organisms forming chromosomes as the universal genetic material. Unfortunately, only Watson and Crick received the Nobel Prize in 1962 for this monumental discovery. Studying chromosomes, DNA and specific diseases is difficult and complex science, and it has taken many decades to uncover genetically based diseases. Most of those that have been worked out are rare metabolic diseases or specific chromosome abnormalities e.g. Down's syndrome. The development of advancing technologies for genetic analysis over the last half century has been quite impressive.

In 2003, after nearly 15 years, the world's largest collaborative study, *The Human Genome Project* (HGP) published its first nearly complete genetic map (92%) of human DNA. Interestingly and somewhat bizarrely, it was spurred along and completed its work early due to direct competition from a private company, Celera, doing DNA sequencing more rapidly with a different technology. The HGP put its data online as open source for anyone to use while Celera attempted to patent some of its findings for its own commercial benefit but fortunately lost out after the public sequenced data was released. It took nearly 10 more years for HGP to fill in the gaps of the last eight percent due to the complexity of those last pieces. The medical world was extremely excited about having a definitive tool to potentially unlock the mystery of diseases. While much has been discovered and advanced in the generation since its release including specific genetics of certain diseases, gene mutations and chromosomal abnormalities, the anticipated answers to the genetic underpinnings of disease have only been partially revealed. What has been found is that nearly all diseases do not have a *single* gene responsible for their cause and that the vast majority of diseases are due to an interplay of many genes. A good example has been the search for genes that cause type 2 diabetes (the most common form in the world) which has several dozen genes causing an increased *risk* (10-30% chance) instead of a single cause. In type 2 diabetes, genetics is not the only factor as environmental and lifestyle factors are equally important in determining who gets it. The overall message of medical genetics is that disease processes are *very* complex and there are very few simple, direct answers.

However, the advances of medical genetics continue forward in impressive fashion. Advanced genetic sequencing techniques can do the same individual human genome sequencing as the HGP did in only a few days and for a few hundred dollars instead of the 15 years and 3 billion dollars it previously took! This method is being increasingly used to evaluate the changes in cancers and is beginning to give insights into specific treatments that are effective, now labeled *precision medicine.*

A recent astounding accomplishment in genetic medicine is with the 2023 approval of the first direct gene treatment to correct the defect in *sickle cell disease* which is a single gene, single amino acid change. The discovery of a natural gene editing technique (removing one gene and replacing it with another) known as Crispr-Cas9 by two women scientists, Emmanuelle Charpentier and Jennifer Doudna, who jointly won the Nobel Prize in 2020 has now opened up this new field of medicine. The future of treating genetic disorders is just in its infancy.

The final section of our historical journey will be concerned with mental health. There are many parallels with general medicine. There has always been a small percentage of the population afflicted with serious psychotic mental disorders (1-2%) such as schizophrenia and bipolar disorders along with the more common problems of depression and anxiety. Hippocrates put "madness" or insanity into the construct of humoral theory, assuming it was caused by an imbalance similar to those of physical illness. However, other ancient cultures and Greek philosophers attributed insanity to an affliction caused by the gods. Treatments included spiritual exorcism, rebalancing of humors by bloodletting, purging agents, starvation, and various torture techniques attempting to correct psychosis. Spiritual and religious attribution to madness continued through the Middle Ages. From the 16th to 18th centuries, the insane were often taken out of society and put in workhouses or jailed where they were often restrained, some were subject to witch-hunts. The evolution of thinking about the insane during the Enlightenment began with the concept that they were "insensitive animals" which justified continued harsh and restraining treatments and the start of "madhouse" institutions such as the infamously nick-named *Bedlam* in London in the 17th century. With the expansion of the industrial age in the 19th century, the rise of the "insane asylum era" developed in the western world. Legislation was adopted to compel authorities to deal with the insane which coincided with the concept of "moral" treatment. In reality, insane asylums were simply a place to take the "crazies" out of sight from society. The previous assumptions of the insane being "possessed by the devil" began to recede and a more humanistic model was slowly adapted. The science of psychiatry still had no scientific backing and even classification of diseases as all were lumped together. Asylums made attempts to cure insanity by teaching the "correct" way to behave to no avail. Also, many disparate groups of unfortunate sufferers were locked up together including the demented, neurologically impaired from diseases such as tertiary syphilis, the mentally retarded, autistic and anyone whose behavior was significantly outside the norm including homosexuals. The growth of the asylum industry in the US in the second half of the 19th century saw patient numbers rise from 5,000 in 1850 to 150,000 by 1904. Increasing attempts to classify and define mental disorders started in the later part of the 19th century and included behaviors such as excess alcohol intake and various "perversions". Sigmund Freud and Carl Jung's theories of the psyche having various unconscious components at the turn of the 20th led to their belief and development of *psychoanalysis* or "talk therapy" as a way to cure the more common problems of anxiety. It's important to note that they both admitted they had *no* help for the insane or psychotic individual. The world of asylums and institutionalization continued through most of the 20th century.

Extreme treatments were adopted as medical and technological advances came into use in the 20th century. *Insulin shock therapy* was adopted (after the therapeutic use of insulin for diabetes was established) as a way to treat schizophrenics in 1927 until the late 1950s. This cruel method was performed by giving a large dose of insulin to induce a hypoglycemic coma with the inaccurate assumption it would "shock" the patient back to a normal state of thinking. In the mid-1930s using a similar thread of assumption, *electro-shock therapy* (ECT) became a popular method to "cure" schizophrenics by inducing a seizure. While this treatment had no effect on psychosis, it was found to have a significant and dramatic effect on improving those with severe depression and is still used today in some patients who do not respond to medications. For all other psychiatric diseases other than depression, ECT fell out of favor by the 1970s. Between 1940 and 1960 the rise of a specific crude brain surgery known as *lobotomy* came into favor for treating psychotic patients. With the increasing understanding of the frontal lobes of the brain having a significant impact on behavior, this brutally invasive procedure was developed. By simply cutting into and destroying this part of the brain, aggressive and psychotic behavior became docile, eliminating all emotion. It was used for all sorts of mental conditions including homosexuality and more often in women than men. In modern culture it was exposed for its mind numbing effect in the book (1962) and movie (1975) *One Flew over the Cuckoo's Nest*.

Fortunately, with the arrival of an entire new class of antipsychotic medications, the *neuroleptics,* in the early 1950s, treatment could safely control psychotic behavior without destroying personalities. *Chlorpromazine* was developed in France first as an aide for anesthesia but also found to have significant calming effects and improved rational thought properties. After positive clinical trials in psychotic psychiatric patients, it was approved for use in schizophrenia and other psychotic disorders in the US in 1954. The psychopharmacological revolution began with this medication and was remarkable in allowing severely psychotic patients to return to clearer, more coherent thinking and functioning in daily life activities. It quickly replaced all the above harsh procedures done on psychotic patients. Of course, like any medication it was not perfect and not without significant side effects, but its overall transformation was similar to that of penicillin in that it allowed many psychiatric patients to not need hospitalization or institutionalization, and they could finally live on their own in society. This first antipsychotic medication was used widely in the 1950s and '60s with great benefit for many patients. These antipsychotics work in the brain to reduce the effects of dopamine in certain areas that produce delusional thoughts including hearing voices common to the schizophrenic experience.

The dramatic and definitive effect of chlorpromazine spurred researchers to develop antidepressant medications. One of the firsts, *imipramine,* was developed as a derivative from chlorpromazine and was found to profoundly help depressed patients with "motor retardation" (physical lethargy and low level of activity) and started the class of medications known as "tricyclic" antidepressants due to their chemical structure. Other early antidepressants came out of drug development for treating tuberculosis, the *monoamine oxidase inhibitors.* While effective for depression these medications could cause serious hypertension and their use has always been limited. Both of these were approved in the late 1950s. The 1960s saw the first benzodiazepine tranquilizers come to market which were quickly overprescribed for various types of anxiety conditions. The popularity of *Valium* as a treatment for anxiety became a symbolic icon of the new psychopharmacological age of the 1960s and 1970s. Many patients became addicted and its use even became a stereotype reflecting the societal changes of those times. The Rolling Stones' infamous hit song "Mother's Little Helper" (1966) portrays its common use.

Advances and new additions in all three classes of psychiatric medications continued with the introduction of *Prozac* as a new type of antidepressant in 1987, the first SSRI (selective serotonin reuptake inhibitor). This led to developing various antidepressants and antipsychotics that focus on modulating different neurotransmitter systems in the brain that have effects on the mental state of humans. Variations of benzodiazepine tranquilizers have evolved as well, targeting specific types of anxiety but they still possess addictive potential making their prescription with caution and in need of close oversight. All of this drug development in the past half century has made psychiatry a significantly pharmacologically oriented specialty.

The development of psychology as a discipline and evolution of treatment of what is known as "talk therapy" started in the late 19th century and was built on work done a century previously during the age of Enlightenment. In parallel to the popularity of Freud's theories of *psychoanalysis* emerging at the turn of the 20th century in Europe were the American psychology academic investigators such as William James who actually attempted to bring scientific study of the mind in the late 19th century. Many large universities developed departments specifically for psychological study. In America the rise of *behaviorism* as a school of thought grew from the 1920s significantly led by BF Skinner. Behaviorism explains human action in terms of reflexes from previous experience in context with a person's motivations and possible rewards or punishments. A well-known example is Pavlov's *conditioning response* experiments with dogs. This theory was gradually replaced in the second half of the 20th century with *cognitive* psychology which brings together the mental processes of attention, language, memory, perception, problem solving, creativity and reasoning as influencing behavior. Specifically, *Cognitive-Behavioral Therapy (CBT)* has become the dominant method for psychological treatment in the modern age. Psychologists and therapists are the ones mostly at the front lines today providing counseling and guidance to those with mental distress. However, it remains (as it always has) that actual *access* to mental health providers is problematic and limited. Besides the social stigmata and hesitance of patients, most insurances today have restricted coverage, along with a limited number of available providers that often represent a significant out of pocket expense. Most patients who need help never see a psychologist or psychiatrist. In my career I have worked alongside excellent psychiatrists and psychologists, however, getting patients to them has always been difficult. This issue is far from solved in our current world.

The advances of medicine over the last century can be seen with the increase of lifespan. A baby born in the U.S. in 1900 could expect to live only forty-seven years in contrast to a baby born today would expect to live seventy-seven years. Most of that improvement in life expectancy is due to reduction of child mortality (1 in 5 children died before age 10 in 1900), improved sanitation (e.g. clean water), nutrition, health education and immunizations. Modestly, it has been estimated that medical treatment advances account for only about 30% of the improvements in life expectancy from the start of the 20th century.

My personal perspective researching this review is feeling quite grateful to have been able to practice medicine during the "modern age of medicine", the last 50 years. Prior to that, medicine had serious limitations other than antibiotics for infections and surgery for a select number of conditions. I truly appreciate the significant humbling experience it must have been for practicing physicians in previous eras. In my career, I've been fortunate to take advantage of the scientific and technological advances that have become available and see them work to successfully treat and cure patients of terrible diseases. Only relatively recently has medical science been able to figure out the human body, what makes it ill, and what can make it better. There remain significant limitations in knowledge and treatments, which continues to make practicing medicine a truly humbling experience. With continued advances in human genetics, diagnostic technology, development of precision drug treatment and the probable importance of artificial intelligence (AI) in medical care over the next fifty years, there will likely be a transformation in medicine greater than the last fifty.

CHAPTER 30

The Best Prescription

Over the course of nearly 40 years of seeing patients in the office, I've often been asked at the end of visits that were for non-acute or serious problems: "Doctor, what's the best vitamin pill to take to become healthier?" It's natural to want to feel better, live longer and keep disease away especially if your doctor can give you some secret insights. I've also received related questions about various supplements that flood the market. The answers are always disappointing to patients. While sufficient vitamins and minerals keep one from getting ill from a deficiency, the thinking that "if a little is good, a lot must be better" is not only false but has been proven dangerous in taking too much especially with certain vitamins such vitamin A and E. Supplements, generally, have no strong scientific backing to improve health or fend off disease. So, what can I say to the vast majority that are asking for help to prevent disease and to improve their overall health? Read on, please!

OK then, I am going to go through in detail a *real, verifiable, scientifically proven* recommendation that will help prevent serious medical diseases, improve your health both physically and mentally and may prolong your life. "What's that?", you say. "Tell me, tell me," you beg. "Please and now," you demand. Warning! It's not a drug, device, or supplement that you can buy on Amazon. It's not a secret, it's not expensive, it's not covered by insurance and can be used by *anyone, anytime!* Huh…, now I've got you confused?

OK, let's go. It's called *bodily movement, physical activity,* or *exercise*. I put that word last as many folks don't like it! Yes, moving your own body regularly in any method, pattern or length of time can have more powerful effects on your health than nearly anything.

With skeletal muscles comprising 40% of our body weight, one might imagine that there is an overall impact to health by keeping that large amount of tissue in proper order. In the past 70 years, this topic has been researched by over 100,000 published articles on the effects of physical activity on health and medical conditions. This massive amount of research includes many studies on the negative health effects of inactivity. Let's look into both sides of this data as it relates to modern life.

To start with the negative, there have been identified forty medical conditions that are made worse or increased in probability with an inactive or sedentary lifestyle. This large-varied list includes: premature death, heart disease, diabetes, arthritis, liver disease, cancers of the colon and ovary, fragile bones, obesity, immune dysfunction, cognitive dysfunction, depression, anxiety and many others. Lotsa serious stuff! What's important is that all of these conditions are *significantly* lessened or prevented with an active lifestyle.

Why and how do these effects occur with just moving your muscles regularly? Let's dive into this fascinating physiology of how our metabolism works to improve your body as it is designed by evolution—as a mobile, responsive active organism able to do physical stuff naturally, with the ability to improve strength and endurance while enhancing the body and spirit!

First, let me say to those that hate to be active and can't stand the idea of exercise and haven't done much and are not fit and have no motivation to change one's sedentary lifestyle that *you, yes you,* have the most to gain from doing anything and even doing just a little bit of increased movement. You will gain significant advantages in health, disease prevention and reducing your risk of death! Now that may be something to take into account instead of getting yet another pill from your doctor for another chronic condition that has been identified.

Unfortunately, the general population of western cultures have become less physically active over the past half century to the extent that at least 50% of the population engages in less than the *minimum* amount needed for basic health. What is a sedentary lifestyle and what is the minimum recommended from medical research to ensure good health? Being *sedentary* means engaging in little movement throughout one's waking day, such as sitting >6-11 hours per day but, also, when one does movement it involves minimal effort, energy expenditure, cardiovascular stimulation, or increase of blood flow to muscles. Let's clarify and define different levels of physical activity. *Sedentary activity* is basically doing nothing like sitting in a chair or lying on the couch. *Light activity* includes slow walking at 2 mph or less, light household chores and cooking, picking up materials that weigh less than 10 pounds, and not using multiple muscle groups at one time (such as going up and down stairs). *Moderate activity* includes many different activities such as walking >3 mph, bicycling ~7 mph, calisthenics, yoga, rowing machines, lifting weights, dancing, doubles tennis, swimming, hopscotch, skateboarding, various yard work such as raking or weeding, housework such as sweeping and scrubbing the bathroom, washing the car, painting the house, even playing with children and pushing a stroller counts here as moderate. Examples of *vigorous or intense activity* are aerobic dancing, water aerobics, martial arts, jumping rope, walking or running >5 mph, sports such as basketball or handball, shoveling snow, splitting logs, concrete or masonry work, loading or unloading a truck, and many other activities that involve many muscle groups at one time and increase heart rate and respiratory rate.

Hopefully, these practical examples will give you a proper understanding of these categories. Here, I want to avoid explaining the scientific measurement jargon. In real terms how much time is recommended per week? About 2.5 hours (150 minutes) at the moderate level, which is best done spread out over many days (5 days/week is a good reference). It's important to know that there are no rules regarding time and intensity. One could do three times seven minutes of brisk walking a day to fulfill this greatly beneficial activity. Also, the type of movement can be almost anything such as walking up and down stairs, moderate yard work, moderate cleaning or more structured, such as cycling, weight training, dance fitness, etc. There are clear benefits from doing a combination of aerobic activity and weight resistance activity.

409

Let's dive into specifically what benefits regular physical activity does for the body and why. First we'll look at regular exercise and the risk of cancer. There are many cancers where being physically fit compared to sedentary folks have a reduced risk. The strongest data is in breast and colon cancer resulting in about a 15% lower risk. There is also reasonably good associative data for reducing cancers of the bladder, uterus, kidney and stomach for about the same benefit (15% less risk). The mechanisms for these reductions are attributed to several factors. A reduction of hormones, such as estrogens, for breast cancer and also reduced insulin for colon cancer are likely factors. The reduction of general inflammation with regular exercise is known to suppress cancer growth. Also, being physically fit enhances the immune system which monitors and suppresses early cancer development. For colon cancer reduction, regular exercise improves transit time of food through the gut and reduces exposure of carcinogens. Lastly, reducing obesity, which is a known risk for many cancers, also lessens cancer risk.

For premature death analysis, there is clear data that one's risk of dying from any cause is reduced with regular moderate exercise (150 minutes/week). Interestingly, this effect does not plateau out and there are continuous gains and risk reductions with qualitatively and quantitatively more exercise. The highest group of fitness predicts a 30% risk reduction of death from any cause. The mechanisms for this protection are similar to those listed above, with the reduction of general inflammation and the protection against cardiovascular disease leading the way.

The most studied and still the leading cause of death in the USA is cardiovascular disease with over 700,000 deaths per year. Heart disease is responsible for 1 in 5 of all deaths and has been determined to be fully 80% preventable with healthy living habits and quitting smoking. The effects of exercise on the cardiovascular system is the most studied area of disease alteration. There are many beneficial physiological adaptations that occur in the cardiovascular system in response to exercise that causes the heart to have increased performance, improved resilience, increased circulation and protection against damage. With regular exercise, the heart muscle gets stronger. Also, the volume of the heart appropriately expands to pump more blood throughout the body lowering mechanical stress on the heart and blood pressure. The blood vessels that feed the heart muscle grow and form collateral networks which protects the heart from blockages. Electrical system efficiency is improved resulting in a lower resting heart rate. The blood vessels throughout the body are expanded to areas that need more blood (muscles, skin, etc.) and the lining of the blood vessels become resistant to build up of cholesterol plagues that cause blockages. Also, regular exercise has significant benefits on lipids by lowering the "bad" cholesterol (LDL) and raising the "good" cholesterol (HDL) which results in less cholesterol plaque buildup that causes heart attacks and strokes. Since the first published study over 70 years ago (1953) showing that physically active train conductors had significantly less cardiovascular events than passive bus drivers, there has been a plethora of well-done scientific studies proving the beneficial effects of exercise for the heart and circulation. There is a dose response for the benefits and reduced death from cardiovascular disease, the more the better. One estimate is that if folks aged 40-85 increased their exercise by 10 minutes per day there would be 6.9% less deaths per year (110,000 less) in the USA! In one of the few areas of medical care where an exercise program is a covered benefit, patients qualify for cardiac rehabilitation if they have had a heart attack, heart failure, valve replacement or a stent placement. The simple reason is that exercise therapy with these conditions has been proven to have a significant impact on preventing future heart attacks and to strengthen the heart so patients can lead a normal functioning life.

Type 2 Diabetes Mellitus (T2DM) has a very strong genetic component. However, it can be successfully modulated, treated and prevented by lifestyle changes in diet, weight control and most importantly by exercise. A significant and telling study from China on prevention of T2DM in prediabetics separated patients into either dietary changes or exercise, the exercise group had reduction to full blown T2DM by 46% compared with 31% reduction in the diet only group. In a related study from Finland, they combined diet and exercise interventions and found a whopping 58% reduction in developing T2DM after 3 years. The biology of T2DM is quite complex, so let's look at the ways that exercise treats it. One of the early and significant problems with T2DM is "insulin resistance" which means that insulin is not working as well as it should be in moving sugar (glucose) into cells by its direct action on insulin receptors in various tissues of the body, most significantly in muscles. Therefore, blood glucose can continue to rise in the blood even as more insulin is secreted, both of which are bad for the body. Exercise does two direct actions to counteract this. One, muscles can directly absorb glucose by a different pathway that is opened up with muscle contractions (increasing by 40%), and also that exercise improves the insulin receptor functioning in muscles. Evidence has been accumulating that the increased inflammation in the body in T2DM causes higher levels of inflammatory proteins which inflict damage to the body that eventually inhibit insulin from being released as the disease progresses. Exercise has a powerful effect on reducing these inflammatory proteins as one of its effects on taming T2DM. Patients can literally physically work themselves out of having this disease by redirecting their physiology back into a healthier direction!

The immune system is also improved with regular physical activity although at first this may seem unclear. The immune system has two main components: the white blood cells that circulate and monitor for infection and abnormal cell growth (early cancer) and by producing antibodies that are specific for neutralizing foreign substances like bacteria and viruses. With exercise, there is increased release of white cells from their storage areas in the lymph nodes and spleen into the circulation. This increases their patrolling activity for many hours after exercise. In addition, the immune system has a crucial role in regulating inflammation in the body. During exercise, there is a temporary increase in muscle inflammation that results in breakdown which is then repaired during recovery. With regular exercise, the activated immune system reduces overall inflammation and also promotes muscle rebuilding and faster recovery. In studies of the elderly, those more physically fit had greater robust measures of their immune system health and a greater response to vaccines. These significant effects are why exercise promotes a stronger body and reduces our chances for illnesses!

Our endocrine system is quite complex and is largely involved with maintaining and balancing the functioning of our bodies during times of rest and stress. With regular physical activity our hormonal system adapts to allow our bodies to do more physical work while improving recovery and repair after exercise. From the endocrine perspective, exercise can be looked at as a form of stress imposed on the body that it must react to for its current and future health. Different types of exercise elicit specific and prolonged adaptations to allow greater capacity. Initially, the hormones of stress such as cortisol and adrenaline are increased but are then reduced as the body becomes more fit. Growth hormone is increased after exercise from the brain which stimulates recovery, repair and building of muscle tissue while enhancing energy use of glucose. Testosterone is a powerful hormone in men and women (although in much less amounts) that stimulates muscle tissue to repair and grow. In both men and women, levels of testosterone increase after a session of moderate exercise for nearly 24 hours. Insulin, the hormone produced by the pancreas, works better after moderate exercise for several hours by adaptive mechanisms in the muscles which can help fend off T2DM.

As we age, so do our bones which get thinner and break easier. Regular movement that involves using gravity such as walking keeps our bones stronger and reduces the chance of fractures.

Beneficial effects of exercise on our nervous system are well documented and include improving balance, preserving nerve tissue, promoting neuroplasticity (growing new nerves and connections) and significantly preventing cognitive decline as we age. Specifically, the neurodegenerative diseases, Parkinson's and Alzheimer's, are improved with regular exercise.

The enormous benefits of regular moderate activity on maintaining and improving our mental state is one of its most remarkable and notable effects. By helping to rebalance neurotransmitters in the brain that are responsible for depression and anxiety, exercise has been found in many studies to be a more effective treatment than medications for these serious common problems. Improvement in cognitive functioning with better decision making and improved memory have been shown in many well-done studies. Memory is improved by the increase in volume of the part of the brain known for storing memories, the hippocampus. For those reluctant and unmotivated to move one's body because "I'm not in the mood," I offer an important truism that is worth remembering: "Feeling follows action" which is an improved mental state that persists after a workout.

Finally, let's look at what happens to your muscles themselves when they are used regularly. Muscles respond dramatically to regular use both structurally and metabolically. Stimulation of muscles causes various adaptive changes to improve performance triggered by increased gene expression in the muscles themselves. Structurally, muscle fibers increase in number and size to be able to handle more mechanical work (lifting, pushing, endurance). Inside muscles, adaptations result in higher energy production, mechanical power and fatigue reduction by increasing muscle size, blood supply and metabolic enzymes. Mitochondria are little organelles that generate energy from sugar and fat metabolism using oxygen. They increase in numbers in response to exercise. Since oxygen is a crucial factor for metabolizing fuel in the muscles, growth of blood vessels and capillaries to and throughout muscle tissue bring more oxygen where it can be utilized. Muscle tissue adapts to the type of exercise with strength training increasing the fibers that move more mass and with endurance training increasing the capacity to generate energy from oxidative metabolism of sugar and fats. Regular exercise results in the ability of muscles to store more carbohydrate energy for use on demand. An amazing discovery over the past 20 years regarding muscle physiology is that besides adapting internally to the demands of exercise, they also secrete hormones into the blood for effects all over the body. These hormones named *myokines* are a varied group of mostly proteins that control inflammation, signal repair mechanisms and help regulate the flow of fuel and circulation. The most known are those that regulate inflammation such as *IL-6* but also many others that carry on crosstalk between organs and muscles. This is an expanding field of scientific inquiry that is just starting to be unraveled. A component of aging made worse with inactivity is the continual loss of muscle tissue that can result in *sarcopenia* where one's strength, endurance and balance are significantly reduced resulting in falls and the inability to do regular activities. This is entirely preventable with a regular program of exercise.

While doctors often will suggest and recommend patients to start exercising to help control and treat various medical conditions such as high blood pressure, diabetes, obesity, etc., it is usually an afterthought at the end of the discussion of treatments in which medications are prescribed. This is due to the perceived difficulty patients have in adopting new lifestyle changes and limited time to explain what is needed as well as the limited understanding of exercise physiology that many doctors possess. It is my view that this approach is a bit backward and that exercise prescription should be more front and center in the active treatment of the 40 medical problems that have been shown to be important. In 2007, the American Society of Sports Medicine started an important initiative and challenge to the medical profession by declaring, defining and promoting the concept that "Exercise is medicine".

In the above review, I've included selected examples of the extensive research done on how regular exercise improves our bodies and minds. What about the practical application in everyday life? Many people are unmotivated, uninterested and have no life pattern for incorporating regular exercise into their busy, time limited lives. What to do? Here I will offer a way to get started and maintain increased movement in one's life. First and simply, I recommend starting small and short and include activities that can be done and fit into one's day. This can be just going out for a 5-minute walk at a pace that feels like you are making some effort. Doing this a couple or a few times a day before work, lunch, after dinner or with any free time can reap huge benefits to those starting out and is not daunting nor needs any equipment. Adding stairs is a great way to get an efficient use of your time. The important point is that it is doable. You might be surprised how much better you feel, how much more energy you have in the period afterward along with reduced stress and appetite for snacks. If you are looking to do something more specific, pick something that gives you pleasure such as dancing, gardening, hiking in the woods, etc. Enjoyment is the reinforcing factor that keeps you going. A crucial component is habit. Pick times for activities that are available or possible. A very frustrating aspect for many folks is deciding to "go to the gym every day after work" and finding out there are other commitments and that you are tired at the end of the day and just want to relax at home. Pick times where your availability and energy are in line. Carving out small periods of movement for your body during the day will leave you with a better mood and better sleep at night. Having a set committed schedule of doing exercise takes away the decision making and figuring out if and when you can. Put it in your life as something important like brushing your teeth and there will be less stress on whether to do something or not. There are many alternative short exercise regimens that one can do as well. Some popular ones such as the "Seven-minute workout" and its variations are excellent for those who are time-strapped where one can do varied workouts at home or the office with the only equipment needed is a chair. The aim is at least 5 days a week of doing something and doing different types of exercise is excellent for your body. Incorporating some resistance or weight training greatly helps especially as we age. Something simple like having 5-10 pounds hand weights by your front door and doing curls, overhead lifts and squats for 10 reps takes only 2 minutes. Fun, doable and consistency will pay off by greatly improving your health and well-being, guaranteed! OK then, let's get out there and get going! Enjoy!

About the Author

George F. Smith, M.D., is a board certified General Internal Medicine physician. He graduated from Jefferson Medical College in Philadelphia in 1982. He completed a residency in Internal Medicine at the Faulkner Hospital in Boston in 1985 which was a teaching hospital for Tufts and Havard medical schools. He spent his early career working in emergency rooms and urgent care clinics in the Boston area and then in Southern California. He relocated to Northern California in 1988 to work at a multidisciplinary spine clinic and then started a solo private practice in Daly City, California in 1995. In 2018, he and his practice became incorporated into a large organization owned by Sutter Health. He retired from full-time work in early 2021. Since then he has done volunteer work at a free clinic in San Francisco and works part time at a local primary care facility near his home in Menlo Park, California. He enjoys traveling, reading and visiting Italy with his wife. He is an avid cyclist. He plans on continuing writing about the world of medicine and life on his Substack page. This is his first and only book.

About this Book

Come along for the professional life journey of Dr. Smith as he weaves together the world of medicine from medical school through the crucial years of internship and training into the work world taking him from Boston to the West Coast. For several years he treats patients in clinics and emergency rooms before joining a multi-specialty group treating spine disorders. He spends the last 25 years in solo private practice in a working class, ethnically diverse area south of San Francisco, dealing with all the issues related to medical care. He dives deeply into the major medical epidemics of the past forty years with personal accounts and interactions of the HIV/AIDS epidemic, the obesity epidemic, the increasing diabetes epidemic, the opioid crisis, the advance of dementia in society and a detailed first-person account of the Covid-19 pandemic. He chronicles the history of medicine from ancient times to the present allowing the reader to understand that current medical practice is a very recent development since the mid-20th century. Dr. Smith's in-depth patient stories allows readers to understand the doctor-patient relationship, how doctors really think and the challenges of complex diseases from a humanistic and compassionate viewpoint. This comprehensive account of the life of a primary care physician during the past 40 years will serve as a reference for future doctors to accurately understand the profession during this period in history. He hopes you enjoy his honest perspective, observations and humor!

www.ingramcontent.com/pod-product-compliance
Lightning Source LLC
Chambersburg PA
CBHW051746040426
42446CB00007B/246